P. E. Petrides · H. L. Pahl (Eds.)
Molecular Basis of Chronic Myeloproliferative Disorders

P. E. Petrides (Editor) · H. L. Pahl (Coeditor)

Molecular Basis of Chronic Myeloproliferative Disorders

With 72 Figures in 95 Parts and 32 Tables

Springer

Petro E. Petrides, M.D., Ph.D.
Hematology Oncology Center, Zweibrückenstr. 2, 80331 Munich,
and University of Munich Medical School, Munich, Germany

Heike L. Pahl, Ph.D.
Department of Experimental Anaesthesiology, University Hospital Freiburg,
Center for Clinical Research, Breisacher Strasse 66, 79106 Freiburg, Germany

ISBN 978-3-642-62271-7 ISBN 978-3-642-18738-4 (eBook)
DOI 10.1007/978-3-642-18738-4

Library of Congress Control Number: 2004111462

http://www.springeronline.com

Originally published by Springer-Verlag Berlin Heidelberg New York in 2004
Softcover reprint of the hardcover lst edition 2004

Cover Design: E. Kirchner, 69121 Heidelberg, based upon Fig. 21.1
Typesetting: FotoSatz Pfeifer GmbH, D-82166 Gräfelfing
Printed on acid-free paper – 21/3150 – 5 4 3 2 1 0

Preface

In these times when the common format for scientific exchange is large meetings with 20,000 or more participants, where it is easy to be anonymous and isolated, bringing together like-minded thinkers in a quieter and more intimate setting is a refreshing, and civilized, innovation. So it was that international meetings at Frauenchiemsee in Upper Bavaria were inaugurated, luring a small group of scientists to a secluded island in beautiful surroundings for a few days to spark and catalyze interpersonal communications, stimulate the fruitful exchange of ideas, and foster future collaborations. The first proof of principle for this concept was an international collaboration between the universities of Munich/Berlin and Iowa City that led to the "Peroxidase Multigene Family of Enzymes" meeting. Scientists from 19 nations enjoyed the serenity of the site and lively interactions which spawned multiple subsequent collaborations. The proceedings were summarized in a volume published by Springer [Petrides PE, Nauseef WM (eds) (2000) The peroxidase multigene family of enzymes. biochemical basis and clinical applications. Springer, Berlin Heidelberg New York]. The event was so successful that it was followed by subsequent international meetings on the peroxidases held in Vienna (2000) and Kyoto (in 2004).

A second Frauenchiemsee meeting focused on chronic myeloproliferative disorders (cMPDs), including essential thrombocythemia, polycythemia vera, myelofibrosis, mastocytosis and hypereosinophilic syndrome. Although such disorders were first described in the late 19th century, clinical decisions and therapy were primarily based on clinical experience, as laboratory data were limited. Consequently, progress in the understanding of the molecular basis of these diseases was slow. To correct this shortcoming, interested hematologists and other scientists from 10 countries were invited to exchange their ideas and to cooperate on defining the molecular biology of these diseases. Organized in collaboration with Heike L. Pahl from the University of Freiburg, the meeting was held at the end of September 2000. As in 1998, the meeting was made possible with the support of a peer-reviewed grant from the Deutsche Forschungsgemeinschaft (DFG) and with additional funds provided by AOP Orphan Pharmaceuticals, Vienna, Austria. As proof of the success of this gathering, there were several international collaborations and subsequent meetings in Italy, the Netherlands and Portugal.

In 2002, in collaboration with Ernest Beutler of the Scripps Research Institute in San Diego, California, a third Frauenchiemsee meeting was convened, this time to discuss the molecular biology and clinics of iron overload and deficiency. Although many of the attending international scientists knew each other from their publications, few had met personally. Since iron was hotly debated, the proceedings were published within a few months after the meeting [Petrides PE, Beutler E (eds) (2002) Molecular and clinical aspects of human iron metabolism. Blood Cells Molec Dis 29:296 – 573].

Perhaps reflecting the ordered differentiation of hematopoietic cells, the lag time between the cMPD meeting and the publication of its proceedings has been somewhat longer. Nonetheless, generous support from Shire Pharmaceuticals, Inc., UK, InnovaMedBiotech, Munich and from Dr.Stephan and Susan Hausknecht, Aachen has brought these exciting proceedings to fruition.

The manuscripts submitted by each of the participants in the cMPD meeting were updated in January 2004 for the publication of this book. Since the meeting many exciting new developments have occurred in this field, including the identification of the FIP1L1-PDGFA fusion gene in hypereosinophilic syndrome, the first gene expression profiling studies using microarray technology in polycythemia vera and essential thrombocythemia, the description of c-mpl Baltimore, the elucidation of the molecular basis of Chuvash polycythemia and the rapidly expanding role of proteomic and transcriptome analysis of platelets. Most of these have been included in this publication. Since cMPDs are rare and relatively heterogeneous, research into their molecular basis and coordinated clinical trials are best performed in an international framework. The collective aim of the meeting and the resulting publication is to spark such projects.

Our thanks again also to our host at Frauenchiemsee, Mother Scholastika of the Benedictine Abbey, and to Dörthe Mennecke-Bühler, Joachim W. Schmidt and John Nicholson of Springer, whose efforts have ensured the high quality of this book. Thanks also to Chuanbing Zang and Hongyu Liu as well as to my wife Maria Beykirch for their support with the organization of the meeting.

The next Frauenchiemsee meeting will take place on 23–28 September 2005. Those interested in the program are referred to our website (www.innova-med.de).

Petro E. Petrides, Munich

Contents

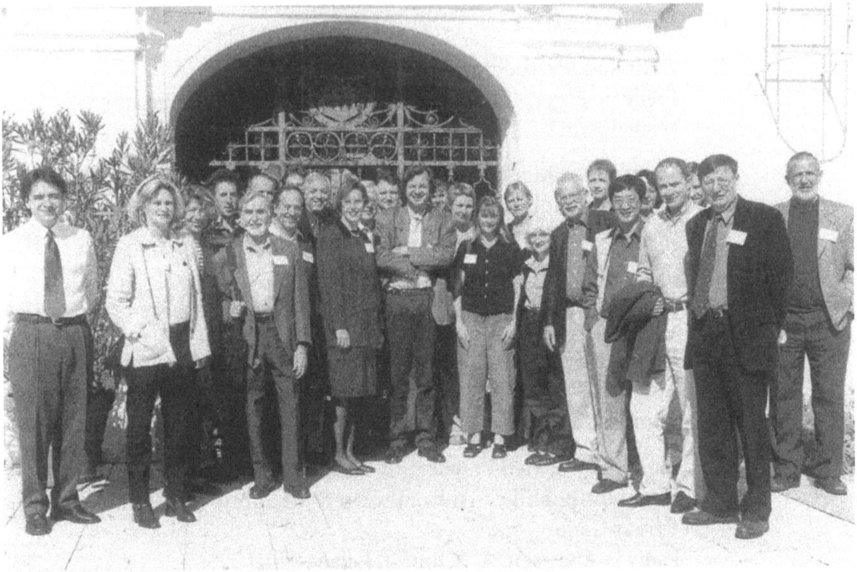

Participants of the CMPD Meeting at Frauenchiemsee, Bavaria

Contributors

Arthur A. Axelrad (e-mail: a.axelrad@utoronto.ca)
Department of Anatomy and Cell Biology, University of Toronto, Toronto, M5S 1A8, Canada

Sylvia Bellucci (e-mail: sylvia.bellucci@lrb.ap-hop-paris.fr)
Laboratory of Hematology, Hospital Lariboisière, 2 rue Ambroise Paré, 75010 Paris, France

Anthony J. Bench (e-mail: anthony.bench@addenbrooks.nhs.uk)
University of Cambridge, Department of Haematology, Cambridge Institute for Medical Research, Addenbrooke's Hospital, Hills Road, Cambridge, CB2 2XY, UK

Marie C. Le Bousse-Kerdilès (e-mail: lebousse@infobiogen.fr)
INSERM Research Network on Myelofibrosis with Myeloid Metaplasia, INSERM U268; Institut André Lwoff, Hôpital Paul Brousse; 14 Avenue Paul-Vaillant Couturier, 94800 Villejuif, France

Elisabeth M. Cramer (e-mail: elisabeth.cramer@cochin.inserm.fr)
INSERM U.567, Département d'Hématologie, Institut Cochin, Maternité 5ème étage, Hôpital de Port Royal, 123 Boulevard de Port-Royal, 75014 Paris, France

Frédéric Féger (e-mail: michel.arock@psl.ap-hop-paris.fr)
CNRS Unit FRE 2444, 4, Ave de l'Observatoire, 75006 Paris, France

Jose L. Fernandez-Luna (e-mail: inmflj@humv.es)
Unidad de Genetica Molecular, Hospital Universitario Marques de Valdecilla, Edificio, Scuela Universitaria Enfermeria, Av. Valdecilla s/n, 39008 Santander, Spain

Rosemary E. Gale (e-mail: rosemary.gale@ucl.ac.uk)
Department of Haematology, University College London, 98 Chenies Mews, London, WC1E 6HX, UK

Pedro Gascon (e-mail: gascon@clinic.ub.es)
Servei d'Oncologia Médica, Institute de Malalties Hemato-Oncológiques, ICMHO, Hospital Clínic Villarroel 170, 08036 Barcelona, Spain

Hermann Heimpel (e-mail: hermann.heimpel@med-uni.ulm.de)
Department of Hematology/Oncology, University of Ulm, Robert Kochstrasse 5, 89081 Ulm, Germany

Amy D. Klion (e-mail: aklion@nih.gov)
Laboratory of Parasitic Diseases, National Institutes of Health, Bethesda, MD; The Whitehead Institute/MIT Center for Genome Research, Cambridge, MA, USA

Robert Kralovics (e-mail: r.kralovics@unibas.ch)
University Hospital Basel, Experimental Hematology 312, Hebelstrasse 20, Basel, Switzerland

Szu-Hee Lee (e-mail: shlee@nus.edu.sg), Department of Pathology, National University of Singapore, Singapore 119074

Daniel I.H. Linzer (e-mail: dlinzer@northwestern.edu)
Department of Biochemistry, Molecular Biology, and Cell Biology, Northwestern University, Evanston, IL 60208, USA

Dagmar Ludolph-Hauser (e-mail: christa.wandschneider@lrz.uni-muenchen.de), Department of Dermatology, University of Munich, Frauenlobstrasse 2, 80331 Munich, Germany

Hans D. Menssen (e-mail: HansDietrich.Menssen@schering.de)
Department of Hematology, Universitätsklinikum Benjamin Franklin der Freien Universität Berlin, Hindenburgdamm 30, 12200 Berlin, Germany

Heike L. Pahl (e-mail: heike.pahl@klinikum.uni-freiburg.de)
Department of Experimental Anaesthesiology, University Hospital Freiburg, Center for Clinical Research, Breisacher Strasse 66, 79106 Freiburg, Germany

Petro E. Petrides (e-mail: petrides@onkologiemuenchen.de)
Hematology Oncology Center, Zweibrückenstr. 2, 80331 Munich; InnovaMedBiotech, Rumfordstrasse 57, 80469 Munich, Germany

Josef T. Prchal (e-mail: jprchal@bcm.tmc.edu)
Section of Hematology/Oncology, Baylor College of Medicine, One Baylor Plaza, MS 525D, Houston, TX 77030, USA

Florence Roufosse (e-mail: froufoss@ulb.ac.be)
Departments of Immunology and Internal Medicine, Hôpital Erasme, Université Libre de Bruxelles, 1070 Brussels, Belgium

Radek C. Skoda (e-mail: skoda@unibas.ch)
University Hospital Basel, Experimental Hematology 312, Hebelstrasse 20, Basel, Switzerland

Christian P. Sommerhoff (e-mail: sommerhoff@lmu.de)
Department of Clinical Chemistry and Biochemistry, Ludwig-Maximilians-Universität, Nußbaumstrasse 20, 80336 Munich, Germany

Jerry L. Spivak (e-mail: jlspivak@jhmi.edu), Division of Hematology, Departments of Medicine and Pathology, Johns Hopkins University School of Medicine, Baltimore, Maryland, USA

Jürgen Thiele (e-mail: j.thiele@uni-koeln.de)
Department of Pathology, Universität Köln, Joseph-Stelzmannstrasse 9, 50931 Cologne, Germany

Brigitte Wittmann-Liebold (e-mail: wittmannliebold@wita.de)
Wita GmbH, Warthestr. 21, 14513 Teltow/Berlin, Germany

A Basics

Introduction: Towards a Molecular Classification of Chronic Myeloproliferative Disorders

Petro E. Petrides

1.1 Chronic Myeloid Leukemia as a Paradigm for Chronic Myeloproliferative Disorders (cMPDs)

Chronic myeloid leukemia (CML) was the first hematological malignancy in which a chromosomal alteration (the Philadelphia chromosome) was identified. This alteration results from a translocation with the formation of a fusion gene. The elucidation of the underlying molecular process has not only allowed a precise diagnosis and the monitoring of residual disease but has also paved the way for the development of imatinib, a therapeutic agent which directly targets the molecular alteration [1].

Until very recently the diagnosis Philadelphia chromosome-negative cMPDs (Fig. 1.1) was based entirely on morphological criteria in peripheral blood and bone marrow samples [2, 3].

1.2 The Evolution of the WHO Criteria for the Classification of cMPDs

1.2.1 Polycythemia Vera, Essential Thrombocythemia and Chronic Idiopathic Myelofibrosis

To identify patients with polycythemia vera (PV) the Polycythemia Vera Study Group (PVSG) devised nearly 30 years ago a set of criteria (categories A and B) which allowed the diagnosis to be established and which were used as standard entry criteria for the PVSG protocols (Table 1.1). After the accumulation of new knowledge, the criteria were modified – some were deleted (leukocyte alkaline phosphatase, vitamin

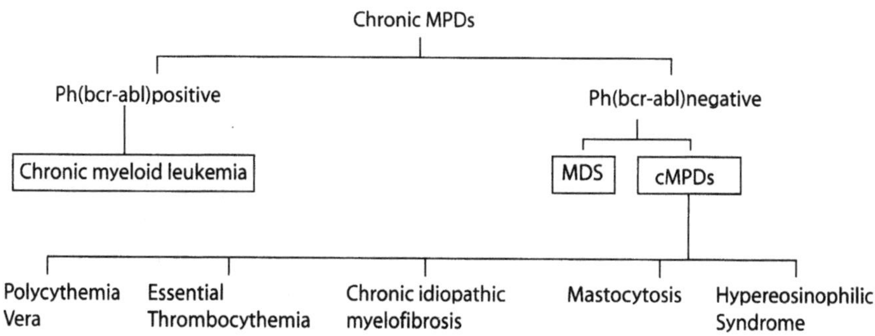

Fig. 1.1. Classification of chronic myeloproliferative disorders

Table 1.1. PVSG criteria for the diagnosis of polycythemia vera [4]

A1	Increased red cell mass: males ≥36 ml/kg, females ≥32 ml/kg
A2	Normal arterial O2 saturation (≥92%)
A3	Splenomegaly
B1	Thrombocytosis: platelet count ≥400,000/µl
B2	Leukocytosis: leukocyte count ≥12,000/µl (no fever or infection)
B3	Increased leukocyte alkaline phosphatase (LAP > 100) in the absence of fever or infection
B4	Increased serum vitamin B12/binders B12: > 900 pg/ml Unbound B12 binding capacity: > 2200 pg/ml

Diagnosis of PV virtually certain in the presence of A1 and A2 and A3 or A1 and A2 and any two from category B

Table 1.2. Updated diagnostic criteria for polycythemia vera [5]

A1	Hematocrit > 60% or raised red cell mass (> 125% of mean normal predicted value)
A2	Absence of cause of secondary polycythemia
A3	Palpable splenomegaly
B1	Platelet count > 400,000/µl
B2	Neutrophil count > 10,000/µl
B3	Definite splenomegaly demonstrated on isotope/ultrasound scanning
B4	Reduced serum erythropoietin
B5	Typical histology of bone marrow biopsy

Diagnosis is acceptable if A1 and A2 and A3 or A1 and A2 and any of B are present

Table 1.3. WHO diagnostic criteria for polycythemia vera [9]

A1	Elevated RBC mass > 25% above mean predicted value or hemoglobin > 18.5 g/dl in men or > 16.5 g/dl in women
A2	No cause of secondary erythrocytosis, including: Absence of familial erythrocytosis No elevation of erythropoietin (EPO) due to: Hypoxia (arterial pO2 < 92%) High oxygen affinity hemoglobin Truncated EPO receptor Inappropriate EPO production by tumor
A3	Splenomegaly
A4	Clonal genetic abnormality other than Philadelphia chromosome or bcr/abl fusion gene in marrow cells
A5	Endogenous erythroid colony formation in vitro
B1	Thrombocytosis > 400,000/µl
B2	White blood cell count > 12,000/µl
B3	Bone marrow biopsy showing panmyelosis with prominent erythroid and megakaryocytic proliferation
B4	Low serum erythropoietin levels

Diagnose PV when A1 and A2 and any other category A are present or when A1 and A2 and any two of category B are present

B12) and others such as serum erythropoietin and bone marrow histology were added (Table 1.2). In the light of progress in the field, convincing arguments were presented [6, 7, 8] for further modifications: in 2001 these were implemented in the proposed WHO classification and included possible causes of secondary polycythemia, cytogenetic alterations and spontaneous erythroid colony formation as well as refining changes in bone marrow morphology (Table 1.3).

Table 1.4. Diagnostic criteria for essential thrombocythemia [14, 15]

1	Platelet count > 600,000/µl
2	Hemoglobin < 13 g/dl or normal red cell mass (males < 36 ml/kg, females < 32 ml/kg)
3	Stainable iron in marrow or failure of iron trial (< 1 g/dl rise in hemoglobin after 1 month of iron therapy)
4	No Philadelphia chromosome
5	Collagen fibrosis of marrow (a) absent or (b) less than one-third of biopsy area without both splenomegaly and leuko-erythroblastic reaction
6	No known cause for reactive thrombocytosis

Table 1.5. WHO diagnostic criteria for essential thrombocythemia [16]

Positive criteria		
1	Sustained platelet count of > 600,000/µl	
2	Bone marrow biopsy specimen showing proliferation mainly of the megakaryocytic lineage with increased numbers of enlarged mature megakaryocytes	
Exclusion criteria		
1	No evidence of polycythemia (PV)	Normal red cell mass or hemoglobin < 18.5 g/dl in men, < 16.5 g/dl in women Stainable iron in marrow, normal serum ferritin or normal MCV If the former condition is not met failure of iron trial to increase red cell mass or hemoglobin levels to the PV range
2	No evidence of chronic myeloid leukemia (CML)	No Philadelphia chromosome and no bcr/abl fusion gene
3	No evidence of chronic idiopathic myelofibrosis	Collagen fibrosis absent Reticulin fibrosis minimal or absent
4	No evidence of myelodysplastic syndrome	No del(5q), t(3;3)(q21;q26),inv(3)(q21q26) No significant granulocytic dysplasia; few if any micromegakaryocytes
5	No evidence that thrombocytosis is reactive due to:	Underlying inflammation or infection Underlying neoplasm or prior splenectomy

Although some molecular criteria for the exclusion of secondary polycythemia were included, only recently have potential molecular diagnostic tools for PV become available. Overexpression of the hematopoietic receptor polycythemia rubra vera-1 (PRV-1) in neutrophils may provide a specific tool for the diagnosis of PV to discriminate it from secondary polycythemia [10] (see Chap. 6). Quantifying neutrophil PRV-1 mRNA is, however, not sufficient for the diagnosis of PV [11, 12].

In the latter half of the 1970s the PVSG also established criteria for the identification of a subset of patients with essential thrombocythemia (ET). These criteria were directed primarily at the exclusion of PV, CML and chronic idiopathic myelofibrosis (CIMF). In addition to thrombocytosis, megakaryocytic hyperplasia was an absolute requirement for the diagnosis of ET. Initially, a platelet count in excess of 1,000,000/µl, megakaryocytic hyperplasia and abundant platelets in bone marrow smears in the absence of any other cMPD were thought to be indicative for ET [13]. Later, however, the minimum platelet count was adjusted to 600,000/µl (Table 1.4). Thus, the diagnosis of ET was one of exclusion and only marginally considered bone marrow morphology.

Distinction between myelodysplastic syndrome (MDS) with cytogenetic alterations and the phenotype of the megakaryocyte became important features when the criteria were updated in the proposed WHO classification in 2001 (Table 1.5). In the present classification, however, there is no information given for how patients with platelet counts between 400,000 and 600,000/μl and a characteristic bone marrow morphology should be classified.

With regard to CIMF, prefibrotic and fibrotic stages are distinguished in the 2001 WHO classification (Table 1.6). The prefibrotic stage is also called IMF-0 and the various stages of the fibrotic stage IMF-1, IMF-2 and IMF-3 [17]. From this classification it becomes evident that patients with thrombocytosis and an absence of bone marrow fibrosis could either have ET (Table 1.5) or prefibrotic CIMF (Table 1.6). The differential diagnosis is primarily based upon the morphology of megakaryocytes which may form clusters in both entities but show bizarre, highly atypical forms only in CIMF (see Chap. 3).

In a histopathological study to compare the updated PVSG criteria and the WHO classification in 483 patients with the PVSG diagnosis of ET, only 162 (34%) fulfilled

Table 1.6. WHO diagnostic criteria for prefibrotic and fibrotic stages of chronic idiopathic myelofibrosis [18]

Stage	Clinical findings	Morphological findings		
	Spleen and liver	*Hematology*	*Blood*	*Bone marrow*
Prefibrotic (IMF-0)	No or mild spleno- or hepatomegaly	Variable, but often mild anemia Mild to moderate leukocytosis, mild to marked thrombocytosis	No or mild leukoerythroblastosis No or minimal red blood cell poikilocytosis; few if any dacrocytes	Hypercellularity Neutrophil proliferation Megakaryocytic proliferation and atypia (clustering of megakaryocytes, abnormally lobulated or naked megakaryocytic nuclei) Minimal or absent reticulin fibrosis
Fibrotic (IMF-1, -2, -3)	Moderate to marked spleno- and hepatomegaly	Moderate to marked anemia Low, normal or elevated WBC Platelet count decreased, normal or elevated	Leukoerythroblastosis Prominent red blood cell poikilocytosis with dacrocytes	Decreased cellularity Dilated marrow sinuses with intraluminal hematopoiesis Prominent megakaryocyte proliferation and atypia (clustering of megakaryocytes, abnormal lobulated or naked megakaryocytic nuclei) New bone formation (osteosclerosis) Reticulin and/or collagen fibrosis

the WHO criteria (true ET or thrombocythemia vera). The others were classified as IMF-0 (184, 38%) and IMF-1 (137, 28%) [19]. This indicates that bone marrow morphology can contribute important information to a better classification of cMPDs [20].

1.2.2
The Hypereosinophilic Syndrome and Chronic Eosinophilic Leukemia

The hypereosinophilic syndrome (HES) was first defined in 1975 as a condition in which there was unexplained eosinophilia (>1500/μl) persisting for at least 6 months and causing tissue damage. HES is distinguished from chronic eosinophilic leukemia (CEL) by a clonal chromosomal abnormality and/or the presence of blast cells (Table 1.7). If all of the requirements, including conditions 1–4, are met, and if the myeloid cells demonstrate a clonal chromosomal abnormality or are shown to be clonal by other means, or if blast cells are present in the peripheral blood (>2%) or increased in the bone marrow (>5% but less than 19% of nucleated bone marrow cells) then a diagnosis of CEL can be made.

The clinical observation that imatinib, an inhibitor of the BCR-ABL, c-kit and PDGF tyrosine kinases, is active in patients with HES and that lower dosages than those used in CML are required implicated a novel tyrosine kinase in their pathogenesis [22]. This led to the identification of a constitutively activated fusion tyrosine kinase on chromosome 4q12 that fuses the platelet-derived growth receptor-alpha (PDGFA) gene to an uncharacterized human gene FIP1-like 1 (FIP1L1) [23] (Fig. 1.2). This fusion results from an approximately 800 kb interstitial chromosomal deletion that includes the cysteine-rich hydrophobic domain 2 (CHIC2) locus. Since not all HES and CEL patients respond to imatinib, disease heterogeneity is suggested. Furthermore, 40% of responding patients lack FIP1L1-PDGFA fusion which indicates further heterogeneity. Since this molecular alteration is also present in patients with

Table 1.7. WHO diagnostic criteria for hypereosinophilic syndrome (HES) and chronic eosinophilic leukemia (CEL) [21]

Required	Exclude
Persistent eosinophilia (>1500/μl) in blood, increased numbers of bone marrow eosinophils and myeloblasts <20% in blood or marrow	1. All cases of reactive eosinophilia secondary to allergy, parasitic or infectious disease, pulmonary disease (hypersensitivity pneumonitis, Löffler's etc), collagen vascular diseases
	2. All neoplastic disorders with secondary reactive eosinophilia (T-cell lymphoma, including mycosis fungoides, Sézary's syndrome), Hodgkin's lymphoma, ALL, mastocytosis
	3. Other neoplastic disorders in which eosinophils are part of the neoplastic clone: Ph-positive CML, AML (including inv(16),t(16,16)(p13;q22), other myeloproliferative disorders (PV, ET, CIMF), MDS
	4. T-cell population with aberrant phenotype and abnormal cytokine production

If there is no demonstrable disease that could cause the eosinophilia, no abnormal T-cell population, and no evidence of a clonal myeloid disorder, then a diagnosis of HES can be made

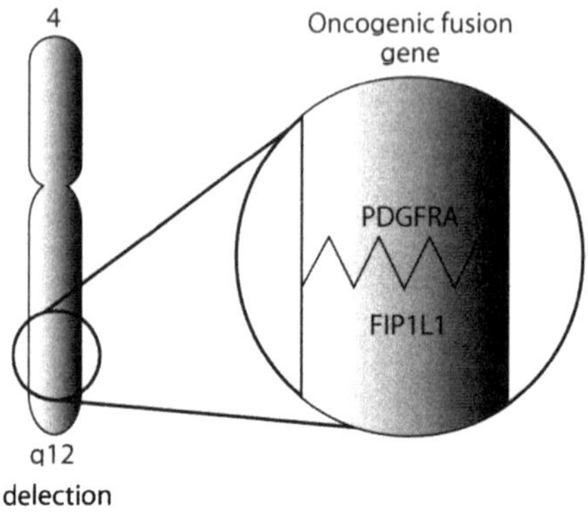

Fig. 1.2. Chromosomal aberration in HES and CEL. Deletion of a region in the long arm of chromosome 4 (q12) is repaired by the joining of pieces of two genes PDGFA and FIP1L1. The product of the fusion gene is a constitutively active tyrosine kinase

CEL, it cannot be used to discriminate the two entities [24]. Interestingly, it has also been found in imatinib-responsive patients diagnosed with systemic mastocytosis and eosinophilia [25].

The screening for the FIP1L1-PDGFA gene fusion by RT-PCR or interphase/metaphase FISH may therefore become important for an improved diagnostic workup and tailoring molecular therapy [26, 27, 28].

1.3 Summary

During the development of classification systems over the last decades, improvements have been made in the incorporation of clinical, biochemical and morphological data. As in the case of CML, the ideal classification system of cMPDs will, however, ultimately be based on the underlying molecular alterations.

Such knowledge is not available yet, but the aim of this book is to spark communication between clinicians, biochemists and pathologists in order to initiate research on the key players in the myeloproliferative processes (stem cells, megakaryocytes, platelets, erythrocytes, granulocytes) with the help of genomic and proteomic methodology.

References

1. Goldman JM, Melo JV (2003) Chronic myeloid leukemia – advances in biology and new approaches to treatment. N Engl J Med 349:1451–1464
2. Tefferi A (1998) The Philadelphia chromosome negative chronic myeloproliferative disorders: a practical overview. Mayo Clin Proc 73:1177–1184
3. Petrides PE, Gisslinger H (2004) Chronisch myeloproliferative Erkrankungen (CMPE). Booklet prepared for German-Austrian-Swiss Annual Hematology-Oncology Meeting, Innsbruck, October 2004
4. Berlin NI (1975) Diagnosis and classification of the polycythemias. Semin Hematol 12:339–351
5. Pearson TC, Missinezy M (1996) The diagnostic criteria of polycythemia rubra vera. Leuk Lymphoma 22:87–93
6. Michiels JJ, Juvonen E (1997) Proposal for revised diagnostic criteria of essential thrombocythemia and polycythemia vera by the Thrombocythemia Vera Study Group. Semin Thromb Hemost 23:339–347
7. Murphy S (1999) Diagnostic criteria and prognosis in PV and ET. Semin Hematol 36:9–13

8. Pearson TC (2001) Evaluation of diagnostic criteria in polycythemia vera. Semin Hematol 38 [Suppl 2]:21–24
9. Pierre R, Imbert M, Thiele J, Vardiman JW, Brunning RD, Flandrin G (2001) Polycythemia vera. In: Jaffe ES, Harris NL, Stein H, Vardiman JW (eds) WHO classification of tumours: tumours of haematopoietic and lymphoid tissues. IARC Press, Lyon, pp 32–34
10. Klippel S, Strunck E, Temerinc S, et al (2003) Quantification of PRV-1 mRNA distinguishes polycythemia vera from secondary erythrocytosis. Blood 102:3569–3574
11. Tefferi A, Lasho TL, Woilanskyi AP, Mesa RA (2004) Neutrophil PRV-1 expression across the chronic myeloproliferative disorders and in secondary or spurious polycythemia. Blood 103:3547–3548
12. Teofili L, Martini M, Luongo M, et al (2002) Overexpression of the polycythemia rubra vera-1 gene in essential thrombocythemia. J Clin Oncol 20:4249–4254
13. Laszlo J (1975) Myeloproliferative disorders (MPD). Semin Hematol 12:409–432
14. Murphy S, Iland H, Rosenthal D, Laszlo J (1986) Essential thrombocythemia: an interim report from the Polycythemia Vera Study Group. Semin Hematol 23:177
15. Murphy S, Peterson P, Iland H, Laszlo J (1997) Experience of the Polycythemia Vera Study Group with essential thrombocythemia: a final report on diagnostic criteria, survival and leukemic transition by treatment. Semin Hematol 34:29–39
16. Imbert M, Pierre R, Thiele J, Vardiman, JW, Brunning RD, Flandrin G (2001) Essential thrombocythemia. In: Jaffe ES, Harris NL, Stein H, Vardiman JW (eds) WHO classification of tumours: tumours of haematopoietic and lymphoid tissues. IARC Press, Lyon, pp 39–41
17. Thiele J, Kvasnicka HM, Fischer R (1999) Histochemistry and morphometry on bone marrow biopsies in chronic myeloproliferative disorders – aids to diagnosis and classification. Ann Hematol 78:495–506
18. Thiele J, Pierre R, Imbert M, Vardiman JW, Brunning RD, Flandrin G (2001) Chronic idiopathic myelofibrosis. In: Jaffe ES, Harris NL, Stein H, Vardiman JW (eds) WHO classification of tumours: tumours of haematopoietic and lymphoid tissues. IARC Press, Lyon, pp 35–38
19. Thiele J, Kvasnicka HM (2003) Chronic myeloproliferative disorders with thrombocythemia: a comparative study of two classification systems (PVSG, WHO) on 839 patients. Ann Hematol 82:148–152
20. Michiels JJ (2004) Bone marrow histopathology and biological markers as specific clues to the differential diagnosis of essential thrombocythemia, polycythemia vera and prefibrotic or fibrotic agnogenic myeloid metaplasia. Hematol J 5:93–102
21. Bain B, Pierre R, Imbert M, et al (2001) Chronic eosinophilic leukemia and the hypereosinophilic syndrome. In: Jaffe ES, Harris NL, Stein H, Vardiman JW (eds) WHO classification of tumours: tumours of haematopoietic and lymphoid tissues. IARC Press, Lyon, pp 29–34
22. Gleich GJ, Leiferman KM, Pardanani A, et al (2002) Treatment of hypereosinophilic syndrome with imatinib mesylate. Lancet 359:1577–1578
23. Cools J, deAngelo DJ, Gotlib J, et al (2003) A tyrosine kinase by fusion of the PDGFA and FIP1L1 genes as a therapeutic target of imatinib in idiopathic hypereosinophilic syndrome. N Engl J Med 348:1201–1214
24. Vandenberghe P, Wlodarska I, Michaux L, et al (2004) Clinical and molecular features of FIP1L1-PDGFRA(+) chronic eosinophilic leukemias. Leukemia 18:734–742
25. Pardanani A, Ketterling RP, Brockman SR, et al (2003) CHIC2 deletion, a surrogate marker for FIP1L1-PDGFalpha fusion, occurs in systemic mastocytosis associated with eosinophilia and predicts response to imatinib mesylate therapy. Blood 102:3093–3096
26. Gotib J, Cools J, Malone JM III, et al (2004) The FIP1L1-PDGFRalpha fusion tyrosine kinase in hypereosinophilic syndrome and chronic eosinophilic leukemia: implications for diagnosis, classification and management. Blood 103:2879–2891
27. Bain B (2004) The idiopathic hypereosinophilic syndrome and eosinophilic leukemias. Haematologica 89:133–136
28. Cortes J, Kantarjian H (2004) Beyond chronic myelogenous leukemia. Potential role for imatinib in Philadelphia negative myeloproliferative disorders. Cancer 100:2064–2078

Chapter 2

Chronic Myeloproliferative Disorders: A Clinician's View

Hermann Heimpel

2.1 Introduction

The term "myeloproliferative disorders" was originally used by W. Dameshek [1] to describe the similarities between acute myeloid leukemias and chronic phenotypes of malignant blood diseases such as chronic myeloid leukemia (CML), polycythemia vera (PV), essential thrombocythemia (ET) and primary chronic (idiopathic) myelofibrosis (IMF). For the three latter conditions he proposed the more restrictive term of chronic myeloproliferative diseases (cMPDs). After CML was shown to be the consequence of the ABL/BCR-fusion gene, the term "Philadelphia-negative cMPDs" became popular to define the entities discussed in this book. Although the identification of the bcr/abl-translocation clearly separates CML from any of the Ph-negative cMPDs, the clinical phenotypes overlap and observations on CML are useful to understand the cellular events of other cMPDs as well.

2.2 Diagnosis and Classification

In contrast to CML, the diagnosis of the different entities or subtypes of cMPDs still relies on the clinical phenotype. Different sets of definition criteria have been proposed (see Chap. 1). The classical criteria were published by the Polycythemia Vera Study Group (PVSG) [2]. Alternative sets of diagnostic criteria have been proposed [3–5]. Two methods, namely the endogenous growth of erythropoietic colonies in EPO-free semisolid media (EECs) and the determination of serum erythropoietin (EPO) concentration are of high predictive value for the diagnosis of PV [6]. Together with bone marrow morphology, they have been included in the recent WHO classification [7], which no longer requires the determination of red cell mass. Their diagnostic power is explained by the EPO-independent proliferation of red cell precursors, and the retained regulation of EPO concentration by the red cell mass, irrespective of whether red cells are derived from a normal or transformed precursor pool. Retrospective classification of our own cases originally matched to the PVSG criteria without considering red cell mass but using a low or normal EPO concentration as a mandatory parameter did not change the diagnosis. Different results have been reported by others [8], and red cell mass determination as an obligatory diagnostic criterion is still a matter of debate [8, 9].

In clinical practice, direct measuring of the red cell mass is often neglected. One reason for this is the inaccuracy of the predicted "normal" red cell volume as related to body weight, set as >36 ml/kg for males and >32 ml/kg for females by the PSVG. A red cell mass of greater than 125% of normal as related to body surface or to lean body mass has been proposed as an alternative. However, the variance of the predicted normal value is still large, in particular in obese patients [10]. Exclusion of secondary erythrocytosis is still a problem in patients with early stages of PV, but has become easier as a result of improved techniques for laboratory diagnosis and imaging (see Chap. 5).

The diagnosis of ET still relies on the exclusion of conditions responsible for secondary thrombocytosis. In ET, serum thrombopoietin (TPO) concentrations are higher and serum EPO concentrations lower than in patients with secondary thrombocytosis or in healthy controls [11, 12], but the large variance precludes its utility for differential diagnosis [13]. Also, clinical and histopathological features of ET, including long-term evolution in individual patients are heterogeneous. In contrast to PV, clonality cannot be shown in all informative females with ET [14–16].

Bone marrow histology is of high diagnostic utility if the specimens are properly processed and well interpreted [17] (see Chap. 3). This is particularly true distinguishing cMPDs from secondary erythrocytosis and/or reactive thrombocytosis. Without information on clinical findings and peripheral blood counts, the diagnostic power of histology to differentiate subtypes within the group of cMPDs is limited. There are patients who have, at least initially, to be diagnosed as "Ph-negative cMPD, unclassified". Phenotypic transitions may occur in particular from ET to PV, but rarely vice versa. Patients who initially fulfill the criteria for ET, in particular with hemoglobin and hematocrit in the upper range or normal, may later be recognized as having PV [18, 19]. One study showed that EECs, which were found in about one-third of patients initially diagnosed with ET, are indicative of subsequent transition to PV [20].

Of course, bone marrow histology is a mandatory test for IMF. Both subtle myelofibrosis and myeloid metaplasia may be present in the early phases and may become prominent features in the late phases of all subtypes of cMPD. Bone marrow histology is of definite value if interpreted in context with other observations, in particular if follow-up biopsies are obtained [21], and the morphology of megakaryocytes is of major importance in recognizing the prefibrotic stage of IMF [22]. When experimental data or new diagnostic tests are to be attributed to particular subtypes, true primary IMF should be clearly separated from phenotypically similar states of myelofibrosis after PV or ET. Thus, both follow-up in patients early stages of suspected IMF, and a careful

Table 2.1. An extended classification of acquired cMPDs

Polycythemia vera (PV)
Essential thrombocythemia (ET)
Thrombocythemia vera, clonal
Non-clonal thrombocythemia?
Idiopathic
Primary myelofibrosis
Osteomyelofibrosis/osteomyelosclerosis (IMF; OMF, OMS)
Myelofibrosis with myeloid metaplasia (MMM)
Chronic myeloproliferative disorder, unclassified
Early Stage of PV, ET, IMF
Others, unclassified e.g., Ph-CML
(Agnogenic myeloid metaplasia)
8p11 chronic myeloproliferative syndrome
Chronic eosinophilic leukemia

Table 2.2. Phenotypes of Ph-negative cMPDs: some questions

Is clonality a definition criterion for Ph-negative cMPDs?
Is clonality of prognostic relevance?
Are the different phenotypes of Ph-negative cMPDs different genotypes?
Is essential thrombocythemia one disease, or two, or more?
Are there new features for early definition of PV versus ET versus CIMF?
Are high TPO concentrations enhancing non-clonal thrombocytopoiesis?
Which are the risk factors for thromboembolic events, not dependent on the phenotype?

history in all patients with more advanced myelofibrosis are complementary to the interpretation of the histology and blood counts obtained at the time of biopsy.

Table 2.1 shows the current classification of the cMPDs commonly used for clinical diagnosis and decision making. The term of agnogenic myeloid metaplasia as known from the Anglo-American literature should no longer be used to describe a distinct phenotype of the cMPDs. The vast majority of patients with extramedullary hematopoiesis as an early manifestation of a variety disorders are in a prefibrotic stage of primary myelofibrosis that can be recognized by appropriate techniques of bone marrow histology [21]. Rare patients with extramedullary hematopoiesis at atypical sites and bone marrow histology not suggesting a cMPD represent a problem of differential diagnosis: carcinoma or hereditary anemias should be considered.

Recent progress in molecular genetics may allow some questions of both pathophysiological and clinical interest to be answered, as shown in Table 2.2. Previous attempts to define potential genotypes by morphological cytogenetics have given inconclusive results [23, 24]. The reduced expression of c-MPL on platelets and the presence of RNA of the recently described PRV-1 in mature neutrophils [25, 26] are concordant in definite cases of PV, but not so in other types of cMPD. This discrepancy, however, is based on a rather small number of patients and it is of high priority to compare the presence of these potential new diagnostic markers in a series of identically classified patients with MPDs. Inclusion of patients with early disease could also improve decision making in patients with disease now attributed to the group of "MPDs, unclassified".

2.3 Prognosis and Therapy

The prognosis for all types of cMPDs as determined by the natural course of the disease is definitely better than that for CML, with ET having the highest and IMF the lowest life expectancy [18, 27, 28]. In all subtypes, the risk of terminal myelodysplastic syndrome and acute myeloid leukemia is significantly greater than in the general population. No curative treatment is known, except for allogeneic stem cell transplantation in the rare cases recognized in adolescence or young adults [29]. Prognosis, as defined by survival, is better in younger patients, but worse as defined by the appropriate parameter, namely excess mortality [30]. Life expectancy is definitely improved by treatment in PV [31], and probably in other cMPDs. Treatment modalities include prevention of major thromboembolic events, and cytoreductive measures to delay the progress towards progressive splenomegaly and myelofibrosis with ultimate pancytopenia. As well as 32-P and cytostatics such as hydroxyurea or pipobroman, interferon-α is effective in all cMPDs, but its utility and details such as the start of treatment and its optimal dose have still to be determined. The same is true for anagrelide, a novel agent which exerts cytoreductive effects on platelet production (see Chap. 15).

2.4 Summary

Many details which are essential for therapeutic decision making are still not understood. Further prospective trials are needed (see Chap. 15). However, due to the low incidence and the long natural course of the cMPDs, these will not be able to adequately answer all questions. Some open questions are listed in Table 2.3. Again, only a better insight into the chain of events leading from the unknown genetic alteration(s) to the clinical phenotypes will allow us to define a limited number of therapeutic hypotheses, which can then be tested in prospective cooperative clinical studies.

Table 2.3. Therapy of the cMPDs: questions

Can better prognostic scores be established?
Support novel molecular markers clinical decision making?
When to start cytoreductive therapy?
Does hydroxyurea increase the risk of secondary leukemia?
Interferon-alpha: better life expectancy, and in which group of patients?
Anagrelide in ET and other cMPDs with an elevated platelet count: impact on survival?
New drugs: Thalidomide, Imatinib, others? Monoclonal antibodies?
Hematopoietic stem cell transplantation: Allogeneic only? Which patients? Which age?

References

1. Dameshek W, Gunz F (1964) Leukemia, 2nd edn. Grune and Stratton, New York London
2. Wasserman LR, Berk PD, Berlin NI (1995) Polycythemia vera and the myeloproliferative disorders. Saunders, Philadelphia
3. Tefferi A (1999) Diagnosing polycythemia vera: a paradigm shift. Mayo Clin Proc 74:159–162
4. Pearson TC, Messinezy M (1996) The diagnostic criteria of polycythaemia rubra vera. Leuk Lymphoma 22 [Suppl 1]:87–93
5. Murphy S (1999) Diagnostic criteria and prognosis in polycythemia vera and essential thrombocythemia. Semin Hematol 36:9–13
6. Westwood N, Dudley JM, Sawyer B, Messinezy M, Pearson TC (1993) Primary polycythaemia: diagnosis by non-conventional positive criteria. Eur J Haematol 51:228–232
7. World Health Organisation (2001) Tumours of the hemopoietic and lymphoid tissues. IARC Press, Lyon
8. Balga I, Solenthaler M, Furlan M (2000) Should whole-body red cell mass be measured or calculated? Blood Cells Mol Dis 26:25–31
9. Fairbanks VF (2000) Myeloproliferative disease: polycythemia vera: the packed cell volume and the curious logic of the red cell mass. Hematology 4:381–395

10. Leslie WD, Dupont JO, Peterdy AE (1999) Effect of obesity on red cell mass results. J Nucl Med 40:422–428
11. Griesshammer M, Hornkohl A, Nichol JL, Hecht T, Raghavachar A, Heimpel H, Schrezenmeier H (1998) High levels of thrombopoietin in sera of patients with essential thrombocythemia: cause or consequence of abnormal platelet production? Ann Hematol 77:211–215
12. Messinezy M, Westwood NB, El Hemaidi I, Marsden JT, Sherwood RS, Pearson TC (2002) Serum erythropoietin values in erythrocytoses and in primary thrombocythaemia. Br J Haematol 117:47–53
13. el Kassar N, Hetet G, Briere J, Grandchamp B (1998) Clonality analysis of hematopoiesis and thrombopoietin levels in patients with essential thrombocythemia. Leuk Lymphoma 30:181–188
14. Anger B, Janssen JWG, Schrezenmeier H, Hehlmann R, Heimpel H, Bartram CR (1990) Clonal analysis of chronic myeloproliferative disorders using X-linked DNA polymorphism. Leukemia 4:258–261
15. Mitterbauer G, Winkler K, Gisslinger H, Geissler K, Lechner K, Mannhalter C (1999) Clonality analysis using X-chromosome inactivation at the human androgen receptor gene (Humara). Evaluation of large cohorts of patients with chronic myeloproliferative diseases, secondary neutrophilia, and reactive thrombocytosis. Am J Clin Pathol 112:93–100
16. Chiusolo P, La Barbera EO, Laurenti L, Piccirillo N, Sora F, Giordano G, Urbano R, Mazzucconi MG, De S, V, Leone G, Sica S (2001) Clonal hemopoiesis and risk of thrombosis in young female patients with essential thrombocythemia. Exp Hematol 29:670–676
17. Thiele J, Kvasnicka HM (2001) Clinicopathology and histochemistry on bone marrow biopsies in chronic myeloproliferative disorders – a clue to diagnosis and classification. Pathol Biol (Paris) 49:140–147
18. Heimpel H, Haug U, Seidler R, Anger B (1993) Chronic myeloproliferative syndromes: initial findings, evolution and prognosis in 489 cases. In: Fleischer J (ed) Leukemias. Springer, Berlin Heidelberg New York, pp 467–475
19. Jantunen R, Juvonen E, Ikkala E, Oksanen K, Anttila P, Ruutu T (1999) Development of erythrocytosis in the course of essential thrombocythemia. Ann Hematol 78:219–222
20. Shih LY, Lee CT (1994) Identification of masked polycythemia vera from patients with idiopathic marked thrombocytosis by endogenous erythroid colony assay. Blood 83:744–748
21. Thiele J, Kvasnicka HM, Fischer R (1999) Histochemistry and morphometry on bone marrow biopsies in chronic myeloproliferative disorders – aids to diagnosis and classification. Ann Hematol 78:495–506
22. Thiele J, Kvasnicka HM, Zankovich R, Diehl V (2001) Clinical and morphological criteria for the diagnosis of prefibrotic idiopathic (primary) myelofibrosis. Ann Hematol 80:160–165
23. Carbonell F, Ganser A, Heimpel H (1983) Cytogenetic studies in chronic myeloproliferative diseases. Acta Haematol 69:145–151
24. Diez Martin JL, Graham DL, Petitt RM, DeWald GW (1991) Chromosome studies in 104 patients with polycythemia vera. Mayo Clin Proc 66:287–299
25. Moliterno AR, Hankins WD, Spivak JL (1998) Impaired expression of the thrombopoietin receptor by platelets from patients with polycythemia vera [see comments]. N Engl J Med 338:572–580
26. Temerinac S, Klippel S, Strunck E, Roder S, Lubbert M, Lange W, Azemar M, Meinhardt G, Schaefer HE, Pahl HL (2000) Cloning of PRV-1, a novel member of the uPAR receptor superfamily, which is overexpressed in polycythemia rubra vera. Blood 95:2569–2576
27. Tefferi A (1998) The Philadelphia chromosome negative chronic myeloproliferative disorders: a practical overview. Mayo Clin Proc 73:1177–1184
28. Brodmann S, Passweg JR, Gratwohl A, Tichelli A, Skoda RC (2000) Myeloproliferative disorders: complications, survival and causes of death. Ann Hematol 79:312–318
29. Jurado M, Deeg H, Gooley T, Anasetti C, Chauncey T, Flowers M, Myerson D, Storb R, Appelbaum F (2001) Haemopoietic stem cell transplantation for advanced polycythaemia vera or essential thrombocythaemia. Br J Haematol 112:392–396
30. Heimpel H (1996) The present state of pathophysiology and therapeutic trials in polycythemia vera. Int J Hematol 64:133–165
31. Rozman C, Giralt M, Feliu E, Rubio D, Cortes MT (1991) Life expectancy of patients with chronic nonleukemic myeloproliferative disorders. Cancer 67:2658–2663

Chapter 3

Chronic Myeloproliferative Disorders: A Pathologist's View

Jürgen Thiele, Hans Kvasnicka

3.1 Introduction

Regarding chronic myeloproliferative disorders (cMPDs) controversial issues include: (1) discrimination between essential thrombocythemia (ET) and concomitant thrombocythemia, (2) initial (prefibrotic) and early stages of chronic idiopathic myelofibrosis (IMF), (3) differentiation of reactive-secondary polycythemias (SP) from early-stage polycythemia vera (PV), and (4) proliferation and apoptosis.

Based on a synoptical approach, which implies a comparative evaluation of laboratory data and histopathology of the bone marrow, an attempt is made to unravel certain aspects of these issues with the aim of improving diagnostic validity.

3.2 Thrombocythemias in cMPDs

An elevated platelet count exceeding 500,000/µl warrants a differentiation of reactive causes from cMPDs. In addition to clinical findings, especially evolution of laboratory data during follow-up examinations, histopathology exerts a significant diagnostic impact [1, 2, 3]. The diagnosis of ET is still the subject of controversy and discussion, probably due to the fact that it has been predominantly approached by exclusion of other eventually thrombocythemic disorders. Moreover, in leading clinical trials the updated diagnostic criteria of the Polycythemia Vera Study Group (PVSG) [4] have been generally acknowledged, although histopathology is considered only marginally [5, 6]. This ambiguous situation was greatly improved by the introduction of certain bone marrow features into the revised set of diagnostic requirements [7, 8]. Usually patients with (true) ET present with no or borderline splenomegaly and without anemia or a leukoerythroblastic blood picture. These findings contrast with those in other patients with questionable or false ET who show clinical signs and symptoms suggesting initial-early IMF associated with severe thrombocythemia [8, 9].

Bone marrow features are significantly different in the two entities (Table 3.1) which, however, according to the postulates of the PVSG may erroneously be regarded as ET [1, 2, 3, 9, 10, 11]. In true ET, the bone marrow is normocellular or slightly hypercellular (Fig. 3.1a). The predominant abnormality is a marked proliferation of giant to large mature megakaryocytes showing quite frequently the phenomenon of emperipolesis and also (endo)mitotic figures. Usually the megakaryocytes are dispersed or occur in loose clusters in the marrow (Fig. 3.1b). They have abundant amounts of mature cytoplasm and deeply lobulated and hyperlobulated (staghorn-

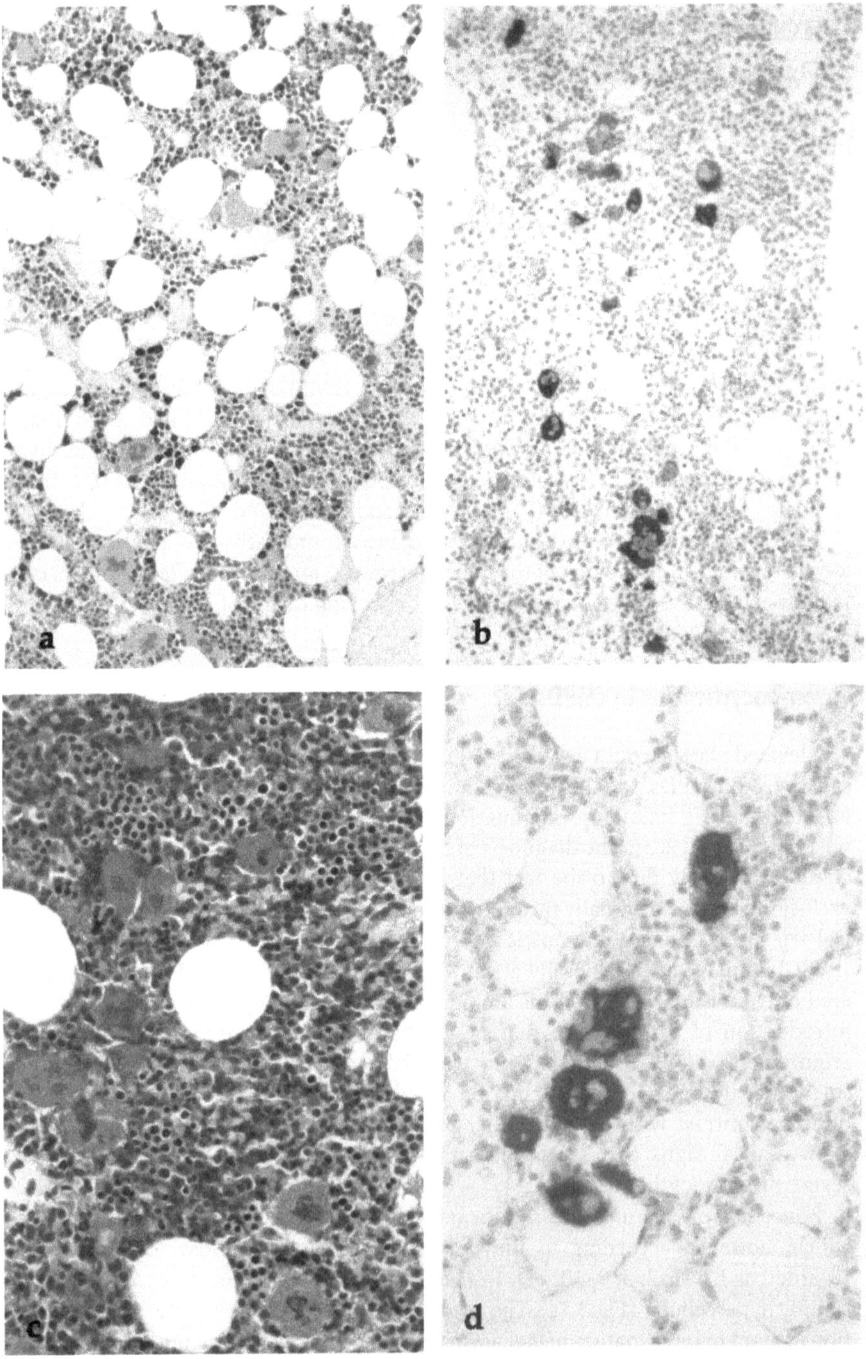

Fig. 3.1a–d. Essential thrombocythemia (ET). **a** Normal cellularity with dispersed large to giant megakaryocytes and no significant proliferation or immaturity of granuloerythrocytopoiesis. **b** Megakaryocytes are either scattered or arranged in loose clusters throughout the marrow. **c** and **d** A conspicuous slender nuclear lobulation of giant to large mature megakaryocytes is recognizable (**c**), contrasting with the abnormal megakaryocytes with their bulbous nuclei (cloud-like appearance) in IMF – see Fig. 3.2b and c (a, b × 170; c, d × 370; a chloroacetate-esterase; b, d CD61; c PAS)

Table 3.1. Survey of bone marrow features, in essential thrombocythemia (*ET*) and initial (prefibrotic) and classical (fibrotic) idiopathic myelofibrosis (*IMF*) and polycythemia vera (*PV*) (*N* normal in comparison to unaltered bone marrow of healthy individuals)

Bone marrow features	ET	Prefibrotic IMF	Fibrotic IMF	PV
Cellularity	N	Increased	Normal to reduced	Increased
Neutrophil granulopoiesis	N	Increased	Normal to reduced	Increased
Erythropoiesis	N	Reduced	Markedly reduced	Markedly increased
Fibers (reticulin)	N	N	Markedly increased including collagen fibers	Normal to slightly increased
Megakaryopoiesis				
- Quantity	Markedly increased	Increased	Increased	Increased
- Dense clustering	No	Mild	Marked	No to mild
- Size	Large to giant	Medium to giant	Small to giant	Small to giant
- Nuclear features	Staghorn-like, deep lobulation (slender segments)	Reduced and bulbous lobulation, cloud-like features, hyperchromasia	Bulbous and abnormal lobulation with cloud-like features, coarse chromatic pattern	Deep lobulation with normal chromatin pattern
Cytological abnormalities	No relevant nuclear-cytoplasmic aberration	Nuclear-cytoplasmic deviation	Marked nuclear-cytoplasmic deviation (dysplastic aspect)	No relevant nuclear-cytoplasmic maturation defects

like) nuclei showing a relatively slender segmentation without chromatin clumping (Fig. 3.1c,d). Bizarre or atypical forms, such as those observed in IMF with accompanying thrombocythemia, are not encountered [2, 8, 9, 10, 11]. A minimal to slight increase in erythroid precursors may be observed in some patients, particularly if the patient has experienced previous hemorrhage (Fig. 3.1c). Granulocytic proliferation, if present, is usually mild and there is no increase in the amount of myeloblasts or promyelocytes. The network of reticulin fibers is normal or minimally increased, but any significant increase in reticulin or collagen is not compatible with the diagnosis of ET [9, 10, 11, 12].

All these features discriminate ET from secondary thrombocytosis (ST) generated by a variety of underlying disorders. ST normally displays medium-sized to small megakaryocytes with an inconspicuous nuclear appearance [8]. For this reason, these characteristics contrast with those found in the other subtypes of cMPDs, especially IMF.

3.3 Initial (Prefibrotic) and Manifest Idiopathic Myelofibrosis

In contrast to classical IMF in which the patient presents with splenomegaly, leukoerythroblastosis with tear-drop poikilocytosis, anemia and definite reticulin or collagen fibrosis of the bone marrow [13, 14, 15], patients with prefibrotic (initial) and early stages are characterized by a certain set of clinical parameters [16, 17]. These

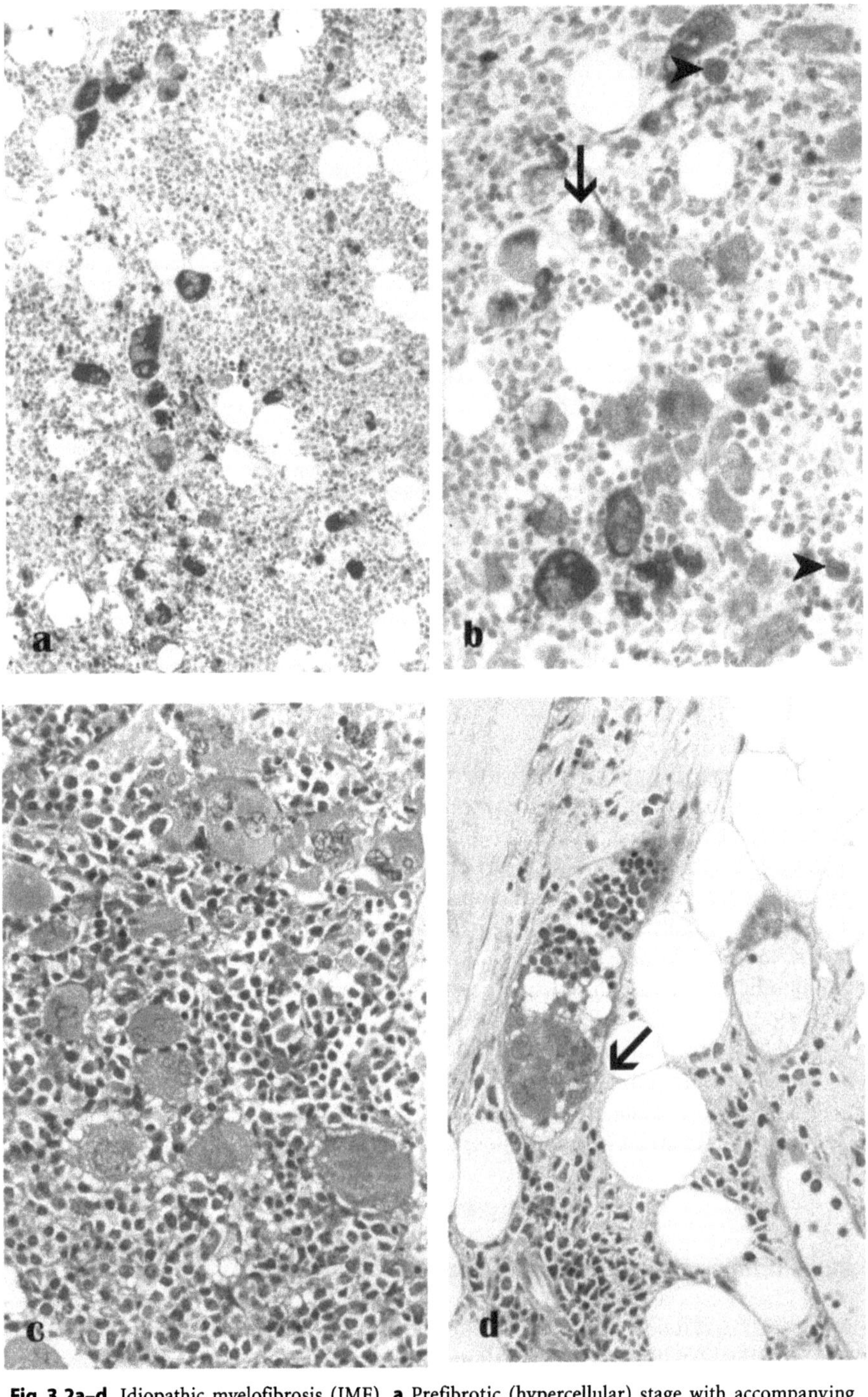

Fig. 3.2a–d. Idiopathic myelofibrosis (IMF). **a** Prefibrotic (hypercellular) stage with accompanying thrombocythemia clinically simulating ET shows clusters of abnormal megakaryocytes (compare with Fig. 3.1b). **b** and **c** Abnormalities of megakaryopoiesis include disturbed histotopography (clustering)

include a borderline to moderate therapy-refractory anemia, minimal to slight splenomegaly and frequently elevated platelet counts [8]. For this reason, these patients are often referred with the presumptive diagnosis of ET, therapy-refractory anemia or unclassifiable cMPDs [3, 9, 11].

Approximately 20–30% of patients are first diagnosed in the prefibrotic or hypercellular stage [10]. Peripheral blood films reveal only very sparse dacrocytes and large atypical platelets and a few erythroid and myeloid precursors [17]. Bone marrow histopathology is consistent with an increase in age-related cellularity and a prominent left-shifted neutrophil granulopoiesis accompanied by a marked proliferation of megakaryocytes (Fig. 3.2a). These prominent features have been formerly termed chronic megakaryocytic-granulocytic myelosis – CMGM [10]. On the other hand, erythropoiesis shows a slight reduction, because of presenting small to medium-sized islets occasionally with a macrocytic appearance. In this context an arrest of erythroid maturation according to proliferative capacity may be encountered [18].

Megakaryopoiesis is a diagnostic hallmark allowing initial (prefibrotic) IMF to be distinguished from the allied subtypes of cMPDs with thrombocythemia (Table 3.1). The megakaryocytic cell lineage is not only characterized by a severe disturbance of histotopography resulting in a prominent and abnormal clustering (Fig. 3.2b) and a translocation towards the endosteal border, but most importantly also by a pronounced deviation from normal nuclear-cytoplasmic differentiation. The latter causes dysplastic features clearly indicating maturation defects (Fig. 3.2b, c). These anomalies are compatible with a gross variety of size and shape ranging from giant- to micromegakaryocytes showing bulky, cloud-like nuclei due to a bulbous lobulation and an abnormal coarse pattern of chromatin [1, 2, 8, 9, 11, 17].

In contrast to the findings in initial-early IMF, marrow biopsy specimens from patients with full-blown disease according to clinical features [14, 15] demonstrate dense reticulin and/or collagen fibrosis. Hematopoiesis may be hypercellular, but is more often normocellular or hypocellular, with patches of cells separated by strands of loose connective tissue or islets of fat (Table 3.1). Foci of immature cells may be prominent, although myeloblasts are not frequent findings. On the other hand, increased numbers and dilation of marrow sinusoids with intrasinusoidal hematopoiesis are further characteristics [10, 19, 20]. Atypical megakaryocytes with cytological abnormalities as described for the prefibrotic (initial) stages of IMF (Fig. 3.2b, c) are often the most notable marrow elements, and occur in sizeable clusters or sheets, or within dilated sinusoids (Fig. 3.2d).

In terminal stages the bone marrow may be almost devoid of hematopoietic elements and consists mainly of dense reticulin or collagen fibrosis with small islands of hematopoietic precursors situated within the marrow sinusoids (Fig. 3.3a, b). Osteoid or plaque-like appositional new bone formation that can occupy more than 70% of the marrow space (osteomyelosclerosis) may be observed in these advanced stages (Fig. 3.3a).

◁
and cytological anomalies, in particular clumping of nuclear chromatin with bulbous cloud-like nuclei, (endo-)mitotic figures (*arrow*) and naked nuclei (*arrowheads*). **d** During the late stages of IMF the bone marrow becomes hypocellular and shows expanded adipose tissue with dilated sinuses harboring clusters of hematopoiesis including atypical megakaryocytes (*arrow*) (a × 170, b–d × 370; a, b CD61; c, d PAS)

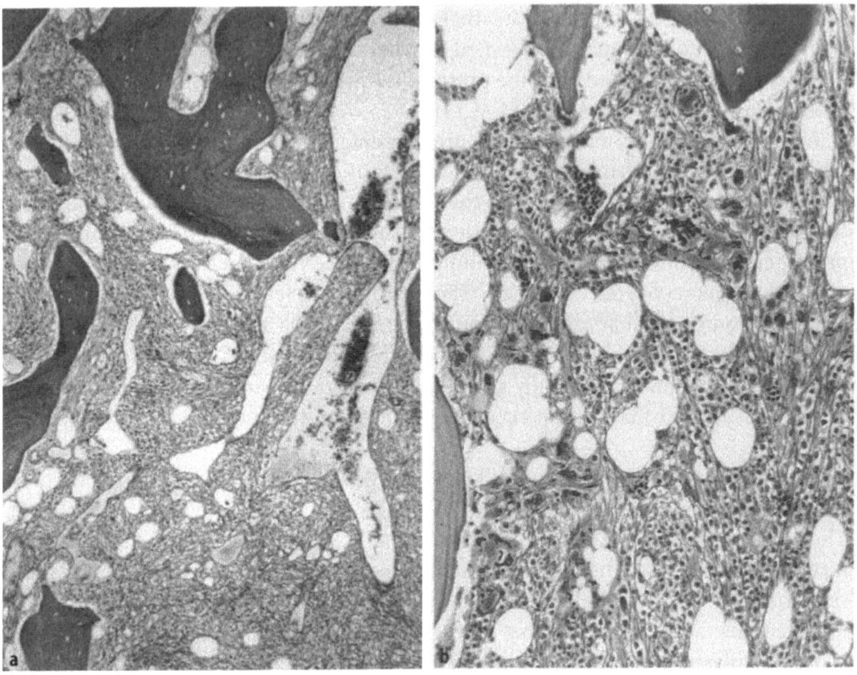

Fig. 3.3a, b. Idiopathic myelofibrosis (IMF). **a** Advanced fibroosteosclerotic (terminal) stage with formation of endophytic (woven) bone and large dilated sinuses containing islets of hematopoiesis (compare with Fig. 3.2d). **b** Clusters of atypical megakaryocytes are grouped between dense bundles of collagen fibers and fat cells (a × 90, b × 170; a, b Gomori's silver impregnation)

Follow-up examination in IMF is in keeping with the assumption that there is a stage-like evolution of the disease process, especially concerning the development of osteomyelosclerotic changes [10, 12, 21, 22]. This feature occurs at a significantly varying speed and its progression is unpredictable [21, 22]. Moreover, it is reasonable to assume that patients present at very different stages to doctors' offices or hospitals. The latter accounts for the occasionally striking heterogeneity of bone marrow morphology (Table 3.1) and clinical data at presentation. In accordance with relevant historical (fatigue, malaise, night sweats, abdominal distress) and characteristic clinical findings (anemia, splenomegaly, erythro- and normoblasts in the peripheral blood), these patients are consistent with more advanced stages [11, 21] and therefore comply with the well-known diagnostic criteria including manifest (so-called agnogenic) myeloid metaplasia [14, 15]. The phenomenon of progressively occurring alterations in IMF is indicated by a corresponding classification of clinical and associated histological features [8].

The first tangible evidence of this disorder is the initial (prefibrotic) and hypercellular stage [17] which about 3 to 5 years later shows an insidious transition into manifest myelofibrosis [1, 10, 16, 22]. Only then are laboratory findings conforming with clear-cut or classical IMF with (agnogenic) myeloid metaplasia according to data in the relevant literature [14, 15] revealed. On the other hand, patients diagnosed at early stages show a more favorable prognosis, in particular when relative survival rates and disease-specific loss of life expectancy are calculated [23]. In the WHO classification of cMPDs [24] (see Chap. 1), this concept of a step-wise evolution of disease features in IMF including the existence of a prefibrotic (initial) stage as precursor lesion has been validated [25].

3.4 Secondary Polycythemia Versus Polycythemia Vera

In patients presenting with a borderline to marked elevation of hemoglobin (> 18 g/dl in men and > 16 g/dl in women, corresponding with hematocrits of about 51% and 48%, respectively), differentiation of PV from reactive-acquired or secondary conditions-SP is a challenging issue. Regarding the diagnostic criteria of the PVSG as a gold standard [4, 6, 26], a number of clinical parameters have proved to be significantly different in both groups of patients presenting with marked erythrocytosis. With exclusion of the red cell mass and cell culture studies [6, 27, 28], which, however, at the beginning are rarely determined in routine practice, erythropoietin (EPO) level, platelet count, LDH, spleen size and leukocyte alkaline phosphatase score are sufficiently discriminating [8].

In this context it should not be overlooked that the value of bone marrow biopsy is still not generally acknowledged and some authors argue that in PV, standardized objective histopathological criteria are not yet well established [6, 26]. Furthermore, until now characteristic bone marrow features have been described in a retrospective fashion, i.e., in patients with PV already diagnosed by reliable clinical criteria [6, 28]. Because there are sufficient clear objective laboratory markers of the disease, the inclusion of bone marrow histology has been assumed to be unnecessary [26]. On the other hand, a more detailed evaluation of histopathology may turn out to be an invaluable aid, in particular to recognizing initial changes as well as the risk of developing myelofibrosis and leukemic transformation.

Features of distinctive value are consistent with a set of specific bone marrow lesions (Table 3.1). In initial-early as well as in so-called polycythemic stages, differentiation from SP is feasible by regarding the trilineage proliferation of myeloid cells or panmyelosis (Fig. 3.4a, b). A diagnostic hallmark is megakaryopoiesis, since in PV there is a conspicuous pleomorphous appearance (Fig. 3.4c). This is in keeping with giant and small megakaryocytes which contain deeply lobulated nuclei and are usually arranged in loose clusters [1, 8, 10, 29]. Contrasting these features, in SP megakaryocytes are small to medium-sized with an inconspicuous cytology [8]. Moreover, in SP distinctive changes of the interstitial compartment may be recognized including iron-laden macrophages, cell debris in the histiocytic reticular cells and a perivascular plasmacytosis [8, 29]. In the full-blown polycythemic stage, there is a predominant normoblastic erythroid proliferation in the marrow [8, 20, 30]. Characteristically, the bone marrow biopsy is hypercellular for the patient's age [8, 10, 19, 20, 29]. Erythroid, megakaryocytic and granulocytic trilineage proliferation (panmyelosis) accounts for the increased cellularity (Table 3.1), but the enhancement in the numbers of nucleated erythroid precursors and of megakaryocytes is usually most prominent [8, 10, 19]. Normoblastic erythropoiesis is not only significantly expanded, but also a pronounced proliferative capacity is seen opposed to SP [31]. Granulopoiesis is mor-

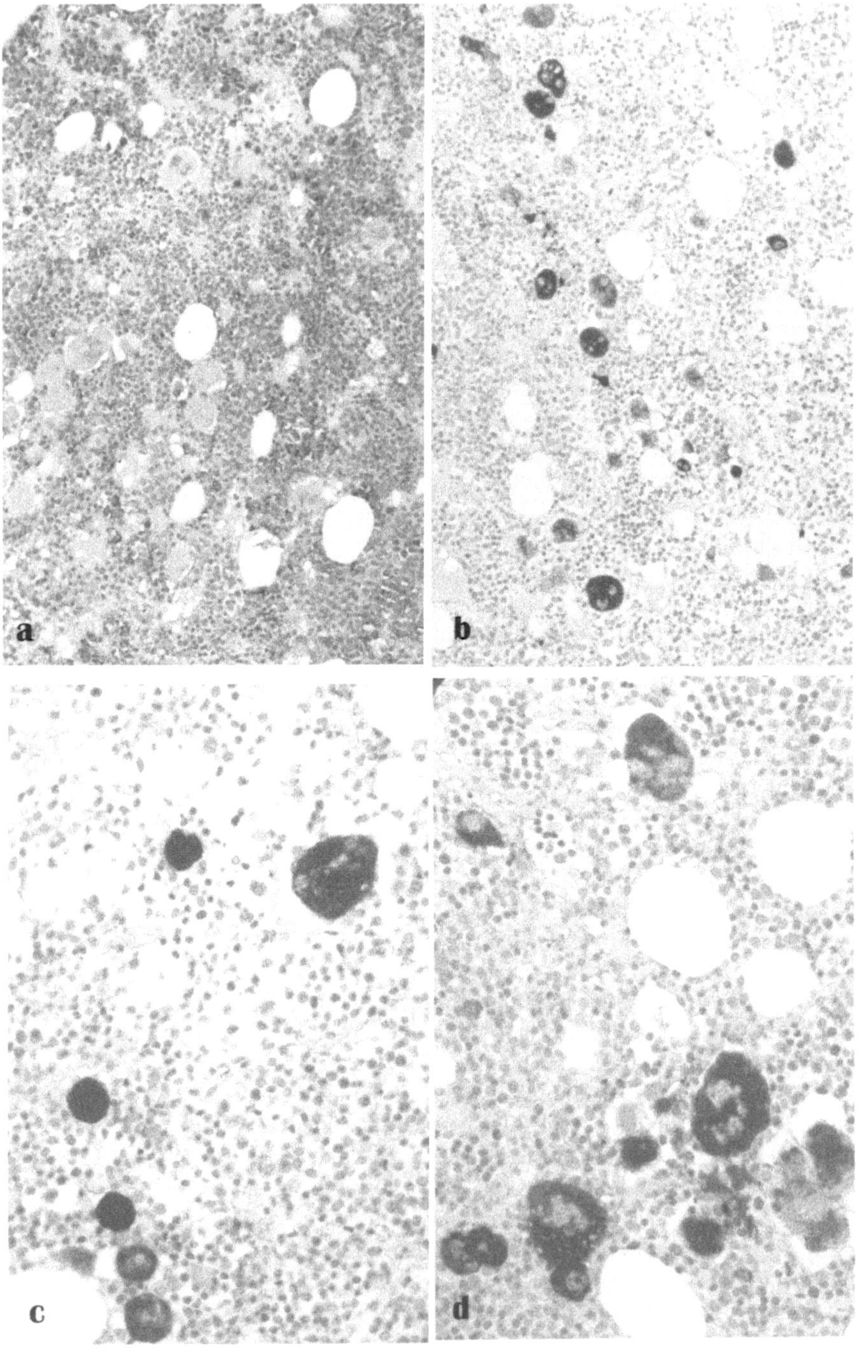

Fig. 3.4a–d. Polycythemia vera (PV). **a** Survey with trilineage proliferation of marrow cells and dilated sinuses. **b** Loose clusters of megakaryocytes reveal a pleomorphous aspect, i.e., giant to large cells are grouped together with small ones. **c** Early-stage PV with small and occasionally giant megakaryocytes indicating a remarkable variability in shape and size. **d** Megakaryocytes may be greatly enlarged (giant forms) in patients with significantly increased platelet counts, but do not display gross cytological anomalies (a, b × 170; c, d × 370; a chloroacetate-esterase, b–d CD61)

phologically normal and the percent of immature precursors is not significantly increased [8, 20]. Contrasting SP, megakaryocytes show a pleomorphous aspect, i.e., small to giant cells are grouped together and usually they have regularly deeply lobulated nuclei without bizarre or dysplastic aspects comparable to those in IMF [1, 8, 10, 11, 29]. Megakaryopoiesis may be very prominent, especially in patients with associated severe thrombocythemia (Fig. 3.4d). Silver stains will show normal reticulin fibers in about 70 to 80% of patients, but the remainder have reticulin fibrosis of variable degrees [10, 20, 30]. Stainable iron (iron-laden macrophages) is not observable in more than 95% of patients [30].

3.5 Proliferation and Apoptosis in cMPDs

In the bone marrow, apoptosis and proliferation are generally held to be important regulators of normal development and homeostasis [32]. While assessment of these variables has been proven to provide useful prognostic information in malignant lymphomas, myelodysplastic syndromes and acute myeloid leukemia, in cMPDs, little in known about the clinical impact of programmed cell death and in particular cell turnover [33, 34]. In this context it is imperative to stress that growth and expansion of the neoplastic hematopoietic cell clone is dependent on both proliferation and cell death and that any situation in which the number of proliferating cells exceeds that of apoptotic cells implies an increase in leukemic tumor burden. Consequently the dynamics of hematopoiesis are characterized by an imbalance of cell death and proliferation [32].

It is reasonable to assume that important biological information may be obtained from applying a combination of proliferation markers in association with an evaluation of apoptosis to extend previous experimental findings on hematopoietic cell kinetics [33]. In bone marrow tissue, proliferative activity is readily detectable by a set of proliferation-associated nuclear antigens such as PCNA (Fig. 3.5a, b). The latter has been to proven by a very reliable method for the identification of cycling cells [18, 31, 35, 36]. In addition, topoisomerase IIα expression can be demonstrated by the monoclonal antibody Ki-S1 [37]. Since both nuclear antigens are expressed in different phases of the cell cycle, the proportion of cells in the G2/M phase is specifically calculable. On the other hand, as has been found that apoptosis can easily be detected by the in-situ end-labeling (ISEL) method (Fig. 3.5c, d).

It is noteworthy that patients with IMF, PV and ET show a normal range of apoptosis (Fig. 3.6), and IMF and PV are characterized by a raised proliferative activity. The PCNA index and topoisomerase IIα expression show significant differences in IMF between prefibrotic-early and advanced fibrosclerotic stages of the disease. Particularly in early (hypercellular) stages of IMF, an imbalance between proliferation and cell death (apoptosis) is present [34]. In patients with a hypercellular bone marrow [17], a normal or enhanced proliferation rate according to PCNA-positivity (late G1 and S phase of the cell cycle) is associated with a higher incidence of apoptosis. It may be speculated that this phenomenon reflects an increase in the regenerative (turnover) capacity of hematopoiesis [34]. The dynamics of hematopoiesis may be readily determined by calculation of the so-called hematopoietic turnover index (HTI), an important indicator of changes in the neoplastic cell burden [33]. In

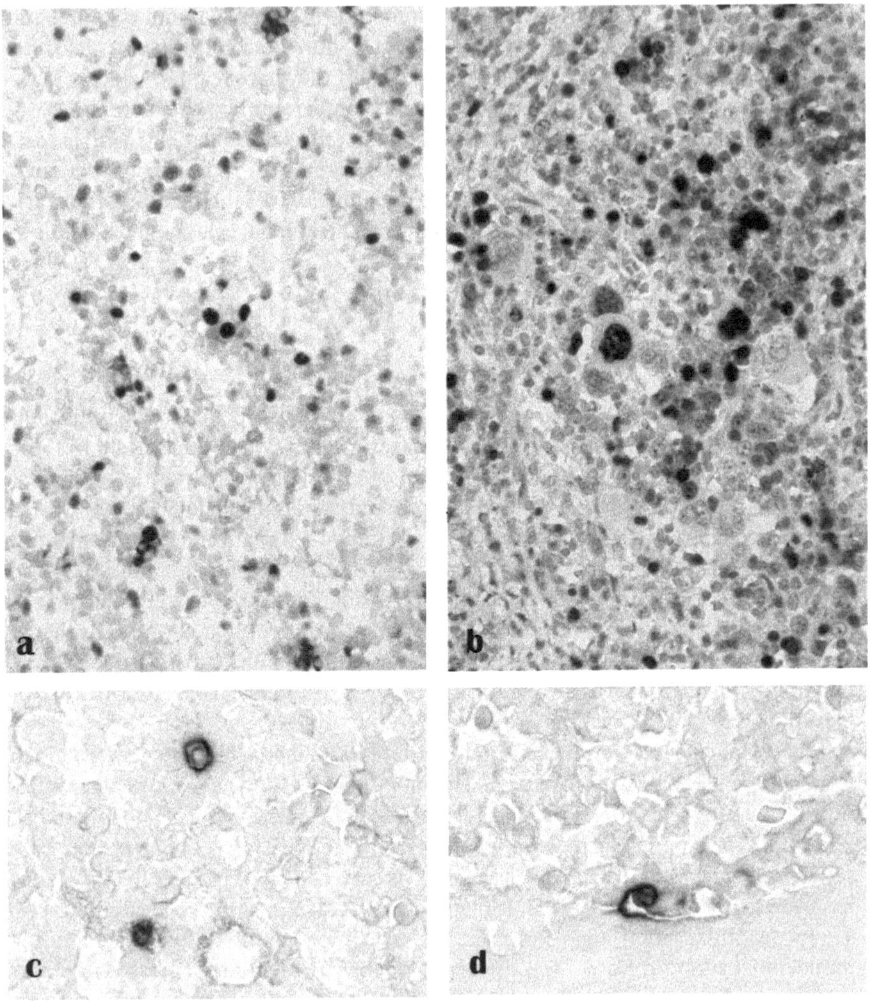

Fig. 3.5a–d. Proliferation and apoptosis in the bone marrow. **a** PCNA-labeling of marrow specimen in PV with distinctively stained nuclei. **b** Increased frequency of positive staining including megakaryocytes for topoisomerase IIα (Ki-S1) in IMF. **c** Single apoptotic bodies are marked in initial IMF in the marrow center. **d** Apoptosis may also occur at the endosteal generation zone (granulopoiesis) in prefibrotic IMF (a, b × 370; c, d × 890)

reactive lesions, such as those in SP or ST, no relevant differences in corresponding values are exhibited, whereas in IMF and PV significant increases are observable (Fig. 3.6).

According to cell culture studies, the proliferation of the neoplastic cell clone in cMPDs depends on deregulated apoptosis, a feature that has been acknowledged especially in PV [38]. Normally, EPO is essential for the survival and proliferation of erythroid lineage progenitors (CFU-E). In PV these precursor cells are hypersensitive to a number of growth factors including this mediator, and therefore they are able to

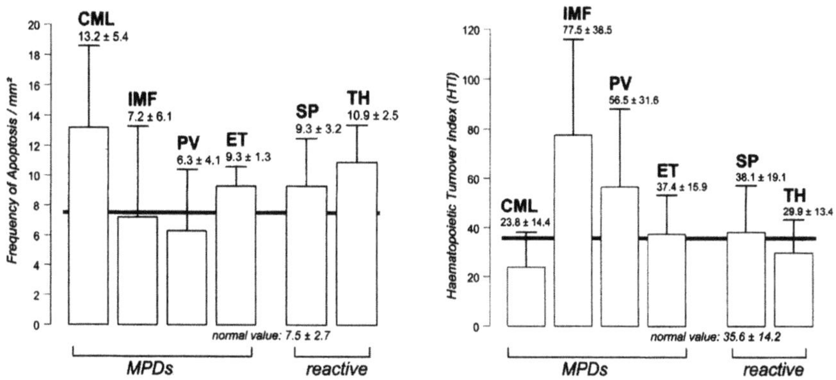

Fig. 3.6. Frequency of apoptosis and hematopoietic turnover index in 400 patients with MPDs according to morphometric evaluation – comparison with chronic myeloid leukemia (CML) as well as reactive lesions, i.e., secondary polycythemia (SP) and reactive thrombocytosis (TH)

survive and differentiate spontaneously [26, 38, 39]. Members of the Bcl-2 family of apoptosis regulators and the Fas-antigen system have been shown to influence their EPO-dependent development [40]. By this mechanisms an enhancement of the erythroid-lineage is generated which is thought to contribute significantly to the pathogenesis of PV that is considered to be a myeloaccumulative disorder [26]. A growing body of evidence stemming from clinical and experimental observations strongly suggests that opposed to the erythroid lineage progenitors, in TH and ET megakaryocyte growth (CFU-MEG) is the predominant feature of cell turnover [41]. Consequently, differences between ET and TH are in line with reduced in vitro formation of CFU-MEG in the latter disorder [42].

3.6 Summary

A more elaborate evaluation of bone marrow features results in certain sets of diagnostic criteria with discriminating capacity in cMPDs, but especially in ET (Table 3.1). In this context assessment of proliferation and apoptosis promotes a better understanding of the underlying hematopoietic cell kinetics. These points should be taken into account in a synoptical approach which should include relevant laboratory data and morphological features from ongoing and prospective clinical trials and have the aim of improving the diagnosis and consequently treatment modalities for cMPDs as has been attempted in the WHO classification cMPD (see Chap. 1).

References

1. Buhr T, Georgii A, Schuppan O, Amor A, Kloutsi V (1992) Histologic findings in bone marrow biopsies of patients with thrombocythemic cell counts. Ann Hematol 64:286–291
2. Thiele J, Kvasnicka HM, Diehl V, Fischer R, Michiels JJ (1999) Clinicopathological diagnosis and differential criteria of thrombocythemias in various myeloproliferative disorders by histopathology, histochemistry and immunostaining from bone marrow biopsies. Leuk Lymphoma 33:207–218

3. Thiele J, Kvasnicka HM, Zankovich R, Diehl V (2000) Relevance of bone marrow features in the differential diagnosis between essential thrombocythemia and early stage idiopathic myelofibrosis. Haematologica 85:1126–1134
4. Murphy S (1999) Diagnostic criteria and prognosis in polycythemia vera and essential thrombocythemia. Semin Hematol 36:9–13
5. Murphy S, Peterson P, Iland H, Laszlo J (1997) Experience of the Polycythemia Vera Study Group with essential thrombocythemia: a final report on diagnostic criteria, survival, and leukemic transition by treatment. Semin Hematol 34:29–39
6. Pearson TC (1998) Diagnosis and classification of erythrocytoses and thrombocytoses. Baillieres Clin Haematol 11:695–720
7. Michiels JJ, Juvonen E (1997) Proposal for revised diagnostic criteria of essential thrombocythemia and polycythemia vera by the Thrombocythemia Vera Study Group. Semin Thromb Hemost 23:339–347
8. Michiels JJ, Thiele J (2002) Clinical and pathological criteria for the diagnosis of essential thrombocythemia, polycythemia vera, and idiopathic myelofibrosis (agnogenic myeloid metaplasia). Int J Hematol 76:133–145
9. Thiele J, Kvasnicka HM, Werden C, Zankovich R, Diehl V, Fischer R (1996) Idiopathic primary osteomyelofibrosis: a clinico-pathological study on 208 patients with special emphasis on evolution of disease features, differentiation from essential thrombocythemia and variables of prognostic impact. Leuk Lymphoma 22:303–317
10. Georgii A, Buesche G, Kreft A (1998) The histopathology of chronic myeloproliferative diseases. Baillieres Clin Haematol 11:721–749
11. Thiele J, Kvasnicka HM (2003) Diagnostic differentiation of essential thrombocythaemia from thrombocythaemias associated with chronic idiopathic myelofibrosis by discriminate analysis of bone marrow features – a clinicopathological study on 272 patients. Histol Histopathol 18:93–102
12. Buhr T, Georgii A, Choritz H (1993) Myelofibrosis in chronic myeloproliferative disorders. Incidence among subtypes according to the Hannover Classification. Pathol Res Pract 189:121–132
13. Reilly JT (1997) Idiopathic myelofibrosis: pathogenesis, natural history and management. Blood Rev 11:233–242
14. Barosi G (1999) Myelofibrosis with myeloid metaplasia: diagnostic definition and prognostic classification for clinical studies and treatment guidelines. J Clin Oncol 17:2954–2970
15. Tefferi A (2000) Myelofibrosis with myeloid metaplasia. N Engl J Med 342:1255–1265
16. Thiele J, Kvasnicka HM, Boeltken B, Zankovich R, Diehl V, Fischer R (1999) Initial (prefibrotic) stages of idiopathic (primary) myelofibrosis (IMF) – a clinicopathological study. Leukemia 13:1741–1748
17. Thiele J, Kvasnicka HM, Zankovich R, Diehl V (2002) Early stage idiopathic (primary) myelofibrosis – current issues of diagnostic features. Leuk Lymphoma 43:1035–1041
18. Thiele J, Windecker R, Kvasnicka HM, Titius BR, Zankovich R, Fischer R (1994) Erythropoiesis in primary (idiopathic) osteomyelofibrosis: quantification, PCNA-reactivity, and prognostic impact. Am J Hematol 46:36–42
19. Bartl R, Frisch B, Wilmanns W (1993) Potential of bone marrow biopsy in chronic myeloproliferative disorders (MPD). Eur J Haematol 50:41–52
20. Dickstein JI, Vardiman JW (1993) Issues in the pathology and diagnosis of the chronic myeloproliferative disorders and the myelodysplastic syndromes. Am J Clin Pathol 99:513–525
21. Buhr T, Buesche G, Choritz H, Langer F, Kreipe H (2003) Evolution of myelofibrosis in chronic idiopathic myelofibrosis as evidenced in sequential bone marrow biopsy specimens. Am J Clin Pathol 119:152–158
22. Thiele J, Kvasnicka HM, Schmitt-Gräff A, Diehl V (2003) Dynamics of fibrosis in chronic idiopathic (primary) myelofibrosis during therapy: a follow-up study on 309 patients. Leuk Lymphoma 44:549–553
23. Kvasnicka HM, Thiele J, Werden C, Zankovich R, Diehl V, Fischer R (1997) Prognostic factors in idiopathic (primary) osteomyelofibrosis. Cancer 15:708–719
24. Vardiman JW, Bain B, Brunning RD, Flandrin G, Harris NL, Imbert M, Pierre R, Thiele J (2001) Chronic myeloproliferative diseases. In: Jaffe ES, Harris NL, Stein H, Vardiman JW (eds) WHO classification of tumours: tumours of haematopoietic and lymphoid tissues. IARC Press, Lyon, pp 16–44
25. Thiele J, Imbert M, Pierre R, Vardiman JW, Brunning RD, Flandrin G (2001) Chronic idiopathic myelofibrosis. In: Jaffe ES, Harris NL, Stein H, Vardiman JW (eds) WHO Classification of tumours: tumours of haematopoietic and lymphoid tissues. IARC Press, Lyon, pp 35–38
26. Spivak JL (2002) Polycythemia vera: myths, mechanisms, and management. Blood 100:4272–4290
27. Eridani S, Sawyer B, Pearson TC (1987) Patterns of in vitro BFU-E proliferation in different forms of polycythaemia and in thrombocythaemia. Eur J Haematol 38:363–369
28. Messinezy M, Pearson TC (1998) Diagnosis of polycythaemia. J Clin Pathol 51:1–4

29. Thiele J, Kvasnicka HM, Zankovich R, Diehl V (2001) The value of bone marrow histology in differentiating between early stage polycythemia vera and secondary (reactive) polycythemias. Haematologica 86:368–374
30. Ellis JT, Peterson P, Geller SA, Rappaport H (1986) Studies of the bone marrow in polycythemia vera and the evolution of myelofibrosis and second hematologic malignancies. Semin Hematol 23:144–155
31. Thiele J, Meuter RB, Titius R, Zankowich R, Fischer R (1993) Proliferating cell nuclear antigen expression by erythroid precursors in normal bone marrow, in reactive lesions and in polycythaemia rubra vera. Histopathology 22:429–435
32. Koury MJ (1992) Programmed cell death (apoptosis) in hematopoiesis. Exp Hematol 20:391–394
33. Thiele J, Zirbes TK, Lorenzen J, Kvasnicka HM, Scholz S, Erdmann A, Flucke U, Diehl V, Fischer R (1997) Hematopoietic turnover index in reactive and neoplastic bone marrow lesions: quantification by apoptosis and PCNA labeling. Ann Hematol 75:33–39
34. Kvasnicka HM, Thiele J, Regn C, Zankovich R, Diehl V, Fischer R (1999) Prognostic impact of apoptosis and proliferation in idiopathic (primary) myelofibrosis. Ann Hematol 78:65–72
35. Pellegrini W, Facchetti F, Marocolo D, Salvi L, Capucci A, Tironi A, Rossi G (1995) Assessment of cell proliferation in normal and pathological bone marrow biopsies: a study using double sequential immunophenotyping on paraffin sections. Histopathology 27:397–405
36. Budke H, Orazi A, Neiman RS, Cattoretti G, John K, Barberis M (1994) Assessment of cell proliferation in paraffin sections of normal bone marrow by the monoclonal antibodies Ki-67 and PCNA. Mod Pathol 7:860–866
37. Kreipe H, Heidebrecht HJ, Hansen S, Röhlk W, Kubbies M, Wacker HH, Tiemann M, Radzun HJ, Parwaresch R (1993) A new proliferation-associated nuclear antigen detectable in paraffin-embedded tissues by the monoclonal antibody Ki-S1. Am J Pathol 142:3–9
38. Fernandez-Luna LJ (1999) Apoptosis and polycythemia vera. Curr Opin Hematol 6:94–99
39. Casadevall N, Vainchenker W, Lacombe C, Vinci G, Chapman J, Breton-Gorius J, Varet B (1982) Erythroid progenitors in polycythaemia vera: demonstration of their hypersensitivity to erythropoietin using serum free cultures. Blood 59:447–451
40. Silva M, Richard C, Benito A, Sanz C, Olalla I, Fernandez-Luna JL (1998) Expression of Bcl-x in erythroid precursors from patients with polycythemia vera. N Engl J Med 338:564–571
41. Juvonen E, Ikkala E, Oksanen K, Ruutu T (1993) Megakaryocyte and erythroid colony formation in essential thrombocythaemia and reactive thrombocytosis: diagnostic value and correlation to complications. Br J Haematol 83:192–197
42. Rolovic Z, Basara N, Gotic M, Sefer D, Bogdanovic A (1995) The determination of spontaneous megakaryocyte colony formation is an unequivocal test for the discrimination between essential thrombocythaemia and reactive thrombocytosis. Br J Haematol 90:326–331

Chapter 4

Cytogenetics of Myeloproliferative Disorders

Anthony J. Bench, Brian J.P. Huntly, Anthony R. Green

4.1 Introduction

Unlike the Philadelphia chromosome in chronic myeloid leukemia (CML), there is no pathognomonic chromosomal abnormality associated with the cMPDs. However, a number of recurrent chromosomal abnormalities have been documented. Chromosomal abnormalities, as detected by G-banding, are seen in 30–40 % of patients with polycythemia vera (PV) and idiopathic myelofibrosis (IMF) (Table 4.1) but are infrequent in patients with essential thrombocythemia (ET).

In PV, an abnormal karyotype is often seen at diagnosis but the proportion of patients with an abnormality increases as the disease progresses, possibly due to clonal progression [1, 2]. A higher incidence of abnormalities is also seen in patients receiving myelosuppressive therapy [3]. This may reflect the leukemogenic effects of the treatment or may indicate that patients whose disease is progressive (and therefore requiring more aggressive treatment) are more likely to develop cytogenetic changes. Indeed, an abnormal karyotype is associated with disease progression to myelofibrosis or leukemia [1, 4]. An abnormal karyotype may be a poor prognostic indicator in PV [1, 2] and IMF [5].

Table 4.1. Summary of karyotypic abnormalities identified by G-banding in the myeloproliferative disorders. Reproduced from [3]

	Polycythemia vera		Idiopathic myelofibrosis		Essential thrombocythemia	
Abnormality	Number of occurrences of abnormality	Percentage of all patients	Number of occurrences of abnormality	Percentage of all patients	Number of occurrences of abnormality	Percentage of all patients
Deletion of 20q	45	8.4	28	7.1	1	0.2
Deletion of 13q	16	3.0	25	6.3	3	0.7
Trisomy 8	37	6.9	20	5.0	4	0.9
Trisomy 9	35	6.6	4	1.0	1	0.2
Trisomy of 1q	19	3.6	14	3.5	0	0
Deletion of 7q or monosomy 7	5	0.9	15	3.8	0	0
Deletion of 5q or monosomy 5	17	3.2	6	1.5	0	0
Total number of patients with one or more abnormality	180	33.7	157	39.5	23	5.0
Total patients	534	–	397	–	456	–

Deletions of part of the long arm of chromosomes 20 [del(20q)] and 13 [(del(13q)], trisomies of chromosomes 8 and 9 and duplication of part of the long arm of chromosome 1 have all been seen in untreated patients and are frequently present as sole abnormalities. They are likely, therefore, to mark the site of genes that play an important role in the pathogenesis of the cMPDs. However, deletions or monosomies of chromosomes 5 and 7 are almost invariably seen after exposure to myelosuppressive therapy and frequently as part of a complex karyotype. It is therefore unlikely that these abnormalities are involved in the etiology of the cMPDs. Balanced translocations are uncommon in MPDs but disorders associated with consistent rearrangements have aided in the identification of genes that contribute to the pathogenesis of rare MPDs.

4.2 Deletions

4.2.1 Deletion of 20q

Deletion of the long arm of chromosome 20 [(del(20q)] was the second most common sole structural abnormality, after t(9;22), seen in a series of almost 3000 consecutive bone marrow samples analyzed by G-banding at the Mayo clinic [6]. In addition to its involvement in the MPDs (Table 4.1), del(20q) is also observed in patients with myelodysplastic syndrome (MDS) and acute myeloid leukemia (AML) and in CML blast crisis, but rarely in lymphoid malignancies. This pattern of disease association suggests that the deleted region of chromosome 20 marks the site of one or more genes, whose loss or inactivation perturbs the behavior of hematopoietic progenitors. There appears to be no difference in the survival of cMPD patients with and without a 20q deletion [7].

MPDs and MDS are thought to result from transformation of a hematopoietic progenitor cell. It was therefore of interest to determine whether 20q deletions arise in a pluripotent progenitor or in a later, committed progenitor. The 20q deletion was detected in clonal granulocytes and monocytes but not in B cells or T cells from one patient [8]. However, it was seen in EBV-transformed B-cell lines from two patients with a 20q deletion [8, 9] and in CFU-GM, CFU-GEMM and BFU-E colonies from one of these patients [9]. Clearly, the 20q deletion can arise in a very early progenitor with both lymphoid and myeloid potential.

The 20q deletion can readily be detected in peripheral blood neutrophils of most patients. However, in a subset of patients, no deletion was detectable in peripheral blood granulocytes despite being present in the majority of bone marrow metaphases [10]. This suggests that granulocytes carrying the deletion may be preferentially destroyed or retained within the bone marrow in some patients. Granulocytes from female patients displayed a clonal pattern of X-inactivation suggesting that either the 20q deletion was not the initiating event or that the clonal X-inactivation pattern in these patients was age-related and not associated with the disease [11].

Molecular and cytogenetic analysis has been undertaken to construct a common deleted region (CDR) spanning 20q12 within which target genes lie. Since MPD and MDS are overlapping but clinically different diseases, it remains possible that different or additional genes are involved in the two disorders. Therefore, two overlapping

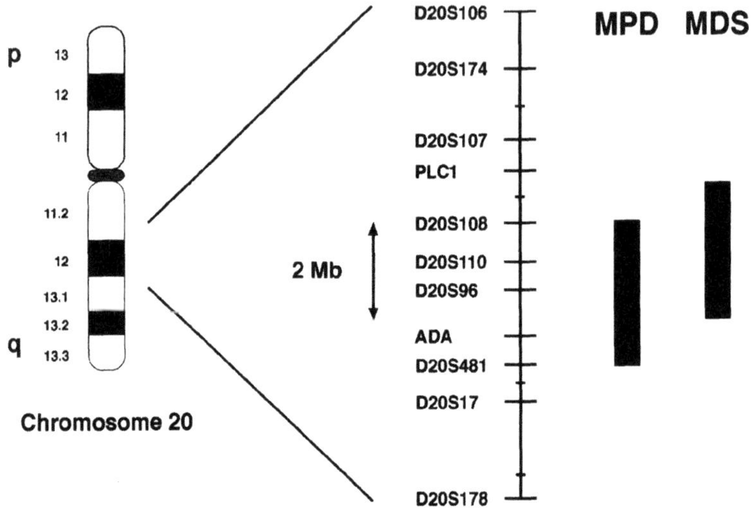

Fig. 4.1. Summary of common deleted regions on 20q for MPD and MDS. The MPD CDR is bordered by D20S108 and D20S481 [12, 13]. The MDS CDR is flanked by PACs 620E11 and 196H17 [13]

CDRs have been defined. Both the MPD CDR and MDS CDR span approximately 3 Mb [12, 13]. The overlapping CDR spans 2 Mb (Fig. 4.1) within which a number of possible target genes have been identified including *SFRS6*, *h-l(3)mbt* and *MYBL2*, although mutations have not yet been identified. However, in the h-l(3)mbt-gene, monoallelic methylation of two CpG islands correlates with transcriptional silencing of this gene and h-l(3)mbt-transcription has been shown to occur from the paternally derived allele in five individuals from two families. Thus, this gene represents a novel imprinted locus, the first vertebrate Polycomb group gene shown to be regulated by this mechanism, which may have implications for the pathogenesis of myeloid malignancies associated with 20q deletions [14].

Despite considerable effort, small deletions of 20q have not been identified [15, 16], with most being many-fold larger than the size of the CDR. It is therefore possible that more than one target gene exists on 20q and different combinations of target genes could account for the different biological characteristics of the myeloid disorders associated with 20q deletions (Fig. 4.2). This concept has important consequences for the strategies used to identify such target genes [17].

4.2.2 Deletion of 13q

Deletion of 13q is more common in IMF than in PV (Table 4.1) and is also associated with post-polycythemic myelofibrosis [1, 2]. Deletions of 13q are also seen in patients with MDS and CML, as well as in a number of lymphoid malignancies. Deletion of 13q is a poor prognostic feature in some lymphoid malignancies, but no data are yet available in cMPDs.

Molecular alterations of 13q may be more common in cMPDs than conventional G-banding results suggest. Firstly, LOH at the *RB1* locus, which maps to 13q14, was

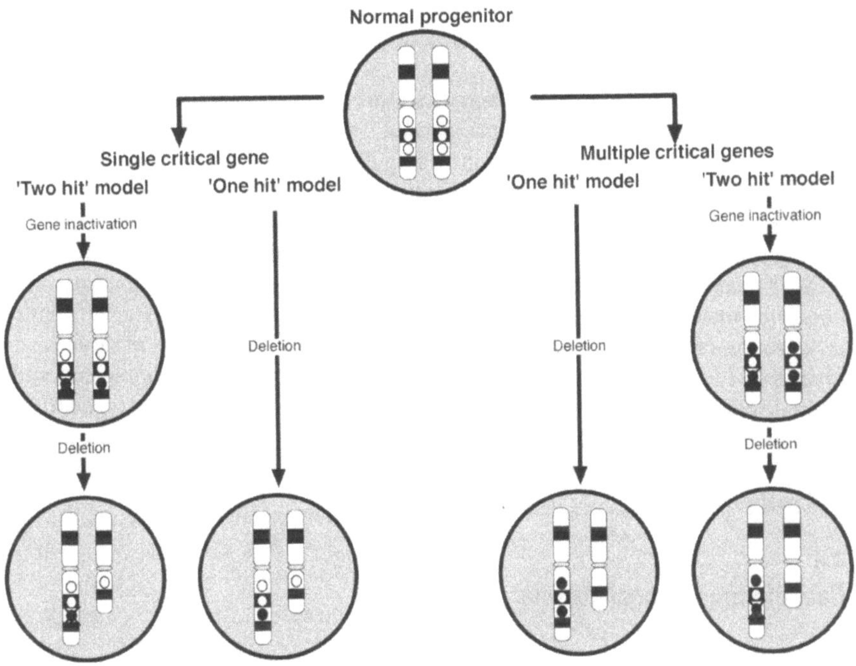

Fig. 4.2. Potential mechanisms of the pathogenesis of deletions in cMPD. If there is a single critical gene (*dark circle*), it may be necessary for both alleles to be deleted or inactivated. Alternatively, loss of a single allele (haploinsufficiency) as mediated by a deletion may be sufficient to produce a phenotypic effect ('one hit' model). If there is more than one target gene, the one hit model could entail haploinsufficiency for two or more target genes, perhaps separated by a large distance. In contrast, the two hit model would involve biallelic inactivation of at least one of the target genes. Reproduced with permission [17]

observed in 13 out of 30 MPD patients [18]. Secondly, loss of loci from 13q14 was demonstrated by FISH in patients with IMF and PV for whom conventional G-banding failed to show a deletion [19, 20]. A CDR spanning 4 cM has been constructed for patients with a myeloid malignancy [21]. This CDR encompasses the small CDRs that have been constructed for CLL. Within the CLL CDRs, a number of candidate genes have been identified, many of which are underexpressed within del(13q) patients compared to normal B cells [22]. However, no genomic mutations have been identified [23] suggesting that downregulation of one or more of these genes by an unknown mechanism may contribute to the pathogenesis of CLL. Whether the same mechanism operates in the pathogenesis of myeloid malignancies with 13q deletions is not known.

4.3 Haploinsufficiency Models

It has been generally assumed that deletions such as del(20q) and del(13q) mark the site of tumor suppressor genes that behave according to Knudson's two hit hypothesis of gene inactivation (Fig. 4.2). In this model, one allele of the gene could be inactivated by a microdeletion or point mutation, or transcriptionally silenced by methylation of the promoter. The second allele is then lost due to a large deletion.

A haploinsufficiency model of tumor suppressor gene inactivation [24] is also possible. The requirement for the presence of two active alleles of a given gene has been noted for a number of genes controlling development as well as for a number of genes implicated in the formation of solid tumors [24]. A number of tumor suppressor genes such as *p27*, *p53* and *p73* do show retention of one active allele in human tumors. Perhaps the best evidence for haploinsufficiency of the tumor suppressor genes *p27* and *p53* has been derived by the generation of heterozygous knockout mice [24]. In these models, tumorigenesis did not necessarily require inactivation of the remaining intact allele implying that haploid loss of these genes is sufficient to contribute towards tumor formation. In myeloid malignancies with a 20q deletion, no evidence of a second inactivating event such as homozygous deletion has been obtained [25]. Hence, inactivation of one copy of the target gene, for example by deletion, could be sufficient to contribute to the pathogenesis of myeloid malignancies.

4.4 Gain of Chromosomal Material

4.4.1 Trisomy 8

Trisomy 8 occurs in approximately 10% of patients with a hematological malignancy, and is therefore the most common numerical autosomal abnormality [6]. Trisomy 8 is also common in MDS and AML and in CML blast crisis. The use of FISH-based techniques to detect trisomy 8 has provided a number of interesting observations [26]. Firstly, in some patients, cells with trisomy 8 may have a proliferative advantage over normal cells in culture [27]. Secondly, trisomy 8 has been detected in minor subclones of some [26] but not all [27] patients for whom conventional karyotyping showed no such aberration, indicating that trisomy 8 may be present in a greater proportion of patients than originally thought. However, initial reports that a quarter of all MPD patients possess a trisomy 8, by FISH, have not been confirmed in larger studies [28].

By combining FISH with immunophenotyping, trisomy 8 has been demonstrated in cells of the erythroid and myeloid origin but not in mature lymphoid cells of PV patients [29]. Furthermore, trisomy 8 was present in the majority of BFU-E and CFU-GM colonies and in CD34+ progenitor cells. Similar restriction of trisomy 8 to mature myeloid and erythroid lineages and its detection in progenitor cells has also been demonstrated in MDS and in CML. Therefore, trisomy 8 usually arises in the stem cell compartment but, like del(20q), is not seen within peripheral blood lymphocytes either due to the inability of cells carrying trisomy 8 to undergo lymphoid differentiation or due to the longevity of peripheral blood lymphocytes. The genetic consequence of trisomy 8 has not been determined.

4.4.2 Trisomy 9

FISH techniques have also been applied to the detection of trisomy 9 in myeloid malignancies. As is the case for trisomy 8, observations that trisomy 9 may be present in a significant number of patients have not been replicated [28]. Despite this, interphase FISH may be useful in identifying abnormalities of chromosome 9 missed by conventional cytogenetics [19]. Trisomy 9p as a result of a supernumerary marker chromosome der(1)t(1;9) is a well-recognized abnormality in cMPD patients [30].

4.4.3 Duplication of 1q

Duplication of part of 1q has been demonstrated in a number of MPD patients [31] as well as in patients with MDS [32] and in those with other myeloid malignancies. It has been found at all stages of disease progression including at diagnosis [5]. Dupl(1q) was found in both erythroid and myeloid precursors of an MPD patient, confirming its origin within a multipotent progenitor [33]. A common duplicated region spanning 1q23-q32 has been identified but no molecular analysis has been undertaken.

Duplication of the long arm of chromosome 1 can also arise as a result of a nonreciprocal translocation. For example, the supernumerary chromosome der(1)t(1;9) described above results in trisomy 1q and trisomy 9p both of which may be pathogenetically significant. A derivative chromosome t(1;7) has been observed along with monosomy 7 [32], the consequence of which is monosomy 7q and trisomy 1q.

4.5 Translocations

Balanced translocations in PV, ET or IMF are very rare [34] but may mark the site of genes important for the pathogenesis of cMPD, further characterization of which could offer a shortcut to the identification of novel fusion genes. Two rare MPDs, each associated with a specific rearrangement, have provided important insights into the underlying pathogenetic mechanisms.

4.5.1 8p11 Myeloproliferative Syndrome

The 8p11 myeloproliferative syndrome (EMS) is a rare atypical MPD with a balanced translocation involving 8p11. The peripheral blood and bone marrow have the appearance of a chronic MPD with prominent eosinophilia. In addition, more than 50% of patients have an associated T-cell NHL. Almost invariably, the disease progresses to AML and has a poor prognosis. The majority of cases possess a t(8;13)(p11;q12) although other translocation partners of 8p11 include 6q27 and 9q33. The same chromosomal abnormality is seen in both the lymphoma and myeloid cells, suggesting transformation of a common myeloid/lymphoid progenitor cell [35]. All these translocations disrupt the fibroblast growth factor receptor-1 gene (FGFR1), a receptor protein tyrosine kinase that maps to 8p11. As a result, *FGFR1* becomes fused to *ZNF198* at 13q12, *CEP110* at 9q33 and *FOP* at 6q27 [36] (Fig. 4.3).

Fusion proteins involving tyrosine kinases are a recurring theme in myeloid malignancies (Fig. 4.4). In EMS, the ZNF198-FGFR1 fusion protein contains the N-terminal portion of ZNF198, including a proline-rich oligomerization domain, fused to the C-terminal portion of *FGFR1*, which contains the tyrosine kinase domain [37]. The TEL-PDGFR fusion resulting from t(5;12) in chronic myelomonocytic leukemia

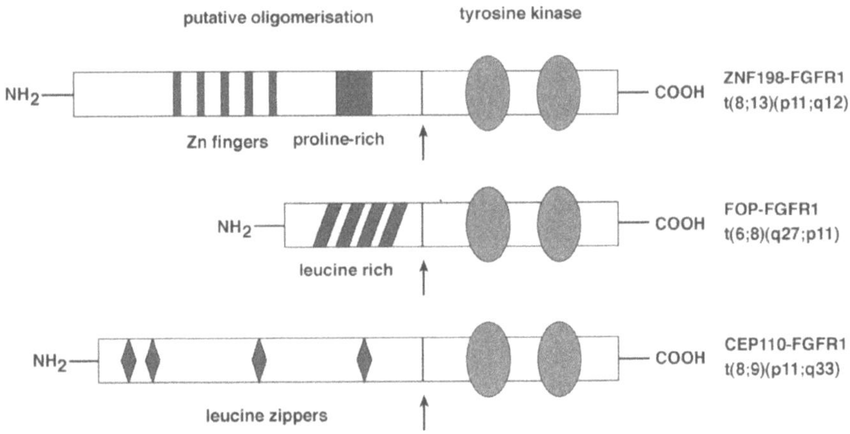

Fig. 4.3. Comparison of the ZNF198-FGFR1, FOP-FGFR1 and CEP110-FGFR1 fusion proteins in 8p11 myeloproliferative syndrome. In each case, the N-terminal portion of the variable partner protein, containing a putative oligomerization signal, is fused with the C-terminal portion of FGFR1, which contains the tyrosine kinase domain. Breakpoints are indicated by *arrows*. Reproduced with permission [34]

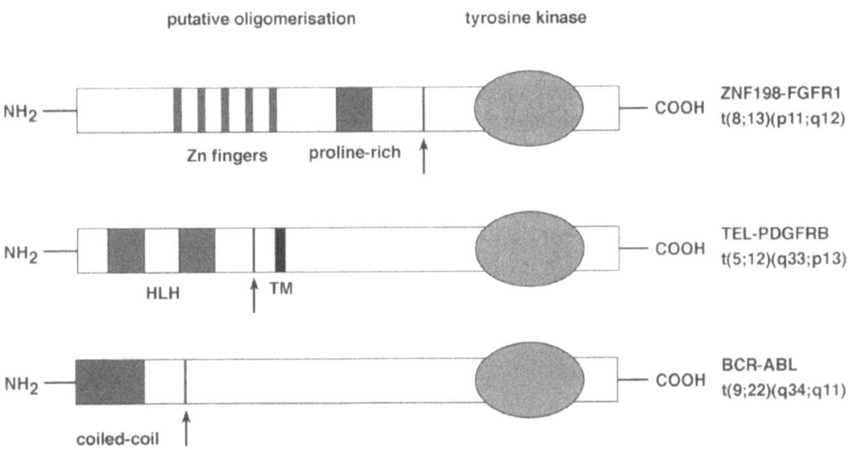

Fig. 4.4. Comparison of fusion proteins involving tyrosine kinase proteins in myeloid malignancies. Each fusion protein includes an oligomerization domain plus a tyrosine kinase domain (*HLH* helix-loop-helix domain, *TM* transmembrane domain). Breakpoints are indicated by *arrows*. Reproduced with permission [34]

contains the helix-loop-helix dimerization domain of TEL and the tyrosine kinase domain of PDGFR [38]. Likewise, the bcr-abl fusion oncogene in CML contains a coiled coil tetramerization motif of bcr fused to the abl tyrosine kinase [39]. In all these cases the fusion protein possesses constitutive, ligand-independent tyrosine kinase activity that is able to mimic activation of signaling pathways resulting in perturbed differentiation and/or proliferation. Indeed, the ZNF198-FGFR1 fusion protein does possess transforming ability in vitro [37].

4.5.2 Idiopathic Hypereosinophilic Syndrome

Recently, a novel fusion gene has been identified in a subset of patients with hypereosinophilic syndrome (HES). A small, cryptic deletion of chromosome 4q12 spanning approximately 800 kb leads to a fusion of 5' exons from a gene termed Fip1-like 1 (*FIP1L1*) with 3' exons of *PDGFRA* [40]. In a similar fashion to ZNF198-FGFR1, the fusion protein, FIP1L1-PDGFRA, is a constitutively active tyrosine kinase. The BCR-ABL inhibitor, imatinib mesylate, is also an inhibitor of FIP1L1-PDGFRA enabling its use for the treatment of FIP1L1-PDGFRA-positive HES patients. The FIP1L1-PDGFRA fusion gene has also been reported in patients with systemic mastocytosis with eosinophilia [41] who were also responsive to imatinib. Thus, knowledge of the underlying pathogenetic change has allowed the treatment of these disorders to be radically improved.

4.6 Summary

Chromosomal abnormalities are seen in approximately one-third of patients with PV and IMF but are rare in patients with ET. In PV and IMF, an abnormal karyotype seems to indicate a poor prognosis. Consistent acquired changes likely to contribute to the pathogenesis of the MPDs include deletion of the long arm of chromosome 20, deletion of 13q, trisomy 8 and 9, and duplication of parts of 1q. Furthermore, del(20q), trisomy 8 and dupl(1q) all arise in multipotent progenitor cells. Molecular mapping of 20q deletions and, to some extent, 13q deletions has identified a number of candidate target genes although no mutations have yet been found. Translocations associated with the rare EMS have permitted the identification of a number of novel fusion genes involving the *FGFR1* gene. Recently, a novel fusion gene, *FIP1L1-PDGFRA*, has been identified in patients with HES who respond to treatment with imatinib, an inhibitor of FIP1L1-PDGFRA.

Acknowledgements. Work in the authors' laboratory is supported by the Leukaemia Research Fund and the Medical Research Council.

References

1. Swolin B, Weinfeld A, Westin J (1988) A prospective long-term cytogenetic study in polycythemia vera in relation to treatment and clinical course. Blood 72:386–395
2. Diez-Martin JL, Graham DL, Petitt RM, Dewald GW (1991) Chromosome studies in 104 patients with polycythemia vera. Mayo Clinic Proc 66:287–299
3. Bench AJ, Nacheva EP, Champion KM, Green AR (1998) Molecular genetics and cytogenetics of myeloproliferative disorders. In: Green AR, Pearson TC (eds) Myeloproliferative disorders. Baillière Tindall, London, pp 819–848
4. Rege-Cambrin G, Mecucci C, Tricot G, Michaux J-L, Louwagie A, Van Hove W, Francart H, Van den Bergh H (1987) A chromosomal profile of polycythemia vera. Cancer Genet Cytogenet 25:233–245
5. Reilly JT, Snowden JA, Spearing RL, Fitzgerald PM, Jones N, Watmore A, Potter A (1997) Cytogenetic abnormalities and their prognostic significance in idiopathic myelofibrosis: a study of 106 cases. Br J Haematol 98:96–102
6. Dewald GW, Schad CR, Lilla VC, Jalal SM (1993) Frequency and photographs of HGM11 chromosome anomalies in bone marrow samples from 3,996 patients with malignant hematologic neoplasms. Cancer Genet Cytogenet 68:60–69
7. Campbell LJ, Garson OM (1994) The prognostic significance of deletion of the long arm of chromosome 20 in myeloid disorders. Leukemia 8:67–71
8. White NJ, Nacheva E, Asimakopoulos FA, Bloxham D, Paul B, Green AR (1994) Deletion of chromosome 20q in myelodysplasia can occur in a multipotent precursor of both myeloid cells and B cells. Blood 83:2809–2816
9. Hollings PE, Rosman I, Beard MEJ (1994) A 20q deletion originating in a pluripotent stem cell. Blood 83:305–306
10. Asimakopoulos FA, Holloway TL, Nacheva EP, Scott MA, Fenaux P, Green AR (1996) Detection of chromosome 20q deletions in bone marrow metaphases but not peripheral blood granulocytes in patients with myeloproliferative disorders or myelodysplastic syndromes. Blood 87:1561–1570
11. Champion KM, Gilbert JG, Asimakopoulos FA, Hinshelwood S, Green AR (1997) Clonal haemopoiesis in normal elderly women: implications for the myeloproliferative disorders and myelodysplastic syndromes. Br J Haematol 97:920–926
12. Wang PW, Iannantuoni K, Davis EM, Espinosa III R, Stoffel M, Le Beau MM (1998) Refinement of the common deleted segment in myeloid leukemias with a del(20q). Genes Chromosomes Cancer 21:75–81
13. Bench AJ, Nacheva EP, Hood TL, Holden JL, French L, Swanton S, Champion KM, Li J, Whittaker P, Stavrides G, Hunt AR, Huntly BJ, Campbell LJ, Bentley DR, Deloukas P, Green AR (2000) Chromosome 20 deletions in myeloid malignancies: reduction of the common deleted region, generation of a PAC/BAC contig and identification of candidate genes. Oncogene 19:3902–3913
14. Li J, Bench AJ, Vassiliou GS, Fourouclas N, Ferguson-Smith AC, Green AR (2004) Imprinting of the human L3MBTL gene, a polycomb family member located in a region of chromosome 20 deleted in human myeloid malignancies. Proc Natl Acad Sci U S A 101:7341–7346
15. Asimakopoulos FA, Holloway TL, Nacheva EP, Scott MA, Fenaux P, Green AR (1996) Deletion constitutes the major mechanism for loss of heterozygosity on chromosome 20q in polycythemia vera. Blood 88:2690–2698
16. Gribble SM, Reid AG, Bench AJ, Huntly BJP, Grace C, Green AR, Nacheva EP (2003) Molecular cytogenetics of polycythaemia vera: lack of occult rearrangements detectable by 20q LSP screening, CGH, and M-FISH. Leukemia 17:1419–1421
17. Asimakopoulos FA, Green AR (1996) Deletions of chromosome 20q and the pathogenesis of myeloproliferative disorders. Br J Haematol 95:219–226
18. Pastore C, Nomdedeu J, Volpe G, Guerrasio A, Cambrin GR, Parvis G, Pautasso M, Daglio C, Mazza U, Saglio G, Gaidano G (1995) Genetic analysis of chromosome 13 deletions in BCR/ABL negative chronic myeloproliferative disorders. Genes Chromosomes Cancer 14:106–111
19. Najfeld V, Montella L, Scalise A, Fruchtman S (2002) Exploring polycythaemia vera with fluorescence in situ hybridization: additional cryptic 9p is the most frequent abnormality detected. Br J Haematol 119:558–566
20. Sinclair EJ, Forrest EC, Reilly JT, Watmore AE, Potter AM (2001) Fluorescence in situ hybridization analysis of 25 cases of idiopathic myelofibrosis and two cases of secondary myelofibrosis: monoallelic loss of RB1, D13S319 and D13S25 loci associated with cytogenetic deletion and translocation involving 13q14. Br J Haematol 113:365–368
21. La Starza R, Wlodarska I, Aventin A, Falzetti D, Crescenzi B, Martelli MF, Van den Berghe H, Mecucci C (1998) Molecular delineation of 13q deletion boundaries in 20 patients with myeloid malignancies. Blood 91:231–237

22. Mertens D, Wolf S, Schroeter P, Schaffner C, Dohner H, Stilgenbauer S, Lichter P (2002) Down-regulation of candidate tumor suppressor genes within chromosome band 13q14.3 is independent of the DNA methylation pattern in B-cell chronic lymphocytic leukaemia. Blood 99:4116–4121
23. Migliazza A, Bosch F, Komatsu H, Cayanis E, Martinotti S, Toniato E, Guccione E, Qu X, Chien M, Murty VV, Gaidano G, Inghirami G, Zhang P, Fischer S, Kalachikov SM, Russo J, Edelman I, Efstratiadis A, Dalla-Favera R (2001) Nucleotide sequence, transcription map, and mutation analysis of the 13q14 chromosomal region deleted in B-cell chronic lymphocytic leukaemia. Blood 97:2098–2140
24. Cook WD, McCaw BJ (2000) Accommodating haploinsufficient tumor suppressor genes in Knudson's model. Oncogene 19:3434–3438
25. Bench AJ, Aldred MA, Humphray SJ, Champion KM, Gilbert JGR, Asimakopoulos FA, Deloukas P, Gwilliam R, Bentley DR, Green AR (1998) A detailed physical and transcriptional map of the region of chromosome 20 that is deleted in myeloproliferative disorders and refinement of the common deleted region. Genomics 49:351–362
26. Jenkins RB, Le Beau MM, Kraker WJ, Borell TJ, Stalboerger PG, Davis EM, Penland L, Fernald A, Esponosa R III, Schaid DJ, Noel P, Dewald GW (1992) Fluorescence in situ hybridization: a sensitive method for trisomy 8 detection in bone marrow specimens. Blood 79:3307–3315
27. Arranz E, Robledo M, Martinez B, Prieto E, Portero JA, Benitez J (1997) Detection of trisomy 8 using conventional cytogenetic techniques and interphase FISH analysis in 34 myeloid disorders: a comparative study. Cancer Genet Cytogenet 94:103–105
28. Westwood NB, Gruszka-Westwood AM, Pearson CE, DeLord CFM, Green AR, Huntly BJP, Lakhani A, McMullin MF, Pearson TC (2000) The incidences of trisomy 8, trisomy 9 and D20S108 deletion in polycythaemia vera: an analysis of blood granulocytes using interphase fluorescence in situ hybridization. Br J Haematol 110:839–846
29. Price CM, Kanfer EJ, Colman SM, Westwood N, Barrett AJ, Greaves MF (1992) Simultaneous genotypic and immunophenotypic analysis of interphase cells using dual-colour fluorescence: a demonstration of lineage involvement in polycythemia vera. Blood 80:1033–1038
30. Rege-Cambrin G, Speleman F, Kerim S, Scaravaglio P, Carozzi F, Dal Cin P, Michaux J-L, Offner F, Saglio G, Van Den Berghe H (1991) Extra translocation +der(1q9p) is a prognostic indicator in myeloproliferative disorders. Leukemia 5:1059–1063
31. Swolin B, Weinfeld A, Westin J (1986) Trisomy 1q in polycythemia vera and its relation to disease transition. Am J Hematol 22:155–167
32. Fonatsch C, Haase D, Freund M, Bartels H, Tesch H (1991) A nonrandom primary chromosomal abnormality in myelodysplastic syndromes? Cancer Genet Cytogenet 56:243–253
33. Knuutila S, Ruutu T, Partanen S, Vuopio P (1983) Chromosome 1q+ in erythroid and granulocyte-monocyte precursors in a patient with essential thrombocythemia. Cancer Genet Cytogenet 9:245–249
34. Bench AJ, Cross NCP, Huntly BJP, Nacheva EP, Green AR (2001) Myeloproliferative disorders. In: Buckle V, Kearney L (eds) Cytogenetics in haematology. Best Practice and Research Clinical Haematology. Baillière Tindall, London, vol 14, pp 531–551
35. Inhorn RC, Aster JC, Roach SA, Slapak CA, Soiffer R, Tantravahi R, Stone RM (1995) A syndrome of lymphoblastic lymphoma, eosinophilia, and myeloid hyperplasia/malignancy associated with t(8;13)(p11;q11): description of a distinctive clinicopathologic entity. Blood 85:1881–1887
36. Macdonald D, Reiter A, Cross NC (2002) The 8p11 myeloproliferative syndrome: a distinct clinical entity caused by constitutive activation of FGFR1. Acta Haematol 107:101–107
37. Xiao S, McCarthy JG, Aster JC, Fletcher JA (2000) ZNF198-FGFR1 transforming activity depends on a novel proline-rich ZNF198 oligomerization domain. Blood 96:699–704
38. Golub TR, Barker GF, Lovett M, Gilliland DG (1994) Fusion of PDGF receptor beta to a novel ets-like gene, tel, in chronic myelomonocytic leukemia with t(5;12) chromosomal translocation. Cell 77:307–316
39. McWhirter JR, Galasso DL, Wang YL (1993) A coiled-coil oligomerization domain of Bcr is essential for the transforming function of Bcr-Abl oncoproteins. Mol Cell Biol 13:7587–7595
40. Cools J, DeAngelo DJ, Gotlib J, Stover EH, Legare RD, Cortes J, Kutok J, Clark J, Galinsky I, Griffin JD, Cross NC, Tefferi A, Malone J, Alam R, Schrier SL, Schmid J, Rose M, Van den Berghe P, Verhoef G, Boogaerts M, Wlodarska I, Kantarjian H, Marynen P, Coutre SE, Stone R, Gilliland DG (2003) A tyrosine kinase created by fusion of the *PDGFRA* and *FIP1L1* genes as a therapeutic target of imatinib in idiopathic hypereosinophilic syndrome. N Engl J Med 348:1201–1214
41. Pardanani A, Ketterling RP, Brockman SR, Flynn HC, Paternoster SF, Shearer BM, Reeder TL, Li CY, Cross NC, Cools J, Gilliland DG, Dewald GW, Tefferi A (2003) *CHIC2* deletion, a surrogate for *FIP1L1-PDGFRA* fusion, occurs in systemic mastocytosis associated with eosinophilia and predicts response to imatinib mesylate therapy. Blood 102:3093–3096

B Polycythemia Vera

Chapter 5

Classification and Molecular Biology of Polycythemias (Erythrocytoses)

Jey Maran, Josef T. Prchal

5.1 Introduction: Definition and Classification of Polycythemias

The name "polycythemia" is derived from the Greek and means literally "too many cells in the blood". Thus, only an increase in red cells constitutes polycythemia. In the clinical setting polycythemia exists when the hemoglobin and red blood cell count are increased, reflecting an elevation of the total red blood cell volume. Polycythemias can be differentiated based on the responsiveness of the erythroid progenitors to circulating cytokines. Primary polycythemias are characterized by an excessive response of the erythroid progenitors to circulating cytokines, as a result of acquired somatic or inherited germline mutations that are expressed within hematopoietic progenitors causing increased proliferation and or decreased apoptosis, resulting in the accumulation of red cells. In terms of oxygen demand and oxygen requirements, primary polycythemias can be viewed as the production of the oxygen carrying capacity (hemoglobin) fully dissociated from the tissue oxygen needs and from the oxygen sensing pathway. In contrast, secondary polycythemias are characterized by a normal responsiveness of the erythroid progenitors to circulating cytokines and an increased level of circulating factors driving erythropoiesis, e.g., erythropoietin (EPO), insulin-like growth factor-I (IGF-I), cobalt, etc. Thus, in terms of oxygen demand, secondary polycythemias can be viewed as a physiological response to satisfy the oxygen needs of the tissues, or the germline or somatic mutations disturbing the oxygen sensing pathway or its target, i.e., EPO.

Primary or secondary polycythemias can be either congenital or acquired. Examples of congenital polycythemias are primary familial and congenital polycythemia (PFCP), high affinity hemoglobins, Chuvash polycythemia, and deficiency of 2,3-bisphosphoglycerate (BPG, previously known as 2,3-diphosphoglycerate) mutase (BPGM). Examples of acquired polycythemias include polycythemia vera (PV) and polycythemia associated with high altitude and lung disease. These conditions can be discriminated by in vitro tests of responsiveness of circulating erythroid progenitors from either peripheral blood BFUE (burst-forming unit–erythroid) or bone marrow CFUE (colony-forming unit–erythroid) [1].

5.2 Primary Polycythemia

5.2.1 Acquired Polycythemias

PV is the most common primary polycythemia characterized by clonal expansion of myeloid cells from an acquired mutation of a single stem cell. Its incidence has been estimated at 2.3 per 100,000 persons, with a median age of presentation at approximately 60 years [2]. PV is associated with significant morbidity and mortality [3], including thrombotic/hemorrhagic events, and a risk of an evolution to leukemia or myelodysplastic syndrome. This contrasts with other polycythemic disorders wherein the progression to leukemia is not part of the disease process and wherein the thrombotic/hemorrhagic events have a lower prevalence. The molecular basis of PV is unknown [4]. The diagnosis of PV is based on criteria established by the Polycythemia Vera Study Group [3] (see Chap. 1), but atypical cases may not be readily discriminated by these criteria.

PV is the result of a clonal expansion of a single hematopoietic progenitor as established by assays based on X-chromosome inactivation [5]. Cytogenetic abnormalities are found in up to one-third of PV patients (deletion of 20q, 13q, trisomy 8, trisomy 9 or trisomy of 1q are the most common); however, none is specific for PV and these abnormalities appear to be more common as the disease progresses. The PV bone marrow progenitor cells are able to form erythroid colonies in the absence of exogenous EPO in the presence of serum. These "endogenous erythroid colonies" (EEC), which can be demonstrated in vitro, are a hallmark of the disease and are a useful for differentiation of PV from secondary polycythemias and primary familial and congenital polycythemia (PFCP) [6]. Anti-EPO and anti-EPO-R neutralizing antibodies completely abolish the formation of EEC in PFCP samples but not in PV samples demonstrating that this PV feature is independent of EPO signaling [7].

In serum-free cultures PV are hypersensitive to IGF-I; hypersensitivity to other cytokines such as GM-CSF, SCF, thrombopoietin (TPO) and interleukin-3 has also been reported. The expression of the TPO receptor has been reported to be decreased in PV. Since the TPO receptor on platelets is the major regulator of circulating TPO it results in an increased TPO level and enhanced platelet production. Recently, increased mRNA of a receptor named polycythemia rubra vera 1 (PRV-1) has been reported in PV granulocytes but not their progenitors (see Chap. 6). The exact function of PRV-1 in normal hematopoiesis is unclear but it likely plays no significant role in PV pathophysiology since there are no differences in the amount of this protein between normal and PV progenitors; however, it may be a useful diagnostic marker of the disease.

Dysregulation of the expression of a number of other genes, including *Bcl-xL* has been observed in PV. A potential localization of PV gene was recently proposed following the demonstration of upregulation of p15 and p16 transcripts [8] and a loss-of-heterozygosity on chromosome 9 [9]. Duplication and other cytogenetic changes of the same chromosome 9 region were reported to be the most frequent cytogenetic abnormalities of PV when more sophisticated techniques are used [10]. Whether PV is due to a mutation of a single gene, or if it is a multigenic disorder or the result of epigenetic abnormalities remains to be established. Taken together, published data suggest that the putative PV defect affects signaling downstream from the cytokine receptors that results in dysregulated responsiveness of PV cells to cytokine stimulation [1].

5.2.2 Primary Familial and Congenital Polycythemia

PFCP is an autosomal dominant disorder present at birth. Many affected patients are incidentally diagnosed by routine blood counts, or when evaluated in the context of familial polycythemia. Characteristic laboratory findings are:

- An increase of the red blood cell mass, without increase in leukocytes or platelet counts
- Normal hemoglobin-oxygen dissociation
- Low serum EPO levels
- In vitro hypersensitivity of erythroid progenitors to EPO
- Normal B12 levels, LAP scores and bone marrow cytogenetics.

To date, 12 mutations of the EPO receptor (EPO-R) have been described, and 9 out of these result in truncation of the EPO-R cytoplasmic carboxyl terminal and only these are convincingly associated with PFCP [11].

The physiological basis for EPO-mediated activation of erythropoiesis is as follows. The interaction of EPO and EPO-R leads to change of conformation of EPO-R dimers/oligomers and signal transduction resulting in the initiation of a cascade of erythroid-specific events. A positive growth-regulatory domain in the cytoplasmic portion of the EPO-R interacts with Janus tyrosine kinase-2 (JAK2) [12] resulting in the phosphorylation of JAK2, EPO-R and other proteins such as STAT-5 (signal transducer and activator of transcription-5), thus initiating a cascade of signaling. This JAK2/STAT-5 signaling plays a nonredundant essential role in the regulation of erythropoiesis mediated by EPO/EPO-R (i.e., EPO "on" signal). The C-terminal cytoplasmic portion of EPO-R also possesses a negative growth-regulatory domain. Hematopoietic cell phosphatase (HCP, also known as SHP1) interacts with this portion of the EPO-R and dephosphorylates JAK2 (i.e., erythropoietin "off" signal). Inactivation of the HCP binding site has been shown to lead to prolonged phosphorylation of JAK2/STAT-5. PFCP-causing mutations result in gain-of-function of the EPO-R by truncating the intracytoplasmic domain with loss of the binding site for the negative regulator HCP.

However, in one study, mutations of the *EPOR* were found in only 5 of 43 unrelated subjects with PFCP, suggesting that mutations of *EPOR* is not the major genetic defect in the pathogenesis of PFCP, and that mutations of other genes cause PFCP in the majority of patients [11]. In a recent study of a family with PFCP, after conclusively excluding *EPOR* mutations, linkage analysis using polymorphic markers showed a region in 7q22.1–7q22.2 as the possible locus [13].

A mouse model bearing a normal human *EPOR* and mutant disease-causing human *EPOR* has been created by *flox-neo* (gene replacement) technology [14]. This mouse model that has the potential for tissue-specific deletion and augmentation of EPO signaling and should help in the understanding of the role of EPO signaling in other tissues such as brain and endothelial cells.

5.3 Secondary Polycythemias

High-EPO secondary polycythemias could be congenital or acquired. High-affinity hemoglobins due to globin gene mutations or BPGM deficiency, and congenital methemoglobinemia are examples of congenital secondary polycythemia.

Chuvash polycythemia (see below) shares features of both primary and secondary polycythemia. Conditions leading to hypoxia, such as high altitude, or underlying diseases (cyanotic heart disease, chronic cor pulmonale, chronic obstructive lung disease, sleep apnea) also result in polycythemia that is a physiological adaptation process to hypoxia mediated by increased EPO.

5.3.1 High Oxygen Affinity Hemoglobin and BPG Deficiency

There are more than 100 mutations of hemoglobin leading to an increase in oxygen affinity and thus decrease oxygen delivery and compensatory polycythemia. Such mutations affect the cooperative binding between the globin subunits (β1/β2 interface) or interfere with the binding of 2,3-BPG. These mutations are dominantly inherited, and such polycythemias are usually benign. Phlebotomies are of no beneficial value and have been shown to decrease exercise tolerance and anaerobic threshold [1] demonstrating the questionable principal role of elevated hematocrit in the pathogenesis of PV. The best initial screening test to detect high oxygen affinity hemoglobin relies on the determination of hemoglobin dissociation kinetics and P50 (pressure of O2 where Hb is 50% oxygenated). If a CO oximeter is not available, P50 can be mathematically estimated from a venous blood gas measurement [15].

5.3.2 BPG Deficiency

A rare cause of congenital polycythemia is 2,3-BPG deficiency, resulting from a deficiency of BPGM. BPG is present in very high concentrations in red blood cells. It binds hemoglobin and allosterically changes its configuration, thereby modulating its ability to bind oxygen. A decreased BPG level shifts the hemoglobin oxygen dissociation curve to the left (increases hemoglobin affinity for oxygen), resulting in decreased delivery of oxygen to the peripheral tissues and compensatory polycythemia. BPGM mutation should be considered in the setting of a low P50 and after globin gene mutations have been conclusively excluded.

5.3.3 Defective Hypoxic Sensing, von Hippel-Lindau Syndrome, and Chuvash Polycythemia

Chuvash polycythemia is an autosomal recessive congenital polycythemia, described in the mid 1970s, and endemic in the Chuvash population of the Russian Federation. It has been alleged that there may be thousands of affected individuals among the 1 million Chuvash people. Although occasionally referred to as familial benign polycythemia, Chuvash polycythemia is associated with a high mortality rate due to thrombotic and hemorrhagic vascular complications [16]. Serum EPO concentration is elevated compared to healthy first-degree family members, although some patients may have a normal serum EPO. However, the erythroid progenitors of patients with Chuvash polycythemia are hypersensitive to EPO, thus Chuvash polycythemia has characteristics of both primary and secondary polycythemia.

A missense mutation in the von Hippel-Lindau (*VHL*) gene was discovered in Chuvash polycythemia patients. This mutation due to a C to T transversion at nucleotide 598 (a R200 W mutation) in both alleles of the *VHL* gene was found to be the molecular defect causing this condition [17]. The demonstration of the mutation within the *VHL* gene indicates that Chuvash polycythemia is a congenital defect of an abnormal oxygen sensing. Interestingly, heterozygote carriers do not seem to be at increased risk for tumors, which contrasts with patients with von Hippel-Lindau syndrome.

Chuvash polycythemia is due to a congenital defect in oxygen homeostasis (Fig. 5.1). The physiological basis is as follows. The principal transcriptional activator of gene expression in hypoxic cells is hypoxia inducible factor-1 (HIF-1). HIF-1 plays a central role in hypoxia sensing and controls the expression of many genes including *EPO (encoding EPO), TF* (encoding transferrin), *TFRC* (encoding transferrin receptor), *SLC2A1* also known as *GLUT1* [encoding solute carrier family 2 (facilitated glucose transporter), member 1] and *VEGF* (encoding vascular endothelial growth factor). It contains α and β subunits which are members of a multigene family. The α subunit (HIF-1α) is regulated in an oxygen-dependent manner at the post-translational level, whereas the expression of the β subunit (HIF-1β) is constitutive.

Accumulation of nondegraded HIF-1α leads to the formation of a heterodimer with HIF-1β forming a transcription factor which results in the expression of hyp-

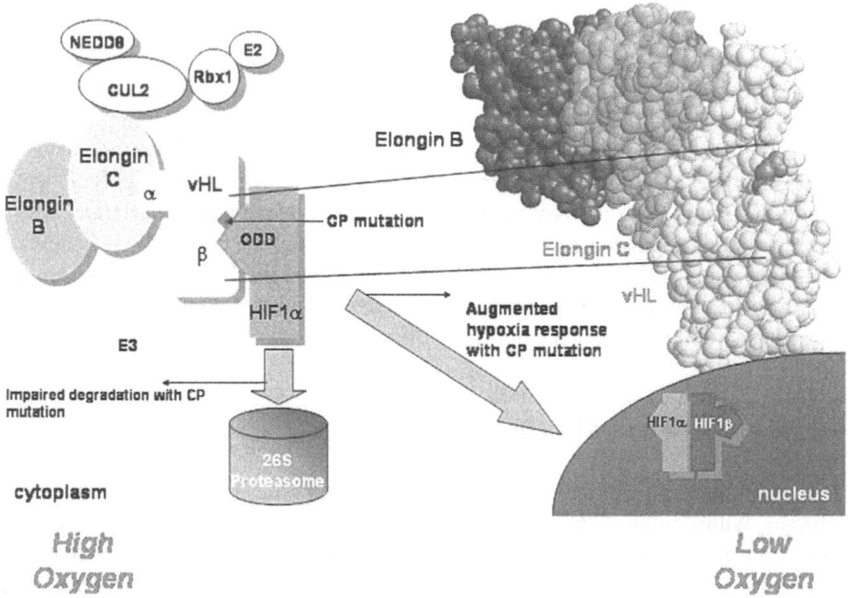

Fig. 5.1. Molecular biology of Chuvash polycythemia

oxia-inducible genes, including *EPO* [17]. HIF-1α is stable under hypoxic conditions but rapidly degraded in normoxia by VHL-mediated ubiquitination and proteasomal degradation by the 26S proteasome resulting in one of the shortest half-lives of any protein. Oxygen-dependent prolyl hydroxylation of HIF-1α is required for its binding to VHL, which is the recognition component of an E3 ubiquitin–protein ligase complex that also includes elongin B, elongin C, ring-box 1, cullin 2, and protein 8. The Arg200Trp substitution in Chuvash polycythemia results in increased HIF-1α expression in normoxic conditions due to decreased interaction between VHL and HIF-1α and a lower rate of ubiquitination. This in turn results in increased expression of a subset of target genes including *EPO, VEGF* and *SCL2A1* under normoxic conditions leading to polycythemia [18].

Germline *VHL* 598C → T mutation, shortly after its identification as a causative mutation responsible for Chuvash polycythemia, was also found in 11 unrelated non-Chuvash patients from diverse ethnic groups including Asians, Caucasians and African-Americans [19, 20, 21]. Haplotype analysis of polymorphic markers showed a strong linkage disequilibrium indicating that the *VHL* 598C → T mutation originated from a single founder 14,000 to 62,000 years ago [22]. Based on its persistence in the Chuvash population and wide dissemination from the original founder, it is possible that this gene has some survival advantages; however, its exact mechanism remains to be proven.

Distinct mutations in the *VHL* gene have been associated with pheochromocytoma, hemangioblastoma and renal cell carcinoma, none of which were observed in any patients with Chuvash polycythemia or obligate carriers of the mutation associated with Chuvash polycythemia. *VHL* mutations associated with VHL syndrome tend to be more severe and are generally 5' to the Chuvash polycythemia mutation. Only one individual has been found to be a homozygote or a compound heterozygote for germline mutations of more than 700 VHL syndromes causing mutations identified thus far [19]; neither this individual, nor his heterozygous relatives, had any evidence of VHL syndrome tumors. Typically the individuals are heterozygous with respect to a germline mutation, and the second hit occurs as a somatic mutation giving rise to sporadic cells with loss of VHL function, which in turn develop into tumors in specific tissues. In contrast, individuals with Chuvash polycythemia are homozygous for a germline *VHL* mutation (expressed in every cell). The Chuvash polycythemia mutation results in a relatively mild defect of oxygen sensing that may affect only a subset of HIF-1-regulated genes consistent with subtle differences in HIF-1-dependent gene expression [18]. This may explain why homozygosity with respect to the Chuvash polycythemia mutation is relatively well tolerated; however, mutations in different positions within the *VHL* gene may have different functional consequences [23].

5.3.4
Polycythemia in Kidney and Liver Diseases

Polycythemia has been reported in association with kidney lesions such as hydronephrosis, Wilms' tumor (adult and children), polycystic kidneys, and in lesions associated with the VHL syndrome (renal cell carcinoma, renal hemangioma). Polycythemia/erythrocytosis has been frequently reported as a complication occurring after kidney transplantation. An entity known as "post-transplant erythrocytosis" (PTE) occurs in up to 20% of renal transplant recipients. The therapeutic effects of angiotensin-converting enzyme (ACE) inhibitors, and losartan (a specific antagonist of the angiotensin type 1, AT1) receptor on PTE/polycythemia in patients with renal failure indirectly links angiotensin II with the regulation of erythropoiesis. AT1 receptor was detected on erythroid progenitors, suggesting that angiotensin II may play a direct role in the regulation of erythropoiesis [24].

Polycythemia is a known paraneoplastic manifestation of hepatocellular carcinoma in 2.5% of patients; polycythemia is secondary to the production of EPO. Polycythemia can also be observed in patients with obstruction of the hepatic venous outflow, the Budd-Chiari syndrome, but these patients may have an overt or latent myeloproliferative disorder.

References

1. Prchal JT (2003) Classification and molecular biology of polycythemias (erythrocytoses) and thrombocytosis. Hematol Oncol Clin North Am 17:1151–1158
2. Ania BJ, Suman VJ, Sobell JL, Codd MB, Silverstein MN, Melton LJ 3rd (1994) Trends in the incidence of polycythemia vera among Olmsted County, Minnesota residents, 1935–1989. Am J Hematol 47:89–93
3. Berlin NI (1975) Diagnosis and classification of the polycythemias. Semin Hematol 12:339–351
4. Spivak JL (2002) Polycythemia vera: myths, mechanisms, and management. Blood 100:4272–4290
5. Prchal JF, Adamson JW, Steinmann L, Fialkow PJ (1976) Human erythroid colony formation in vitro: evidence for clonal origin. J Cell Physiol 89:489–492
6. Prchal JF, Axelrad AA (1974) Bone-marrow responses in polycythemia vera (letter). N Engl J Med 290:1382
7. Fisher MJ, Prchal JF, Prchal JT, D'Andrea AD (1994) Anti-erythropoietin (EPO) receptor monoclonal antibodies distinguish EPO-dependent and EPO-independent erythroid progenitors in polycythemia vera. Blood 84:1982–1991
8. Dai C, Krantz SB (2001) Increased expression of the INK4a/ARF locus in polycythemia vera. Blood 97:3424–3432
9. Kralovics R, Guan Y, Prchal JT (2002) Acquired uniparental disomy of chromosome 9p is a frequent stem cell defect in polycythemia vera. Exp Hematol 30:229–336
10. Najfeld V, Montella L, Scalise A, Fruchtman S (2002) Exploring polycythaemia vera with fluorescence in situ hybridization: additional cryptic 9p is the most frequent abnormality detected. Br J Haematol 119:558–566
11. Kralovics R, Prchal JT (2001) Genetic heterogeneity of primary familial and congenital polycythemia. Am J Hematol 68:115–121
12. Witthuhn B, Quelle F, Silvennoinen O, Ui T, Tang B, Miura O, Ihle J (1993) JAK2 associates with the erythropoietin receptor and is tyrosine phosphorylated and activated following stimulation with erythropoietin. Cell 74:227–238
13. Jedlickova K, Stockton DW, Prchal JT (2003) Possible primary familial and congenital polycythemia locus at 7q22.1–7q22.2. Blood Cells Mol Dis 31:327–331
14. Divoky V, Liu Z, Ryan TM, Prchal JF, Townes TM, Prchal JT (2001) Mouse model of congenital polycythemia: homologous replacement of murine gene by mutant human erythropoietin receptor gene. Proc Natl Acad Sci U S A 98:986–991
15. Lichtman MA, Murphy, MS, Adamson JW (1976) Detection of mutant hemoglobins with altered affinity for oxygen. A simplified technique. Ann Intern Med 84:517–520
16. Gordeuk VR, Sergueeva AI, Miasnikova GY, Okhotin D, Voloshin, Y, Choyke PL, Butman JA, Jedlickova K, Prchal JT, Polyakova LA (2004) Congenital disorder of oxygen sensing: association of the homozygous Chuvash polycythemia VHL mutation with thrombosis and vascular abnormalities but not tumors. Blood 103:3924–3932
17. Ang SO, Chen H, Gordeuk VR, Sergueeva AI, Polyakova LA, Miasnikova GY, Kralovics R, Stockton DW, Prchal JT (2002) Endemic polycythemia in Russia: mutation in the VHL gene. Blood Cells Mol Dis 28:57–62
18. Ang SO, Chen H, Hirota K, Gordeuk VR., Jelinek J, Guan Y, Liu E, Sergueeva AI, Miasnikova GY, Mole D, Maxwell P, Stockton DW, Semenza GL, Prchal JT (2002) Disruption of oxygen homeostasis underlies congenital Chuvash polycythemia. Nat Genet 32:614–621

19. Pastore Y, Jedlickova K, Guan Y, Liu E, Fahner J, Hasle H, Prchal JF, Prchal JT (2003) Mutations of von Hippel-Lindau tumor-suppressor gene and congenital polycythemia. Am J Hum Genet 73:412–419
20. Percy MJ, McMullin MF, Jowitt SN, Potter M, Treacy M, Watson WH, Lappin TR (2003) Chuvash-type congenital polycythemia in 4 families of Asian and Western European ancestry. Blood 102:1097–1099
21. Pastore YD, Jelinek J, Ang S, Guan Y, Liu E, Jedlickova K, Krishnamurti L, Prchal JT (2003) Mutations in the VHL gene in sporadic apparently congenital polycythemia. Blood 101:1591–1595
22. Liu E, Percy MJ, Amos CI, Guan S, Shete S, Stockton DW, McMullin MF, Polyakaova LA, Ang SO, Pastore YD, Jedlickova K, Lappin TR, Gordeuk V, Prchal JT (2004) The worldwide distribution of the VHL 598C>T mutation indicates a single founding event. Blood 103:1937–1940
23. Corn PG, McDonald ER 3rd, Herman JG, El-Deiry WS (2003) Tat-binding protein-1, a component of the 26S proteasome, contributes to the E3 ubiquitin ligase function of the von Hippel-Lindau protein. Nat Genet 35:229–337
24. Mrug M, Stopka T, Julian BA, Prchal JF, Prchal JT (1997) Angiotensin II facilitates erythropoietin mediated proliferation of normal early erythroid progenitors. J Clin Invest 115:508–522

Characterization of PRV-1, a Novel Hematopoietic Cell Surface Marker Overexpressed in Polycythemia Rubra Vera

Heike L. Pahl

6.1 Molecular Markers of Polycythemia Vera

While the pathognomonic mutation causing chronic myeloid leukemia (CML), the "Philadelphia chromosome", is well characterized, and the detection of the bcr/abl fusion transcript, allows a precise, molecular diagnosis of CML, to date there is no characteristic molecular marker for the diagnosis of polycythemia vera (PV). The reason for this is simple: the molecular defects leading to the development of PV have not been elucidated. However, recently, advances towards a molecular understanding of this disorder have been made. Many of these, such as the decreased expression of c-mpl and the overexpression of Bcl-xL are described in Chaps. 7 and 9 of this book. This chapter concentrates on a recently cloned, novel hematopoietic receptor, called PRV-1, which is selectively and consistently overexpressed in patients with PV.

6.2 The Cloning of PRV-1, a Novel Hematopoietic Receptor

One possible approach to elucidating the molecular defect underlying a disease process is to define differences in gene expression between patient cells and normal controls. In the author's laboratory, subtractive hybridization was used to clone cDNAs which are differentially expressed in PV versus healthy control granulocytes. Granulocytes were used in this experiment for practical reasons. Although the terminally differentiated granulocyte is not the disease-eliciting cell, since PV is a disorder of the pluripotent hematopoietic stem cell, as detailed above, peripheral granulocytes are derived clonally from the affected bone marrow stem cell [1, 2]. Therefore, mutations present in the mutant stem cell should be maintained in the clonal, granulocytically differentiated progeny.

Peripheral granulocyte mRNA from 5 PV patients and 20 controls was pooled and submitted to a suppressive subtractive hybridization (Fig. 6.1). The resulting clones were rescreened using the subtracted cDNAs as probes. Only those clones which hybridized to the forward-subtracted cDNA, but not the reverse-subtracted cDNA (Fig. 6.1) were analyzed further. These cloned cDNAs were used as probes in Northern blot experiments and hybridized to total granulocyte RNA of five PV patients and five healthy controls. From the Northern blots, the cDNAs displaying the largest difference in expression between PV patients and healthy controls were chosen for DNA sequence analysis. By databank comparisons, the nature of the sequenced cDNAs was determined. For detailed analysis, we chose a clone, which had appeared in several copies in the initial screen, and which did not code for any known gene then present in the databases (April 1998).

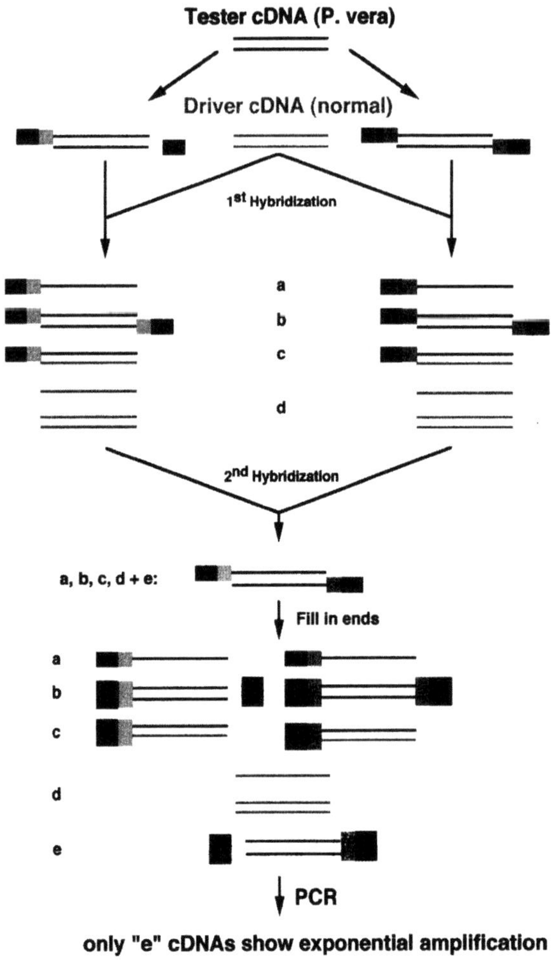

Fig. 6.1. The suppressive subtractive hybridization technique. Briefly, mRNA from healthy controls and PV patients is reverse-transcribed into cDNA. The PV cDNA is split into two pools and two different adaptor molecules are ligated to the ends. Each PV cDNA pool is hybridized to an excess of healthy control cDNA. In a second hybridization the two pools are mixed without denaturation, again in the presence of excess healthy control cDNA. After hybridization, the cDNA fragments are amplified by PCR; only those fragments bearing two different adaptor molecules will be exponentially amplified

Analysis of the polypeptide chain encoded by this cDNA revealed that it represented a novel hematopoietic cell surface receptor, which we named polycythemia rubra vera-1 (PRV-1) [3]. PRV-1 is a member of the uPAR superfamily of cell surface receptors. This family shares very little overall amino acid homology between its individual members [4]. Its defining characteristic is the presence of cysteine residues at precisely defined positions [5]. Individual cysteine pairs form disulfide bridges, defining the three-dimensional structure of the "uPAR-domain" [6, 7] (Fig. 6.2). Unfortunately, because of the lack of amino acid homology, the members of the uPAR superfamily also fulfill diverse biological functions in various cell types. For example, uPAR family members are involved in T-cell differentiation, prevention of erythroid autologous lysis and bone morphogenesis [8, 9]. Therefore, we are currently unable to suggest a function for our novel hematopoietic receptor.

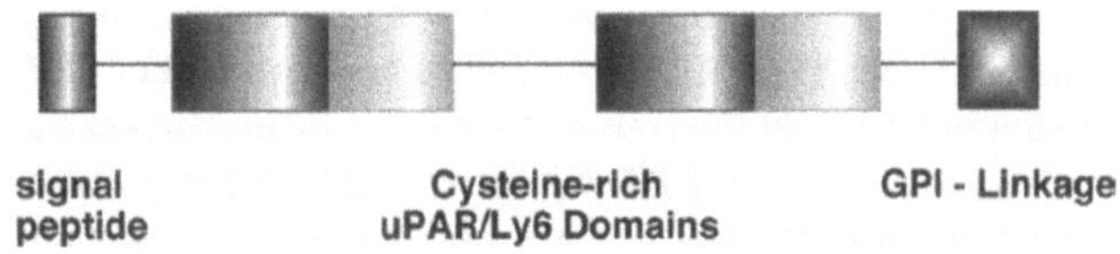

Fig. 6.2. Schematic representation of the PRV-1 protein and its domains (signal peptide, uPAR domains the putative hydrophobic GPI attachment sequence)

6.3
PRV-1 is Consistently and Selectively Overexpressed in Patients with *PV*

Using Northern blots, we investigated PRV-1 expression in patients with PV as well as in patients with other myeloproliferative disorders, patients with acute myeloid leukemia (AML) and patients with secondary or idiopathic erythrocytosis. The latter patient population is especially interesting from a diagnostic point of view, because it is not always trivial to distinguish a PV patient from a patient with secondary erythrocytosis by clinical criteria. PRV-1 is strongly overexpressed in granulocytes from PV patients (27/27), but not expressed in normal control granulocytes (61/61) (Fig. 6.3 and data not shown). Moreover, PRV-1 is not expressed in granulocytes or mononuclear cells from patients with CML or AML [10]. Most importantly, patients with secondary erythrocytosis also do not express PRV-1 [10].

Interestingly, a subset of patients with essential thrombocythemia (ET) also express PRV-1 in their peripheral granulocytes [10]. Shih and Lee have previously

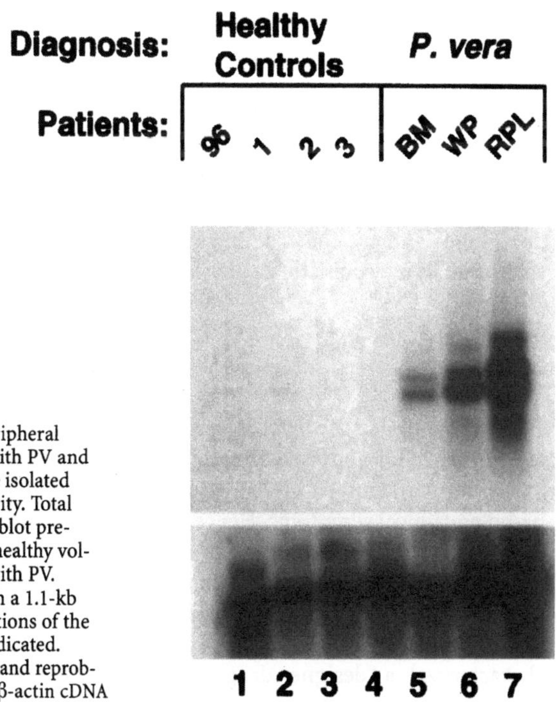

Fig. 6.3. Expression of PRV-1 in peripheral blood granulocytes from patients with PV and normal controls. Granulocytes were isolated from peripheral blood to >98% purity. Total RNA was extracted and a Northern blot prepared using 10 µg RNA. *Lanes* 1–4 healthy volunteer donors, *lanes* 5–8 patients with PV. *Top* The membrane was probed with a 1.1-kb fragment of PRV-1 cDNA. The positions of the 18S and 28S ribosomal RNAs are indicated. *Bottom* The membrane was stripped and reprobed with a 1.2-kb fragment of human β-actin cDNA

reported that a subset of ET patients will progress to develop the full clinical symptoms of PV over time [11]. It remains to be seen whether PRV-1-positive ET patients will develop PV over the course of their disease or whether there are significant clinical differences between PRV-1-positive and PRV-1-negative ET patients. We are currently investigating these hypotheses. If these hypotheses are true, our data suggest that PRV-1 expression in peripheral granulocytes may serve as a molecular marker for PV.

6.4 The Physiological Function of PRV-1

Although PRV-1 overexpression may serve a very useful function as a diagnostic tool for PV, no gene exists that causes the disease. Therefore, the PRV-1 protein must serve a physiological role in healthy tissues. In order to elucidate this function, we investigated PRV-1 expression in healthy volunteers. In these individuals, PRV-1 was selectively expressed in the bone marrow and not in a large variety of other tissues tested [10]. Immunohistochemical staining, using a polyclonal antibody, localized PRV-1 expression to early erythroblasts, as well as megakaryocytes, promyelocytes and myelocytes. These cells represent the precursor cells of all three lineages which are hyperproliferating in PV patients. Although these findings suggest a role for PRV-1 in normal hematopoiesis, the precise function of this molecule remains elusive. We are currently conducting a yeast two-hybrid screen to identify proteins that interact with PRV-1 in healthy bone marrow.

Although all members of the uPAR receptor superfamily are tethered to the cell membrane via a lipid anchor, they nonetheless participate actively in signal transduction [12]. Several groups have shown that uPAR interacts with and can activate protein tyrosine kinases including hck, fyn, lyn, fgr and lck [13, 14, 15) In addition, uPAR has been shown to activate the JAK/STAT pathway [14, 16]. It is therefore likely that PRV-1 also mediates signal transduction in bone marrow cells.

A myriad of further experiments are required to investigate both the physiological function of PRV-1 in healthy bone marrow as well as its role in the pathogenesis of PV. In addition to the yeast two-hybrid assay mentioned above, we have cloned the mouse homologue and are constructing knockout and transgenic mice. The phenotype of such animals may point to the physiological role of this novel hematopoietic receptor.

6.5 Conclusions

To date, the molecular defects leading to the development of PV remain unknown. Seen from a clinical perspective, this has two consequences. First, due to the lack of a molecular marker, the differential diagnosis of myeloproliferative disorders remains based on clinical symptoms. Hence, a small proportion of patients with atypical disease manifestations may initially be misdiagnosed. Of much more concern, however, is the second effect. Because we do not understand the underlying defect, we cannot use rational drug design or molecular medicine to develop a cause-based therapy for these patients. In contrast, because the molecular defect in CML has been extensively characterized, a "designer drug" for this disease was recently developed [17]. This agent, called STI 571, inhibits the Abl-kinase, whose activity is upregulated by the bcr/abl translocation. In clinical trials, this drug has been shown to be very efficacious [17]. Once the molecular cause of PV has been elucidated, the hope is to use a similar strategy to develop a cause-based therapy.

Seen from a scientific perspective, describing the changes which take place in PV, will increase our understanding of hematopoiesis in healthy humans. cMPDs differ in one interesting aspect from acute leukemias. In the latter disorders, the affected cells show both an increased proliferation as well as an arrest in differentiation. Leukemic blast cells are immature. In contrast, in cMPDs, the affected cells hyperproliferate, but they differentiate and mature almost completely. Thus, investigating the molecular pathology of cMPDs may allow us to identify signals regulating cell proliferation and to distinguish these from the processes governing hematopoietic differentiation.

Acknowledgements. The author gratefully acknowledges support by grants from the Deutsche Forschungsgemeinschaft (SFB 364, Teilprojekt A12) and by the Alfred Krupp-Förderpreis für Junge Hochschullehrer.

References

1. Kreipe H, Felgner J, Jaquet K, Heidorn K, Radzun HJ, Parwaresch R (1992) DNA analysis to aid in the diagnosis of chronic myeloproliferative disorders. Am J Clin Pathol 98:46–54
2. Kreipe H, Radzun HJ, Bartels H, von Heyden H-W, Löffler H, Parwaresch MR (1990) Detection of clonality and stem cell mutations in chronic myeloproliferative disorders. Verh Dtsch Ges Pathol 74:49–64
3. Temerinac S, Klippel S, Strunck E, Röder S, Lübbert M, Lange W, Azemar M, Meinhardt G, Schaefer HE, Pahl HL (2000) Cloning of PRV-1, a novel member of the uPAR receptor superfamily, which is overexpressed in polycythemia rubra vera. Blood 95:2569–2576
4. MacNeil I, Kennedy J, Godfrey DI, Jenkins NA, Masciantonio M, Mineo C, Gilbert DJ, Copeland NG, Boyd RL, Zlotnik A (1993) Isolation of a cDNA encoding thymic shared antigen-1. J Immunol 151:6913–6923
5. Ploug M, Kjalke M, Ronne E, Weidle U, Hoyer-Hansen G, Dano K (1993) Localization of the disulfide bonds in the NH2-terminal domain of the cellular receptor for human urokinase-type plasminogen activator. J Biol Chem 268:17539–17546
6. Ploug M, Behrendt N, Lober D, Dano K (1991) Protein structure and membrane anchorage of the cellular receptor for urokinase-type plasminogen activator. Semin Thromb Hemost 17:183–193
7. Meri S, Morgan BP, Davies A, Daniels RH, Olaveton MG, Waldmann H, Lachmann PJ (1990) Human protectin (CD59), an 18,000–20,000 MW complement lysis restricting factor, inhibits C5b-8 catalysed insertion of C9 into lipid bilayers. Immunology 71:1–9
8. Ninomiya H, Sims PJ (1992) The human complement regulatory protein CD59 binds to the alpha-chain of C8 and to the "b" domain of C9. J Biol Chem 267:13675–13680
9. Noel LS, Champion BR, Holley CL, Simmons CJ, Morris DC, Payne JA, Lean JM, Chambers TJ, Zaman G, Lanyon LE, Suva LJ, Miller LR (1998) RoBo-1, a novel member of the urokinase plasminogen activator receptor/CD59/Ly6/Snake toxin family selectively expressed in rat bone and growth plate cartilage. J Biol Chem 273:3878–3883
10. Klippel S, Strunck E, Busse CE, Behringer D, Pahl HD (2002) Biochemical characterization of PRV-1, a novel hematopoietic cell surface receptor, which is overexpressed in polycythemia rubra vera. Blood 100:2441–2448
11. Shih L-Y, Lee C-T (1994) Identification of masked polycythemia vera from patients with idiopathic marked thrombocytosis by endogenous erythroid colony assay. Blood 83:744–748
12. Stefanova I, Horejsi V, Ansotegui IJ, Knapp W, Stockinger H (1991) GPI-anchored cell surface molecules complexed to protein tyrosine kinases. Science 254:1016–1019
13. Bohuslav J, Horejsi V, Hansmann C, Stöckl J, Weidle UH, Majdic O, Bartke I, Knapp W, Stockinger H (1995) Urokinase plasminogen activator receptor b2-integrins, and src-kinases within a single receptor complex of human monocytes. J Exp Med 181:1381–1390
14. Dumler I, Weis A, Mayboroda OA, Maasch C, Jerke U, Haller H, Gulba DC (1998) The Jak/Stat pathway and urokinase receptor signalling in human aortic vascular smooth muscle cells. J Biol Chem 273:315–321

15. Konakova M, Hucho F, Schleuning W-D (1998) Downstream targets of urokinase-type plasminogen-activator-mediated signal transduction. Eur J Biochem 253:421–429
16. Koshelnick Y, Ehart M, Hufnagl P, Heinrich PC, Binder BR (1997) Urokinase receptor is associated with the components of the JAK/STAT1 signalling pathway and leads to activation of this pathway upon receptor clustering in the human kidney epithelial tumor cell line TCL-598. J Biol Chem 272:28563–28567
17. Druker BJ (2003) Imatinib mesylate in the treatment of chronic myeloid leukemia. Expert Opin Pharmacother 4:963–971

Chapter 7

Impaired Expression of the Thrombopoietin Receptor, Mpl, in Polycythemia Vera

Jerry L. Spivak, Alison R. Moliterno, Edward G. Weir, Donna M. Williams

7.1 Introduction

Polycythemia vera (PV) is a clonal disorder of unknown etiology involving a multipotent hematopoietic progenitor cell that is characterized by the accumulation of phenotypically normal red cells, white cells and platelets in the absence of a definable physiologic stimulus. Trilineage hematopoietic cell hyperplasia is the hallmark of PV but erythrocytosis is its most prominent clinical manifestation, the cause of its most common and most serious clinical complications and the only feature that sets it apart from idiopathic myelofibrosis (IMF) and essential thrombocytosis (ET). As a consequence, most research with respect to the pathogenesis of PV has focused on erythropoiesis, but without completely enlightening results.

The lifespan of the red cell is not prolonged in PV [1] nor is the erythroid progenitor cell pool expanded at the expense of the myeloid progenitor cell pool [2]. PV erythroid progenitor cells appear to be hypersensitive to erythropoietin [3] or erythropoietin-independent [4]. However, this behavior is actually an in vitro artifact since in serum-free cultures these cells are not more sensitive to erythropoietin than normal cells; rather, they are more sensitive to insulin-like growth factor-I (IGF-I) [5]. Most importantly, it has recently been observed that PV erythroid progenitor cells, in contrast to normal erythroid progenitor cells, are resistant to apoptosis following growth factor withdrawal [6].

Studies of the erythropoietin receptor have failed to reveal structural abnormalities of its gene (see Chap. 6), of its expression or its ligand-binding behavior in PV erythroid progenitor cells [7]. Importantly, forced expression of a normal erythropoietin receptor in primitive hematopoietic progenitor cells does not lead to autonomous proliferation or stimulate trilineage hematopoietic cell hyperplasia [8] which are essential features of PV. In contrast to the erythropoietin receptor, Mpl, the thrombopoietin (TPO) receptor is a candidate receptor for involvement in the pathogenesis of PV. Mpl is expressed in pluripotent hematopoietic stem cells [9], both the proliferation and survival of which it promotes [10, 11]. As a corollary, TPO or Mpl knockout mice have reduced numbers of multilineage hematopoietic progenitor cells [12]. Overexpression of TPO in mice causes granulocytosis, thrombocytosis, osteomyelofibrosis and extramedullary hematopoiesis [13], while ectopic Mpl expression in vivo is associated with a fatal erythroblastosis [14]. TPO also suppresses apoptosis of erythroid progenitor cells deprived of erythropoietin [15]. Most importantly, however, Mpl is a protooncogene since a truncated Mpl variant is the oncogenic protein of the retrovirus MPLV which in vitro immortalizes hematopoietic progenitor cells [16] and, following in vivo infection, causes a syndrome in mice similar to PV [17].

To examine the behavior of Mpl in the pathogenesis of PV, we exploited the persistence of functional Mpl expression in circulating platelets.

7.2 Studies of Mpl-mediated Signal Transduction in PV Platelets

Exposure of washed normal platelets in vitro to a saturating concentration of TPO for 10 minutes at room temperature stimulated tyrosine phosphorylation of a variety of platelet proteins including JAK2, STAT5 and the TPO receptor, Mpl, itself as demonstrated by immunoblotting of PV platelet lysates using a phosphotyrosine antiserum (Fig. 7.1a) [18]. Exposure of PV platelets under the same conditions or even with a tenfold increase in TPO for up to 30 minutes failed to produce the same degree of protein tyrosine phosphorylation, even though the ability of the same platelets to phosphorylate proteins on tyrosine in response to thrombin was intact. The blunted signal transduction response of PV platelets to TPO was not due to the absence of members of the JAK tyrosine kinase family or substrate proteins such as STAT5 since they were present in the same quantities as in normal platelets determined by immunoblotting (Fig. 7.1b, c).

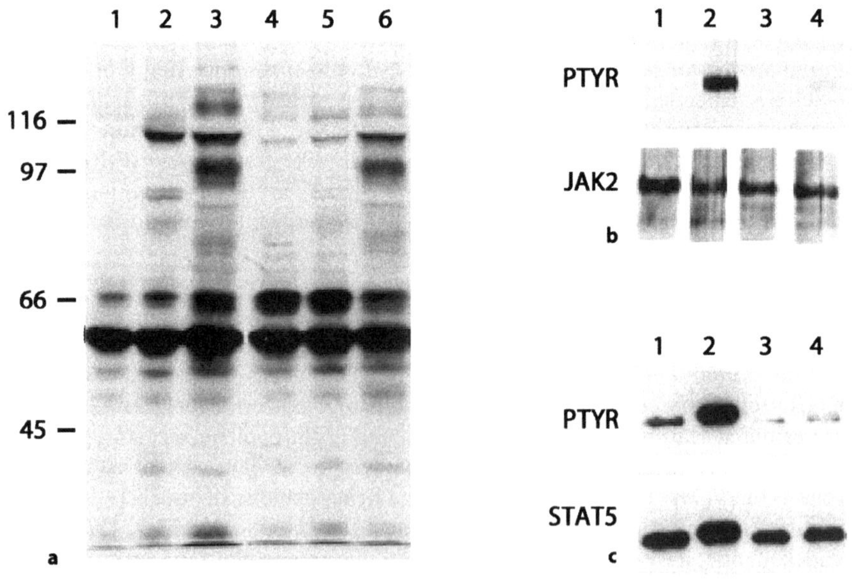

Fig. 7.1. a Immunoblot of normal (*lanes 1–3*) and PV (*lanes 4–6*) platelet lysates using a phosphotyrosine antiserum following exposure of the platelets (*lanes 2 and 5*) to 100 ng/ml of TPO for 10 minutes at room temperature or (*lanes 3 and 6*) to 2 U/ml of thrombin for 2 minutes at room temperature [19]. **b** Immunoblot of JAK2 immunoprecipitates using a phosphotyrosine antiserum from normal (*lanes 1 and 2*) and PV (*lanes 3 and 4*) platelets, unstimulated (*lanes 1 and 3*) or stimulated (*lanes 2 and 4*) with TPO. The blot was stripped and reprobed with a JAK2 antiserum. **c** Immunoblot of STAT5 immunoprecipitates using a phosphotyrosine antiserum from normal (*lanes 1 and 2) and PV (lanes 3 and 4*) platelets, unstimulated (*lanes 1 and 3*) or stimulated (*lanes 2 and 4*) with TPO. The blot was stripped and reprobed with a STAT5 antiserum

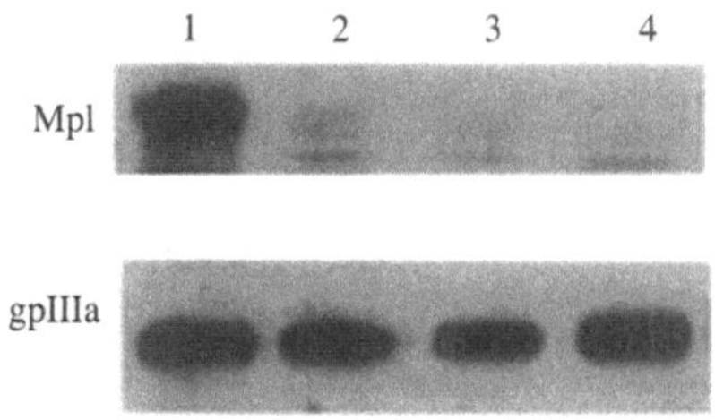

Fig. 7.2. Immunoblot of normal (control, *lane 1*) and PV (*lanes 2–4*) platelet lysates using a polyclonal N-terminal antiserum. The membrane was stripped and reprobed with a gpIIIa antiserum to establish equal loading of platelet lysate protein [21]

Impairment of TPO-induced signal transduction in the cells of a disorder characterized by cell accumulation was a surprising observation. To determine if the interaction of TPO with Mpl in platelets was intact, we studied the binding of 125I-labeled TPO to platelets. Labeled TPO could be crosslinked to normal platelets and its binding was prevented by exposure of the platelets to unlabeled TPO. By contrast, labeled TPO could not be crosslinked to PV platelets [19]. These observations suggested that either PV platelet Mpl was defective or poorly expressed at the platelet surface.

7.3 Studies of Mpl Expression in PV Platelets and Megakaryocytes

To examine the possibility of an abnormality in PV platelet Mpl we assessed PV platelet Mpl expression by immunoblotting and by flow cytometry using an N-terminal Mpl polyclonal antiserum. As shown in Fig. 7.2, for equal quantities of platelet lysate, PV Mpl expression was markedly reduced as compared to its expression in normal platelets. This was not an artifact due to platelet manipulation ex vivo, because flow cytometry of PV and normal platelets after labeling with the same antibody demonstrated reduced Mpl expression only in PV platelets [18]. The possibility that PV platelet Mpl expression was reduced due to proteolysis during platelet isolation or by a factor in PV plasma was excluded by incubating normal platelets in PV plasma over night, by mixing normal and PV platelets in equal quantities before lysis and by incubating normal platelets with saturating concentrations of TPO. In none of these circumstances was there evidence of inappropriate loss of platelet Mpl [19].

To determine whether reduced PV platelet Mpl expression was also characteristic of PV megakaryocytes, we examined the expression of Mpl by bone marrow megakaryocytes using immunohistochemistry. Normal megakaryocytes as identified by Factor VIII staining, reacted strongly with an N-terminal Mpl antiserum. However, the bulk of PV marrow megakaryocytes, while staining strongly for Factor VIII, failed to react with the Mpl N-terminal antiserum, indicating that reduced PV platelet Mpl expression was due to impaired megakaryocyte Mpl expression as opposed to an isolated platelet defect [18].

7.4 Specificity of Impaired Platelet Mpl Expression

The specificity of impaired PV platelet Mpl expression was examined by immunoblotting and quantitative densitometry in patients with IMF, ET, chronic myeloid leukemia (CML), secondary erythrocytosis, iron deficiency anemia, hemochromatosis and normal controls. All 34 patients with PV, 13 of 14 with IMF and 4 of 9 with ET had reduced platelet Mpl expression. None of the patients with secondary erythrocytosis, iron deficiency anemia, CML, hemochromatosis undergoing repeated phlebotomy, or the normal subjects had reduced platelet Mpl expression. To date, three of the ET patients with reduced Mpl expression had developed either PV or IMF [20].

7.5 Mechanism for Impaired PV Platelet Mpl Expression

The impaired response of platelets to TPO as well as reduced platelet Mpl expression as measured by immunoblotting with an N-terminal Mpl antiserum, suggested an abnormality of the Mpl extracellular domain. To examine this possibility we raised a polyclonal antiserum against an Mpl C-terminal peptide. As shown in Fig. 7.3, in contrast to the Mpl N-terminal polyclonal antiserum, immunoblotting of platelet lysates with the C-terminal Mpl antiserum revealed detectable Mpl in PV platelets but the absolute quantity was reduced. The extent of the reduction was proportional to the duration of the PV and was most marked in patients with disease of long duration and substantial splenomegaly [21]. Furthermore, using the C-terminal Mpl antiserum, two forms of Mpl were apparent in PV platelets.

To determine the molecular basis for the differences in PV and normal platelet Mpl, we employed two-dimensional (2-D) gel electrophoresis, using isoelectric focusing in the first dimension and SDS-PAGE in the second. As shown in Fig. 7.4, 2-D gel electrophoresis revealed two Mpl isoforms in PV platelet lysates, but only one in normal platelets and in some PV patients only the faster migrating, less acidic form was present. Since the extracellular domain of Mpl has a reduplicated cytokine receptor module and as a consequence four canonical sites for N-glycosylation, it seemed likely that the two forms of Mpl differed with respect to their glycosylation status and might represent fully and incompletely glycosylated Mpl. Examination of Mpl expression in DAMI cells supported these contentions since on 2-D gel electrophoresis, both

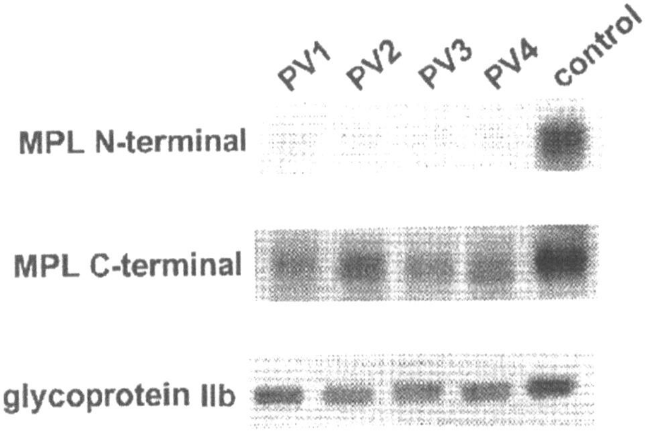

Fig. 7.3. Immunoblot of PV and control platelet lysates using either an N-terminal or a C-terminal Mpl antiserum. The membrane was stripped and reprobed with a gpIIb antiserum to establish equal loading of the platelet lysate protein [21]

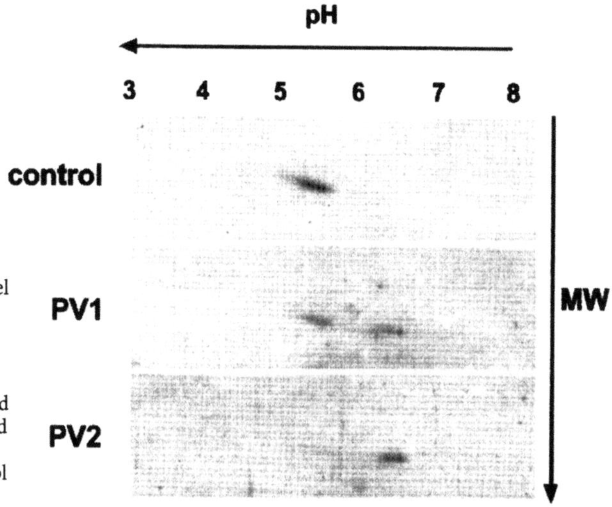

Fig. 7.4. Two-dimensional gel electrophoresis of PV and normal (control) platelet lysates (25 μg) with isoelectric focusing in the first dimension (horizontally) and 10% SDS-PAGE in the second (vertically), followed by immunoblotting with an Mpl C-terminal antiserum [21]

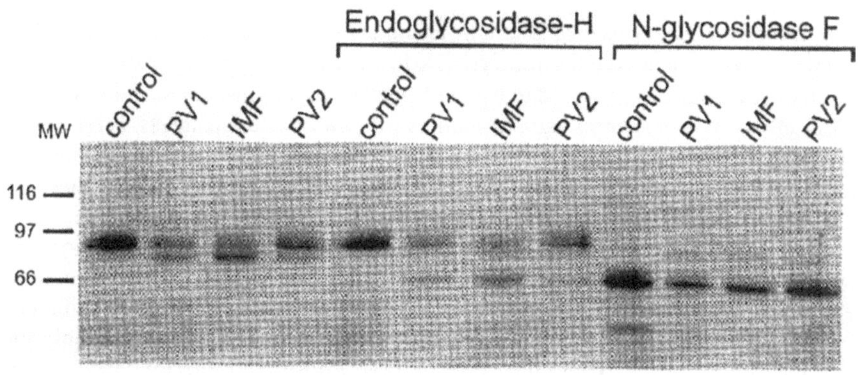

Fig. 7.5. Digestion of normal (control), PV and IMF platelet lysates using endoglycosidase H (*lanes 5–8*) or N-glycosidase F (*lanes 9–12*) followed by immunoblotting with an Mpl C-terminal antiserum [21]

forms of Mpl were present and following digestion of DAMI cell lysates with neuraminidase only the faster migrating, less acidic Mpl isoform was present [21].

Since incompletely glycosylated proteins are sensitive to endoglycosidase H, we digested normal, PV and IMF platelet lysates with this enzyme. As shown in Fig. 7.5, the faster migrating form of PV or IMF platelet Mpl was sensitive to endoglycosidase H. Following digestion of platelet lysate Mpl with N-endoglycosidase F, which cleaves sugar residues at their asparagine linkage, the electrophoretic mobilities of normal, PV and IMF platelet Mpls were identical indicating similarity of their polypeptides. Examination of two other major platelet membrane glycoproteins, gpIIb and multimerin, by 2-D gel electrophoresis failed to reveal impaired glycosylation [21].

To elucidate the expression of the two forms of PV platelet Mpl, we examined platelet Mpl expression serially over time in individual PV patients as well as in PV patients at different stages of the disease. As shown in Fig. 7.6, with increasing dura-

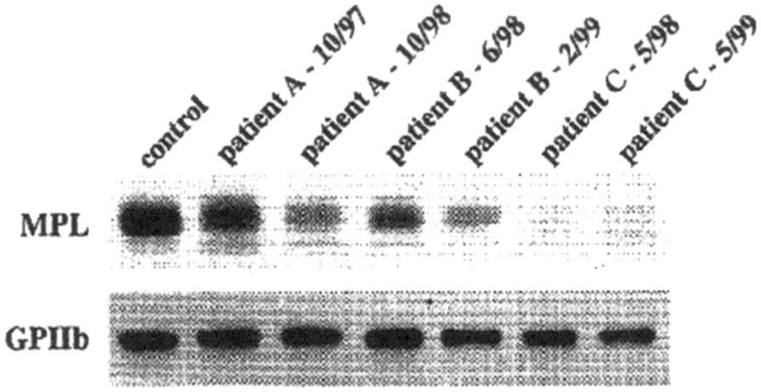

Fig. 7.6. Serial analysis of Mpl expression in platelets from three PV patients by immunoblotting with an Mpl C-terminal antiserum

tion of disease there was a gradual increase in the proportion of incompletely glycosylated Mpl and total platelet Mpl concentration declined as well.

7.6 The Molecular Basis for Impaired PV Platelet Mpl Glycosylation

To investigate the possibility that the abnormality in PV Mpl was due to an abnormality in the Mpl gene or its expression, we examined the Mpl gene by Southern blotting and its expression by Northern analysis. No evidence of Mpl gene deletion, amplification or rearrangement was found using PV leukocyte genomic DNA, and full-length Mpl mRNA was present in equal amounts in PV and normal platelets. Screening of the exon-containing regions of Mpl genomic DNA from eight patients by the MisMatch Detect II Assay (Ambion) also failed to reveal relevant mutations. However, isolates cloned from PCR-amplified platelet Mpl cDNA revealed increases in the proportions of two previously undescribed Mpl splice variants: a 21-base deletion at the beginning of exon 2 in the N-terminal domain present in six of seven patients in up to 50% of the isolates, in contrast to only one of 14 isolates from two normal controls, and a 33–36-base addition from the adjacent intron attached to the upstream end of exon 8 which is also in the extracellular domain [22]. An RNAse protection assay in one patient indicated that the exon 2 deletion splice variant comprised 30% of the Mpl message. No mutations were found in the intervening sequence between exons 1 and 2 indicating that both splice donor and acceptor sites were intact. In addition, in one patient a point mutation at nucleotide 175 was identified that changed a lysine to asparagine at amino acid 39. Studies of the patient's hematologically normal son failed to reveal a similar mutation, suggesting that it may not be a constitutional defect.

To determine if the exon 2 deletion splice variant and the exon 2 point mutation, both of which were in the distal cytokine receptor module, would influence Mpl glycosylation, Mpl variant cDNA was inserted into the IL-3-dependent cell line 32D, using a retroviral vector. Immunoblotting of 32D cells expressing either of the Mpl variants revealed incompletely glycosylated Mpl with impaired expression as compared to wild-type Mpl expression. Furthermore, cells expressing either variant Mpl were less sensitive to the proliferative effects of TPO than wild-type Mpl. These observations indicated that incompletely glycosylated Mpl was expressed at the cell surface and could participate in ligand-mediated signal transduction in a nucleated hematopoietic cell.

7.7 Effect of Impaired Mpl Glycosylation on NF-κB Expression in PV Platelets and Megakaryocytes

Impaired protein glycosylation causes abnormalities in protein folding, as well as endoplasmic reticulum protein overload, both of which are associated with upregulation of NF-κB [23, 24], a transcription factor that activates cytokine gene expression and promotes resistance to apoptosis [25]. We therefore examined NF-κB expression in normal and PV megakaryocytes by immunohistochemistry [26]. NF-κB p65 but not p50 expression was increased in the cytoplasm of PV but not normal megakaryocytes but the expression of IκBα was not different from normal. To determine if the NF-κB was transcriptionally active, we examined its behavior in PV platelets. As in PV megakaryocytes, expression of NF-κB p65 but not p50 was increased in PV platelets as determined by immunoblotting and immunoprecipitation, and this was not a consequence of leukocyte contamination. By EMSA, platelet NF-κB interacted specifically with its consensus DNA-binding site in a concentration-dependent fashion and could be supershifted using p65 antibodies but not p50 antibodies whether used alone or together after complexing NF-κB with p65. Since NF-κB is antiapoptotic, we examined megakaryocyte Bcl-x expression by immunohistochemistry. Total Bcl-x expression was comparable in normal and PV megakaryocytes but Bcl-xl expression was qualitatively more pronounced in PV megakaryocytes [26].

7.8 Discussion

The mechanisms involved in the pathogenesis of PV are undefined but with respect to erythropoiesis appear to involve growth factor hypersensitivity [5], resistance to apoptosis under conditions of growth factor deprivation [6] and accelerated differentiation as compared to normal erythroid progenitor cells [27]. Any explanation for the pathogenesis of PV must also encompass the behavior of pluripotent or multipotent hematopoietic progenitor cells since the hallmark of PV is trilineage hematopoietic cell hyperplasia, of which erythrocytosis is the most dramatic example and the defining diagnostic feature. Based on its role in the survival and proliferation of primitive CD34+ hematopoietic progenitor cells [10], as well as its ability to function as an oncogene capable of conferring growth factor independence on hematopoietic progenitor cells [16, 17], we focused our attention on the expression and behavior of Mpl in PV. Platelets provide a convenient assay system since they express Mpl, although at a low copy number. Our observations pose a conundrum since we have established that Mpl expression is impaired in a disorder characterized by an accumulation of phenotypically normal hematopoietic cells. They also potentially represent a new paradigm for the pathogenesis of a clonal hematopoietic disorder.

Impaired Mpl expression was associated with incomplete Mpl glycosylation and the glycosylation defect appeared to be more severe as the disease progressed. Importantly, impaired PV platelet Mpl glycosylation was associated with the expression of an Mpl splice variant or point mutation involving the distal cytokine receptor module. This module has been demonstrated to be necessary for not only ligand binding, but also downregulation of Mpl signaling [28]. Deletion of the distal cytokine receptor module with or without replacing it with the proximal one, led to constitutive proliferation of cells expressing these Mpl constructs in the absence of ligand binding [28]. The behavior of cells expressing Mpl lacking the distal cytokine receptor module is similar to that of cells expressing the oncogenic Mpl variant, vMpl, which also lacks most of its N-terminal domain and causes a syndrome similar to PV in mice [17].

Thus, changes such as alternative splicing or mutations involving that portion of the Mpl N-terminal domain containing the distal cytokine receptor module could have the potential to alter the behavior of the receptor. Support for this contention comes from the observation that expression of the exon 2 21-base deletion Mpl splice variant or the point mutant in IL-3-dependent cells not only recapitulated the glycosylation defect observed in PV platelet Mpl, but also decreased their sensitivity to TPO as compared to wild-type Mpl. The mechanisms involved are as-yet unknown.

Impaired glycosylation is a second potential mechanism by which the variant Mpl representing alterations in the distal N-terminal domain could influence cell behavior. Proteins that cannot be completely glycosylated trigger a biochemical response [23, 24] that includes the activation of NF-κB, a transcription factor that has antiapoptotic properties. An increase in transcriptionally active NF-κB p65 was evident in PV megakaryocytes by immunohistochemistry without any change in its inhibitor IκBα α [26]. This was associated with an increase in Bcl-xl in these cells. Whether the changes are related and whether they represent a consequence of impaired Mpl glycosylation has not yet been established. Other possibilities for the involvement of variant Mpl in the pathogenesis of PV include uncontrolled intracellular signaling due to the interaction of incompletely glycosylated variant with wild-type Mpl receptors in the cytoplasm or the Golgi apparatus. Alternatively, impaired glycosylation might actually diminish receptor function and render the cell more sensitive to other growth factors. Precedence for this behavior is found in the behavior of cells expressing erythropoietin receptors with C-terminal domain truncations. Although initially thought to be hypersensitive to erythropoietin because of loss of the binding site for the negative regulatory phosphatase SHP-1 [29], we now understand that such cells are actually hyposensitive to erythropoietin and hypersensitive to IGF-1 [30]. IGF-1 hypersensitivity is, of course, a feature of PV [5]. Impaired Mpl expression in PV could, therefore, represent a physiologic cellular response to the process causing PV or be intrinsic to the pathogenesis of the disease. Elucidation of the molecular basis for this defect will provide insight into the regulation of growth factor signaling under normal circumstances and in hematopoietic disorders.

Acknowledgements. Supported in part by NHLBI Grant 58589 (J.L.S.) and a Doris Duke Clinical Scientist Award (A.R.M). The excellent technical assistance of Evelyn Connor and Mary Ann Isaacs is gratefully acknowledged.

References

1. London IM, Shemin D, West R, Rittenberg D (1949) Heme synthesis and red blood cell dynamics in normal humans and in subjects with polycythemia vera, sickle cell anemia, and pernicious anemia. J Biol Chem 179:463–484
2. Eaves AC, Henkelman DH, Eaves CJ (1980) Abnormal erythropoiesis in the myeloproliferative disorders: an analysis of underlying cellular and humoral mechanisms. Exp Hematol 8 [Suppl 8]:235–247

3. Eaves CJ, Eaves AC (1978). Erythropoietin (Ep) dose-response curves for three classes of erythroid progenitors in normal human marrow and in patients with polycythemia vera. Blood 52:1196–1210
4. Prchal JF, Axelrad AA (1974) Bone-marrow responses in polycythemia vera. N Engl J Med 290:1382
5. Correa PN, Eskinazi D, Axelrad AA (1994) Circulating erythroid progenitors in polycythemia vera are hypersensitive to insulin-like growth factor-1 in vitro: studies in an improved serum-free medium. Blood 83:99–112
6. Silva M, Richard C, Benito A, Sanz C, Olalla I, Fernandez-Luna JL (1998) Expression of Bcl-x in erythroid precursors from patients with polycythemia vera. N Engl J Med 338:564–571
7. Hess G, Rose P, Gamm H, Papadileris S, Huber C, Seliger B (1994) Molecular analysis of the erythropoietin receptor system in patients with polycythaemia vera. Br J Haematol 88:794–802
8. Lu L, Ge Y, Li Z-H, Keeble W, Kabat D, Bagby G, Broxmeyer H (1996) Retroviral transfer of the recombinant human erythropoietin receptor gene into single hematopoietic stem/progenitor cells from human cord blood increases the number of erythropoietin-dependent erythroid colonies. Blood 87:525–534
9. Solar GP, Kerr WG, Zeigler FC, Hess D, Donahue C, de Sauvage FJ, Eaton DL (1998) Role of c-mpl in early hematopoiesis. Blood 92:4–10
10. Young JC, Bruno E, Leuns KM, Wu S, Backer M, Murray LJ (1996) Thrombopoietin stimulates megakaryocytopoiesis, myelopoiesis, and expansion of CD34+ progenitor cells from single CD34+ thy-I+ Lin– primitive progenitor cells. Blood 88:1619–1631
11. Borge OJ, Ramsfjell V, Cui L, Jacobsen SEW (1997) Ability of early acting cytokines to directly promote survival and suppress apoptosis of human primitive CD34+ CD38– bone marrow cells with multilineage potential at the single-cell level: key role of thrombopoietin. Blood 90:2282–2292
12. Carver-Moore K, Broxmeyer H, Luoh S-M, Cooper S, Peng J, Burstein S (1996) Low levels of erythroid and myeloid progenitors in thrombopoietin- and c-mpl-deficient mice. Blood 88:803–808
13. Villeval J-L, Cohen-Solal K, Tulliez M, Giraudier S, Guichard J, Burstein SA, Cramer EM,Vainchenker W, Wendling F (1997) High thrombopoietin production by hematopoietic cells induces a fatal myeloproliferative syndrome in mice. Blood 90:4369–4373
14. Cocault L, Bouscary D, Kerdiles CLB, Clay D, Picard F, Gisselbrecht S, Souyri M (1996) Ectopic expression of murine TPO receptor (c-mpl) in mice is pathogenic and induces erythroblastic proliferation. Blood 88:1656–1659
15. Ratajczak MZ, Ratajczak J, Marlicz W, Pletcher CH Jr, Machalinski B, Moore J, Hung H-L, Gewirtz AM (1997) Recombinant human thrombopoietin (TPO) stimulates erythropoiesis by inhibiting erythroid progenitor cell apoptosis. Br J Hematol 98:8–17
16. Souyri M, Vigon L, Penciolelli J-F, Heard J-M, Tambourin P, Wendling F (1990) A putative truncated cytokine receptor gene transduced by the myeloproliferative leukemia virus immortalizes hematopoietic progenitors. Cell 63:1137–1147
17. Wendling F, Varlet P, Charon M, Tambourin P (1986) MPLV: a retrovirus complex inducing an acute myeloproliferative leukemic disorder in adult mice. Virology 149:242–246
18. Moliterno AR, Hankins WD, Spivak JL (1998) Impaired Expression of the thrombopoietin receptor by platelets from patients with polycythemia vera. N Engl J Med 338:572–580
19. Moliterno AR, Siebel KE, Sun AY, Hankins WD, Spivak JL (1998) A novel thrombopoietin signaling defect in polycythemia vera platelets. In: Murphy M Jr, Kuter DJ (eds) Thrombopoietin: from molecule to medicine. AlphaMed Press, Miamisburg, Ohio, pp 185–192
20. Moliterno AR, Silver RT Spivak JL (2000) A diagnostic assay for polycythemia vera. Blood 96 [Suppl 1]:512a
21. Moliterno AR, Spivak JL (1999) Posttranslational processing of the thrombopoietin receptor is impaired in polycythemia vera. Blood 94:2555–2561
22. Moliterno AR, Williams DM, Hankins WD, Spivak JL (1999) An increase in Mpl splice variants in polycythemia vera platelets. Blood 94 [Suppl 1]:112a
23. Kozutsumi Y, Segal M, Normington K, Gething M-J (1988) The presence of malfolded proteins in the endoplasmic reticulum signals the induction of glucose-regulated proteins. Nature 332:462–464
24. Pahl HL, Baeuerle PA (1995) A novel signal transduction pathway from the endoplasmic reticulum to the nucleus is mediated by transcription factor NF-κB. EMBO J 14:2580–2588
25. Pyatt DW, Stillman WS, Yang Y, Gross S, Zhang JH, Irons RD (1999) An essential role for NF-κB in human CD34+ bone marrow survival. Blood 93:3302–3308
26. Spivak JL, Weir E (1999) Upregulation of NF-κB in polycythemia vera megakaryocytes: the platelet as a fossil record. Blood 94 [Suppl 1]:112a
27. Papayannopoulou T, Buckley J, Nakamoto B, Kurachi S, Nute PE, Stamatoyannopoulos G (1979) Hb F production in endogenous colonies of polycythemia vera. Blood 53:446–454
28. Sabath DF, Kaushansky K, Broudy VC (1999) Deletion of the extracellular membrane-distal cytokine receptor homology module of Mpl results in constitutive cell growth and loss of thrombopoietin binding. Blood 94:365–367

29. D'Andrea AD, Yoshimura A, Youssoufian H, Zon L, Koo J-W, Lodish HF (1991) The cytoplasmic domain of the erythropoietin receptor contains nonoverlapping positive and negative growth-regulatory domains. Mol Cell Biol 11:1980–1987
30. Damen JE, Krosl J, Morrison D, Pelech S, Krystal G (1998) The hyperresponsiveness of cells expressing truncated erythropoietin receptors is contingent on insulin-like growth factor-I in fetal calf serum. Blood 92:425–433

Growth Factor Signaling in Polycythemia Vera Cells: Specific Hypersensitivities to Cytokines in the Chronic Myeloproliferative Disorders

Arthur A. Axelrad, in collaboration with Dominick Amato, Paulo N. Correa, Denise Eskinazi, Shereen Ezzat, W.Y. Jia, Amer M. Mirza, Josef T. Prchal, T. Zhang, L. Zhou

8.1 Introduction

Each member of the family of chronic myeloproliferative disorders (cMPDs) is believed to originate as a regulatory defect in a single pluripotential bone marrow stem cell [1–5]. These disorders are characterized by trilineal marrow hyperplasia with the major clinicopathological emphasis usually on a single cell lineage only [6–8]. The basis for this selective emphasis is at present unknown. In polycythemia vera (PV), it has long been known that erythroid progenitor cells grown in cultures containing serum produce colonies in the absence of added erythropoietin (EPO) [9]. The debate that followed as to whether the cells were independent of, or hypersensitive to, the small quantities of EPO in serum, could not be resolved as long as the cells were grown in media containing serum [10]. In 1994, Paulo Correa and I developed a strictly serum-free medium [11] and applied it to this question. We were able to show that the PV erythroid progenitor cells were not hypersensitive to EPO [10]. In the same year, Fisher and associates found that among the erythroid progenitor cells in PV there were those that proliferated and differentiated in the presence of even high concentrations of EPO- and EPO receptor-neutralizing monoclonal antibodies; the cells were clearly independent of EPO [12]. Then we found that the PV progenitor cells were in fact hypersensitive to another growth factor – insulin-like growth factor-I (IGF-I) [10]. IGF-I, like EPO, we now know stimulates erythropoiesis [11, 13].

8.2 Patients, Materials and Methods

Information on these items may be found elsewhere [10, 11, 14].

8.3 Experimental Results and Discussion

To determine relative sensitivities of the progenitor cells to these cytokines, Ficoll-Hypaque-separated peripheral blood mononuclear cells (PBMNC) from PV patients, patients with secondary erythrocytosis, and normal volunteers were seeded in strictly serum-free methylcellulose culture containing various concentrations of IGF-I or EPO, and fixed concentrations of all-*trans*-retinoic acid (ATRA), interleukin-3

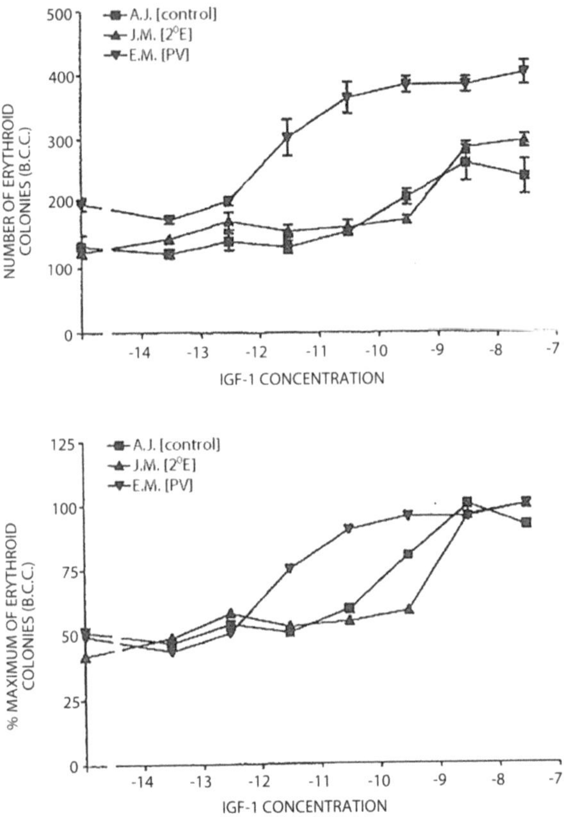

Fig. 8.1. Representative curves of erythroid colony formation by PBMNC from a healthy volunteer (■), a patient with secondary erythrocytosis (▲), and a patient with PV (▼), plotted as a function of rHu IGF-I concentration (mol/L) in strictly serum-free methylcellulose culture. All cultures also contained ATRA (3×10−8 mol/l), hemin (100 μmol/l), and rHu IL-3 (10 ng/ml). *Left* Erythroid colonies scored as number of burst component colonies (BCC) [10, 11] per 7×104 PBMNC per 0.7 ml per well. *Right* Erythroid colony number normalized to percentage of maximum. Note left shift of the PV curve as compared with curves of the normal control and the secondary erythrocytosis patient (experiment no. 213)

(IL-3) and hemin. Erythroid bursts and burst-component colonies (BCCs) were scored, and normalized as percentage of maximum [10, 11]. The curves of erythroid bursts produced by the cells of PV patients under the influence of EPO were not different from those of normal individuals. In contrast, the curves of erythroid bursts of BCCs produced by the cells of PV patients under the influence of IGF-I were shifted to the left of the control curves (Fig. 8.1), and showed that the PV erythroid progenitors were at least 100 times as sensitive to IGF-I as those of the normal volunteers or patients with secondary erythrocytosis.

Investigating larger numbers of patients, we found that the erythroid progenitor cells of PV patients varied in their IGF-I sensitivities over a broad range. Comparison of normal and PV pairs of cultures (Table 8.1) showed that PV erythroid progenitors could reach IGF-I sensitivity ratios as high as 20,000 times normal. The median IGF-I sensitivity ratio for PV was >4000 times normal. No other cytokine of those we have looked at has shown an IGF-I sensitivity ratio even approaching this value.

How specific is the hypersensitivity of PV erythroid progenitors to IGF-I? Several authors have claimed that erythroid progenitor cells in PV are hypersensitive to a number of different cytokines. These have included EPO, stem cell factor (SCF) [15], thrombopoietin (TPO) [16], IL-3 [17, 18], and granulocyte-macrophage colony stim-

Table 8.1. Relative sensitivities of normal and PV erythroid progenitor cells to IGF-I

Experiment no.	IGF-I concentration (*M*) at half-maximal colony number Normal	PV	IGF-I sensitivity ratio
173	7.5×10^{-10}	2.0×10^{-13}	3,750
176	4.3×10^{-10}	$<3.0\times10^{-14}$	>14,300
179	7.0×10^{-10}	1.6×10^{-13}	4,375
180	3.0×10^{-10}	8.0×10^{-13}	375
184	9.8×10^{-9}	6.4×10^{-13}	15,300
192	5.2×10^{-10}	3.3×10^{-13}	1,576
205	9.0×10^{-10}	4.5×10^{-14}	20,000
211	3.5×10^{-10}	$<3.0\times10^{-14}$	1,167
213	2.3×10^{-10}	3.0×10^{-12}	77
247	1.4×10^{-10}	$<3.0\times10^{-14}$	> 4,667
250	1.0×10^{-10}	1.7×10^{-13}	588
254	1.2×10^{-9}	1.8×10^{-13}	6,667
260	2.1×10^{-10}	$<3.0\times10^{-14}$	> 7,000
268	2.1×10^{-10}	2.3×10^{-12}	91
Median	3.9×10^{-10}	1.75×10^{-13}	> 4,063
Range			77–20,000

ulating factor (GM-CSF) [18]. However, the experiments leading to these conclusions were all carried out in media containing serum or serum-derived products. Serum is known to contain IGF-I [19]. This could confound interpretation of data from these experiments, especially since PV erythroid progenitors can be exquisitely sensitive to IGF-I. Damen et al. [20] have shown that inherited or experimentally induced mutations of the EPO receptor gene that cause C-terminal truncations are associated with erythrocytosis, and this turns out to be due to hypersensitivity to IGF-I, and not to EPO. In collaboration with Dr. Josef Prchal, we have also obtained evidence that in familial polycythemia, the hypersensitivity to EPO in the presence of serum is probably due to IGF-I: in the absence of serum, there was hypersensitivity to IGF-I, but not to EPO. We also found that IGF-I increased EPO sensitivity of erythroid progenitor cells of both polycythemic patients and normal individuals (Table 8.2). Thus, to get a reliable assessment of sensitivity to EPO it appears to be necessary to carry out the determinations in strictly serum-free, IGF-I-free medium.

Table 8.2. IGF-I increases EPO sensitivity of erythroid progenitor cells of normal individuals and patients with polycythemia

Group	IGF-I half-maximum (*M*)	IGF-I sensitivity ratio	–IGF-I		+IGF-I	
			EPO half-maximum (U/ml)	EPO sensitivity ratio	EPO half-maximum (U/ml)	EPO sensitivity ratio
Control	1×10^{-10}	–	2.15	–	0.34	5.3
Familial polycythemia	3.8×10^{-14}	263	1.25	1.7	0.23	5.4
PV	$<3.0\times10^{-14}$	3333	1.70	1.3	<0.19	> 8.9
PV	6.6×10^{-14}	1515	2.25	0.96	<0.19	>11.8

Dai and colleagues, using highly purified BFU-E from PV patients, have reported that a marked increase in the number of PV bursts occurs with increasing concentrations of SCF, but they did not show a change in the concentration of the ligand required for this effect. They concluded that the erythroid progenitor cells in PV are hypersensitive to SCF [15]. However, Kahn in 1978 [21] clearly distinguished between a change in the maximal response to a hormone (which he called 'responsiveness') and a shift in the dose-response curve to the right or left (which he called 'sensitivity'), and he provided evidence that the mechanisms underlying the two responses were different. Thus the claim of Dai et al. of hypersensitivity of erythroid progenitors to SCF in PV was not supported by the data. Moreover, the cultures Dai et al. used contained insulin, which would have had the same effect as IGF-I. We have investigated the effect of SCF in strictly serum-free cultures of erythroid progenitor cells from PV patients, but could find no evidence of hypersensitivity to this cytokine. We have also reinvestigated the question of hypersensitivity to megakaryocyte growth and development factor (MGDF)/TPO, to IL-3, and to GM-CSF in PV under strictly serum-free conditions, and could find no evidence of hypersensitivity to any of these cytokines either.

We have not seen hypersensitivity to IGF-I with respect to megakaryocytic (MK) colony formation or GM colony formation in PV (Table 8.3). The progenitor cells in both appeared to be independent of, and insensitive to, IGF-I. Thus the hypersensitivity to IGF-I in PV seems to be restricted to the erythroid lineage.

Why should the emphasis in PV be on the erythroid lineage? A possible answer could be: Because a major characteristic of PV is the pronounced hypersensitivity of erythroid progenitor cells to IGF-I, while there appears to be no hypersensitivity of MK or GM progenitor cells to this growth factor. We are thus left with the conclusion that PV progenitor cells are not hypersensitive to a large number of different cytokines, as was generally believed. They are apparently hypersensitive to one cytokine only, IGF-I, and with a sensitivity up to 20,000 times normal. The molecular mechanism of the specific IGF-I hypersensitivity in PV, however, is still an open question. One wonders whether this bears any relation to the prominent role of IGF-I in normal fetal hematopoiesis [22].

PV was not the first clonal cMPD to show specific hypersensitivity of progenitor cells to a normal endogenous cytokine. Juvenile chronic myelomonocytic leukemia (JMML) is a rare, clonal, fatal pediatric disease, arising at the myeloid stem cell level or earlier. In 1991 Emanuel et al. found that dose-response curves relating GM colony number to concentration of ligand in culture showed hypersensitivity to GM-CSF of around ten times normal, while sensitivities to IL-3 and G-CSF remained unchanged [23].

Table 8.3. Specificity of the IGF-I hypersensitivity in PV with respect to cell lineage

Cell lineage	IGF-I concentration (*M*) at half-maximal colony number		IGF-I sensitivity ratio
	Control	PV	
Erythroid	4.3×10–10	<3.0×10–14	>14,300
Megakaryocytic	1.4×10-8	High and flat [14]	–
Granulocyte/macrophage	Low and flat [14]	High and flat [14]	–

Activation of p21RAS is an essential component of the proliferative response to several hematopoietic growth factors [24], and the GM-CSF hypersensitivity seen in JMML was believed to be a direct consequence of Ras activation in a susceptible myeloid progenitor [25, 26]. This was the first demonstration of a myeloid leukemia in which hypersensitivity to a specific growth factor appeared to be involved in the pathogenesis of the disease.

We have now seen that hematopoietic progenitor cells in two MPDs, JMML and PV, are hypersensitive to the cytokines that control normal progenitor cell proliferation, differentiation, and survival in their respective granulocyte/macrophage and erythroid lineages. Since TPO controls the same functions in the normal megakaryocytic lineage, we sought to determine whether MK progenitor cells in the MPD essential thrombocythemia (ET) are hypersensitive to TPO [14]. PBMNC from patients with ET, or secondary (reactive) thrombocytosis, or healthy volunteers were grown in strictly serum-free agarose culture containing IL-3 and ATRA, with various concentrations of PEG-rHu MGDF, a cytokine closely related to TPO.

We found that the ET MGDF sensitivity curve was shifted to the left of the control curve (Fig. 8.2). The median MGDF sensitivity ratio in ET was about 53 times greater than in controls. Hypersensitivity to PEG-rHu MGDF was arbitrarily defined as a tenfold or more reduction in the concentration of cytokine required for half-maximal MK colony formation. This hypersensitivity, which was also directed to rHu TPO, was

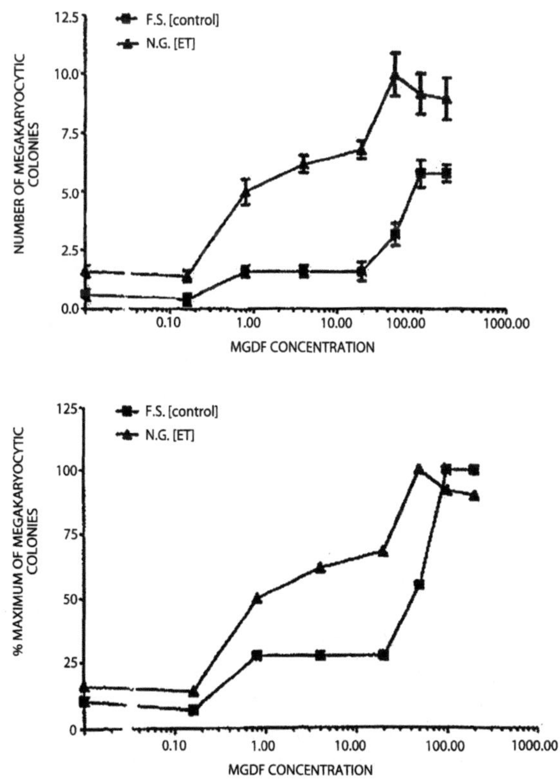

Fig. 8.2. Representative curves of megakaryocytic colony formation by PBMNC from a healthy volunteer (■), and a patient with ET (▲), plotted as a function of PEG-rHu MGDF concentration, in strictly serum-free agarose culture; all cultures also contained ATRA (3×10–8 mol/l) and rHu IL-3 (10 ng/ml). *Left* Number of megakaryocytic colonies produced. *Right* Percentage of maximum number of megakaryocytic colonies produced, both per 4×104 cells per 0.1 ml per well. Sensitivity (concentration of PEG-rHu MGDF at half-maximum colony number): control 50 ng/ml, ET patient 2.3 ng/ml. MGDF sensitivity ratio: control/ET 21.7. Specificity: IL-3 sensitivity ratio 1.8, GM-CSF ratio 1.2 (data not shown). Note left shift of the ET curve as compared with the normal control curve (experiment no. 212)

highly specific with respect to cytokine: cytokine sensitivity ratio (N/ET) for IL-3 + MGDF was 1.1×; for SCF + MGDF it was about 1.5×; for GM-CSF it was 1.3×; but for MGDF + IL-3 it was > 250×. The hypersensitivity was also highly specific with respect to disease: hypersensitivity to PEG-rHu MGDF was found in circulating MK progenitor cells from 18/20 (90%) of informative patients with the presumptive diagnosis of ET, from 1/8 (12.5%) of patients with secondary thrombocytosis, from 0/8 PV patients, and from 0/21 normal individuals. The hypersensitivity was also highly specific with respect to cell lineage: PEG-rHu MGDF, the effect of which on MK colony formation was striking, had no significant effect on GM or erythroid colony formation by normal or ET progenitor cells.

The present study thus brings to three (out of three so far investigated) the number of clonal cMPDs which have in common the property of specific hypersensitivity to a cytokine that is capable of stimulating proliferation, differentiation, and survival of normal progenitors in their respective lineages. It should be noted that in PV [27], JMML [28], and ET [29–31], the levels of endogenous cytokines are usually within the normal range. Thus it is not a high concentration of circulating endogenous cytokine that is responsible for the development of MPDs.

We suggest that a lineage-restricted hypersensitivity of hematopoietic progenitor cells to normal endogenous cytokine may be one mechanism underlying the selective amplification of different progenitor cells in the different myeloproliferative disorders, despite their origin in a single pluripotential stem cell. This notion could also provide an attractive explanation for the unique clinicopathological emphasis seen in each of these clonal disorders if acquisition of the lineage-restricted hypersensitivity to cytokine is brought about amplification of those cells whose progenitors had already become committed to a particular cell lineage.

Again, the molecular mechanisms for these phenomena remain to be worked out. Since in many instances activation of a receptor is associated with activation of the Ras signal transduction pathway, we sought to determine whether in PV or ET there was evidence of activation of the Ras gene. We used an improved method of detecting activation of Ras based on the interaction between Ras-GTP and the Ras binding domain of Raf-1 [32], but found no evidence of Ras activation in PV or ET, while positive controls behaved as expected. It is possible that the failure to activate Ras in PV and ET, although it has been reported to be activated in JMML [25, 26], may be related to the fact that JMML is already a fully developed malignant neoplasm, while the MPDs PV and ET, though sometimes premalignant, are ordinarily not already transformed.

8.4 Idiopathic Myelofibrosis as a Test of the Cytokine Hypersensitivity Hypothesis

We now wished to test our hypothesis that the phenotype in each of the clonal cMPDs depends upon a distinctive lineage-restricted hypersensitivity of progenitor cells to a single normal endogenous cytokine.

Idiopathic myelofibrosis (IMF) is a chronic MPD in which the emphasis is not unilineal; the condition is composed of a clonal extramedullary (splenic) hematopoiesis and a non-clonal bone marrow fibrosis [3], believed to result from inappropriate release from MKs of growth factors that stimulate fibroblast proliferation [33, 34].

Table 8.4. The cytokine hypersensitivity hypothesis

Myeloproliferative disorder	Progenitor cells	Specifically hypersensitive to
PV	Erythroid	IGF-I
JCML/JMML	Granulocyte/macrophage	GM-CSF
ET	Megakaryocytic	MGDF/TPO
IMF	Megakaryocytic	SCF

Since two or more cell lineages (the fibroblast lineage and the MK lineage at least) are involved, this would lead to the prediction that in this disorder there should be hypersensitivity of progenitor cells to more than one lineage-restricted cytokine and/or to a cytokine that is not lineage-restricted but affects more than one cell lineage.

To test this hypothesis, we plated PBMNC from IMF patients and controls in strictly serum-free agarose culture with fixed concentrations of PEG-rHu MGDF and ATRA, and various concentrations of SCF [35] and GM-CSF. At 16–18 days, cultures were harvested, fixed, and stained, and the numbers of MK colonies were scored, normalized, and plotted against the concentration of cytokine. The half-maximum values obtained for SCF were 27 ng/ml for the normal cells, and 0.3 ng/ml for the IMF cells, a SCF sensitivity ratio of about 90 times normal – clear evidence of SCF hypersensitivity. With GM-CSF, in contrast, the half-maximal values were 1.7 ng/ml for the control cells and 0.7 ng/ml for the IMF cells, a GM-CSF sensitivity ratio 2.4 times normal (i.e., below the level at which we consider the cells to be significantly hypersensitive to the cytokine).

Thus, in a MPD that encompasses more than one cell lineage, progenitor cells showed hypersensitivity to a cytokine, SCF [35], that has multilineal proliferation stimulatory activity. This finding provides further evidence in favor of our hypothesis, and is consistent with the notion that the clinicopathological phenotypes of the MPDs are related to, and perhaps determined by, specific hypersensitivities of their progenitor cells to endogenous cytokines (Table 8.4).

8.5 Summary

In the cMPD PV, it has long been clear that erythroid progenitor cells in serum-containing cultures can produce colonies in the absence of added EPO. With dose-response curves in strictly serum-free medium, these progenitor cells have since been shown by us to be not only independent of EPO, but hypersensitive to IGF-I (IGF-I sensitivity ratios up to 20,000 times normal, and specific to IGF-I). In 1991 Emanuel et al. found that GM progenitor cells in juvenile chronic myelogenous/myelomonocytic leukemia (JCML/JMML) were around ten times as sensitive to the cytokine GM-CSF as normal progenitor cells in this lineage, while sensitivities to IL-3 and G-CSF remained unchanged. Since TPO controls the same functions of proliferation, differentiation and survival in the normal MK lineage (as GM-CSF in the GM lineage), we investigated the sensitivity of MK progenitor cells to MGDF (a cytokine closely related to TPO) in ET. Experiments in strictly serum-free agarose cultures showed that MK progenitor cells were hypersensitive to MGDF in 18/20 patients (90%) with ET; median MGDF sensitivity ratios were > 50 times normal. This hypersensitivity, which was also directed to TPO, was highly specific with respect to cytokine, to disease, and to cell lineage. Our results provide compelling evidence that the clinicopathological phenotypes of the clonal cMPDs are related to, and perhaps determined by, specific hypersensitivities of their progenitor cells to individual endogenous cytokines.

References

1. Adamson JW, Fialkow PJ, Murphy S, Prchal JF, Steinmann L (1976) Polycythemia vera: stem cell and probable clonal origin of the disease. N Engl J Med 295:913–916
2. Fialkow PJ, Jacobson RJ, Papayannopoulou T (1977) Chronic myelocytic leukemia: clonal origin in a stem cell common to the granulocyte, erythrocyte, platelet and monocyte/macrophage. Am J Med 63:125–130
3. Jacobson RJ, Salo A, Fialkow PJ (1978) Agnogenic myeloid metaplasia: a clonal proliferation of hematopoietic stem cells with secondary myelofibrosis. Blood 51:189–194
4. Fialkow PJ, Faguet GB, Jacobson RJ, Vaidya K, Murphy S (1981) Evidence that essential thrombocythemia is a clonal disorder with origin in a multipotent stem cell. Blood 58:916–919
5. Busque L, Gilliland DG, Prchal JT, et al (1995) Clonality in juvenile chronic myelogenous leukemia. Blood 85:21–30
6. Adamson JW, Fialkow PJ (1978) Annotation: the pathogenesis of myeloproliferative syndromes. Br J Haematol 38:299–303
7. Croizat H, Amato D, McLeod DL, Eskinazi D, Axelrad AA (1983) Differences among myeloproliferative disorders in the behavior of their restricted progenitor cells in culture. Blood 62:578–584
8. Ogawa M (1984) Annotation: cellular mechanisms of myeloproliferative disorders. Br J Haematol 58:563–565
9. Prchal JF, Axelrad AA (1974) Bone marrow responses in polycythemia vera. N Engl J Med 290:1382
10. Correa PN, Eskinazi D, Axelrad AA (1994) Circulating erythroid progenitors in polycythemia vera are hypersensitive to IGF-I in vitro: studies in an improved serum-free medium. Blood 83:99–112
11. Correa PN, Axelrad AA (1991) Production of erythropoietic bursts by progenitor cells from adult human peripheral blood in an improved serum-free medium: role of IGF-I. Blood 78:2823–2833
12. Fisher MJ, Prchal JF, Prchal JT, D'Andrea AD (1994) Anti-erythropoietin (EPO) receptor monoclonal antibodies distinguish EPO-dependent and EPO-independent erythroid progenitors in polycythemia vera. Blood 84:1982–1991
13. Aron DC (1992) Insulin-like growth factor I and erythropoiesis –mini review. Biofactors 3:211–216
14. Axelrad AA, Eskinazi D, Correa PN, Amato D (2000) Hypersensitivity of circulating progenitor cells to megakaryocyte growth and development factor (PEG-rHu MGDF) in essential thrombocythemia. Blood 96:3310–3321
15. Dai CH, Krantz SB, Green WF, Gilbert HS (1991) Polycythemia vera. III. Burst-forming units-erythroid (BFU-E) response to stem cell factor and c-kit receptor expression. Br J Haematol 86:12–21
16. Martin JM, Gandhi YK, Jackson WR, Dessypris EN (1996) Hypersensitivity of polycythemia vera megakaryocytic progenitors to thrombopoietin. Blood 88 [Suppl 1]:94a
17. Dai CH, Krantz SB, Means RT Jr, Horn ST, Gilbert HS (1991) Polycythemia vera blood burst-forming units-erythroid are hypersensitive to interleukin-3. J Clin Invest 87:391–396
18. Dai CH, Krantz SB, Dessypris EN, Means RT Jr, Horn ST, Gilbert HS (1992) Polycythemia vera. II. Hypersensitivity of bone marrow erythroid granulocyte-macrophage, and megakaryocyte progenitor cells to interleukin-3 and granulocyte-macrophage colony-stimulating factor. Blood 80:891–899
19. Congote LF, Brox A, Lin FK, Lu HS, Fauser AA (1991) The N-terminal sequence of the major erythropoietic factor of an anephric patient is identical to insulin-like growth factor I. J Clin Endocrinol Metab 72:727–729
20. Damen JE, Krosl J, Morrison D, Pelech S, Krystal G (1998) The hyperresponsiveness of cells expressing truncated erythropoietin receptors is contingent on insulin-like growth factor-I in fetal calf serum. Blood 92:425–433
21. Kahn CR (1978) Insulin resistance, insulin insensitivity, and insulin unresponsiveness: a necessary distinction. Metabolism 27 [Suppl 2]:1893–1902
22. Werther GA, Haynes K, Johnson GR (1990) Insulin-like growth factors promote DNA synthesis and support cell viability in fetal hemopoietic tissue by paracrine mechanisms. Growth Factors 3:171–179
23. Emanuel PD, Bates JL, Castleberry RP, Gualtieri RJ, Zuckerman KS (1991) Selective hypersensitivity to granulocyte-macrophage colony-stimulating factor by juvenile chronic myeloid leukemia hematopoietic progenitors. Blood 77:925–929

24. Satoh T, Nakafuku M, Miyajima A, Kaziro Y (1991) Involvement of ras p21 protein in signal-transduction pathways from interleukin 2, interleukin 3, and granulocyte/macrophage colony-stimulating factor, but not from interleukin 4. Proc Natl Acad Sci U S A 88:3314–3318
25. Largaespada DA, Brannan CI, Jenkins NA, Copeland NG (1996) *NF1* deficiency causes Ras-mediated granulocyte/macrophage colony stimulating factor hypersensitivity and chronic myeloid leukemia. Nat Genet 12:137–143
26. Bollag G, Clapp DW, Shih S, et al (1996) Loss of *NF1* results in activation of the Ras signaling pathway and leads to aberrant growth in haematopoietic cells. Nat Genet 12:144–148
27. Mirza AM, Ezzat S, Axelrad AA (1997) Insulin-like growth factor binding protein-1 is elevated in patients with polycythemia vera and stimulates erythroid burst formation in vitro. Blood 89:1862–1869
28. Emanuel PD, Bates LJ, Zhu SW, Castleberry RP, Gualtieri RJ, Zuckerman KS (1991) The role of monocyte-derived hemopoietic growth factors in the regulation of myeloproliferation in juvenile chronic myelogenous leukemia. Exp Hematol 19:1017–1024
29. Harrison CN, Gale RE, Pezella F, Mire-Sluis A, Machin SJ, Linch DC (1999) Platelet c-mpl expression is dysregulated in patients with essential thrombocythemia but this is not of diagnostic value. Br J Haematol 107:139–147
30. Wang JC, Chen C, Nichol J (1996) Serum thrombopoietin (TPO) levels in patients with essential thrombocytosis (ET) and reactive thrombocytosis (RT). Blood 88 [Suppl 1]:212b
31. El-Kassar N, Hetet G, Brière J, Grandchamp B (1998) Clonality analysis of hematopoiesis and thrombopoietin levels in patients with essential thrombocythemia. Leuk Lymphoma 30:181–188
32. Taylor SJ, Shalloway D (1996) Cell cycle-dependent activation of Ras. Curr Biol 6:1621–1627
33. Castro-Malaspina H (1984) Pathogenesis of myelofibrosis: role of ineffective megakaryopoiesis and megakaryocytic components. Prog Clin Biol Res 154:427–454
34. Reilly JT (1998) Pathogenesis and management of idiopathic myelofibrosis. Baillieres Clin Haematol 11:751–767
35. Axelrad AA, Eskinazi D, Amato D (1999) Does hypersensitivity of progenitor cells to normal cytokine(s) play a role in the pathogenesis of idiopathic myelofibrosis with myeloid metaplasia? Blood 94 [Suppl 1]:2886

Role of the Antiapoptotic Protein Bcl-xL in the Pathogenesis of Polycythemia Vera

Jose L. Fernandez-Luna

9.1 Regulation of Apoptosis Within the Erythroid Compartment

Hematopoietic progenitor cell survival is mediated via the interaction of stimulatory and inhibitory hematopoietins (i.e., cytokines, growth factors) and their receptors. Among these, erythropoietin (EPO) is the principal growth factor that promotes the survival of erythroid progenitors. Analysis of mutant mice has clearly established an essential role for EPO and its receptor (EPOR) in erythroid development. In embryos of mice deficient in EPO or the EPOR, definitive erythropoiesis is completely impaired and liver tissue contains increased numbers of nucleated erythroid cells undergoing apoptosis [1]. In addition, in vitro studies show that in the absence of EPO, erythroid progenitors die and their genomic DNA is degraded into oligonucleosomal fragments, a feature of apoptotic cell death [2]. Based on these data, a model has been proposed whereby the concentration of circulating EPO controls the number of erythroid progenitors that survive by inhibiting apoptotic cell death [3]. Although the precise mechanisms by which EPO suppresses apoptosis of erythroid cells remains to be elucidated, several recent publications have thrown some interesting light on this issue.

9.1.1 The Jak2-Stat5 Signaling Pathway Induces Transactivation of the *bcl-xL Gene*

By using a murine erythroid progenitor cell line that requires EPO for proliferation and survival, it has been shown that EPO withdrawal induces downregulation of Bcl-xL at the protein and mRNA levels and the cells undergo apoptosis. Furthermore, enforced expression of a constitutive Bcl-xL protein protects the cells from apoptosis in the absence of EPO; however, endogenous levels of *bcl-xL* are downregulated, suggesting that EPO specifically maintains the expression of *bcl-xL* and that this is an important mechanism to repress apoptosis in erythroid progenitors [4]. But how does EPO connect with Bcl-xL to transduce an antiapoptotic signal? Binding of EPO to its cognate receptor activates Jak2, a member of a subfamily of protein tyrosine kinases, which in turn, converts a latent cytoplasmic transcription factor, Stat5, into its active form by tyrosine phosphorylation. The activated Stat5 dimerizes and translocates into the nucleus, where it binds to specific DNA-response elements of target genes to induce gene transcription [5, 6].

Increasing evidence gives credence to Stat5 as a bona fide antiapoptotic mediator in a number of cell systems [7, 8]. Based on these data, the obvious question is whether EPO can induce the expression of Bcl-xL through Stat5 in erythroid cells.

Recently, an EPO-responsive motif for the binding of a Stat protein has been identified in the untranslated 5' region of the mouse *bcl-x* gene [9]. Furthermore, this consensus sequence specifically binds to Stat5 but not to other Stat family members (i.e., Stat3 or Stat1). In EPO-dependent progenitor cells, the Stat5 binding element found in the *bcl-x* promoter is active in response to EPO, a finding confirmed because mutagenesis of this sequence motif abrogates its promoter activity and overexpression of a dominant negative Stat5 protein blocks transactivation [9]. Stat5 has been also shown to induce the expression of Bcl-xL in hematopoietic progenitor cells in response to other growth factors such as interleukin-3 (IL-3) [10], further confirming that Stat5 act as a mediator of cell survival via transactivation of *bcl-xL*.

These in vitro studies have been confirmed in mice with targeted Stat5 gene disruption [11]. Stat5 knockout embryos are severely anemic and consistently, erythroid progenitors show higher levels of apoptosis and are less responsive to EPO. All these data indicate that EPO-dependent activation of Stat5 is a critical transcriptional pathway to induce the expression of *bcl-xL* and consequently to inhibit apoptosis. However, it remains to be elucidated how the phenotype of adult Stat5 knockout mice demonstrate that the responses to a variety of cytokines, including EPO, are largely unaffected [12]. A likely explanation might be that a different transcriptional activator could account for the expression of *bcl-xL* and survival of erythroid progenitors.

9.1.2
GATA-1 Cooperates with EPO to Stimulate *bcl-xL* Gene Expression

The erythroid factor GATA-1, was initially identified as a zinc-finger-containing nuclear protein that binds to the promoter region of globin genes, but further investigation has revealed the presence of GATA-binding sites in virtually all erythroid-specific genes [13, 14]. Some of these GATA target genes have been linked to regulation of apoptosis; however, none of them can account for the apoptosis of GATA-1-deficient erythroid cells. In fact, mouse embryonic stem cells lacking GATA-1 cannot form mature red blood cells in vivo, which is consistent with the developmental arrest and cell death exhibited by GATA-1-deficient erythroid progenitors [15]. Interestingly, although the EPO receptor is considered a GATA-1 target gene, proerythroblasts deficient in GATA-1 express a normal level of EPO receptor mRNA and protein. Furthermore, the formation of GATA-1-deficient erythroid colonies is EPO-dependent, indicating that the EPO receptor signaling pathway is functionally active in these mutant cells and accounts for the erythroid cell viability. These data suggest that both EPO and GATA-1 may contribute to the inhibition of apoptosis in erythroid progenitors. Consistently, it has been described that GATA-1 strongly induces the expression of *bcl-xL* in erythroid cells, and that EPO cooperates with GATA-1 to stimulate *bcl-xL* gene expression and to maintain erythroid cell viability during terminal differentiation [16].

9.1.3
EPO Can Induce Erythroid Survival Through a Phosphatidylinositol-3-Kinase-Dependent Pathway

Alternative survival pathways of erythroid progenitors include the PI3K-dependent activation of the serine/threonine kinase Akt. In erythroid cell lines, EPO induces phosphorylation of Akt via a PI3K-dependent pathway. Interestingly, when an EPO-independent subclone derived from an erythroid cell line (HCD-57) was analyzed for the activation of antiapoptotic signaling pathways, it was found that both Akt and Stat5 were constitutively active. Treatment with a PI3K inhibitor (LY294002) blocked both constitutive Akt in the resistant clone and EPO-dependent Akt activity in the parental cell line, indicating that PI3K is an upstream activator of Akt [17]. This has been confirmed in another erythroid cell line (UT-7/EPO) in which the EPO-induced phosphorylation of Akt is completely blocked by LY294002. Furthermore, overexpression of the constitutively active form of Akt on UT-7/EPO cells partially inhibits apoptosis induced by EPO deprivation, suggesting that the PI3K-Akt signaling pathway is a mediator of the antiapoptotic activity of EPO [18]. Similar studies have been carried out on primary cultured human erythroid precursors, where treatment with LY294002 induced apoptosis of erythroid progenitor cells and accelerated apoptosis induced by EPO withdrawal [19]. All these findings suggest that PI3K-Akt signaling is important for the survival of erythroid cells, and that it may cooperate with other survival pathways (i.e., Stats) to maintain the viability of erythroid progenitors.

9.2 Pathogenesis of Polycythemia Vera

A number of studies suggest that chromosomal abnormalities, which have long been known to be associated with PV, may be somehow responsible for the polycythemia vera (PV) phenotype [20]. However, structural chromosomal alterations are seen in about 15% of patients with PV at diagnosis, which indicates that the genetic changes responsible for the pathogenesis of PV are likely to be due to DNA mutations which cannot be detected by cytogenetic methods but by DNA sequence analysis.

Because analysis of mutant mice has established an essential role for EPO and its receptor in the development of erythroid progenitors in vivo [1], an attractive hypothesis is that an activating mutation in the EPO receptor gene may render erythroid cells EPO-independent for proliferation and survival. However, despite some encouraging results obtained with cell lines that expressed mutated EPO receptors, mutations in the EPO receptor gene have not been detected in PV [21].

Several authors have reported that both peripheral blood mononuclear cells and purified erythroid burst-forming units (BFU-E) progenitors obtained from patients with PV are hypersensitive to human IL-3, GM-CSF, and stem cell factor [22–24]. In addition, it has been shown that the PV progenitor cells have a markedly increased sensitivity to insulin-like growth factor (IGF-I), which is able to stimulate erythroid colony formation [25]. In the absence of exogenous IGF-I, there is a basal level of tyrosine phosphorylation of the IGF-I receptor much greater in PV than in normal peripheral blood mononuclear cells [26]. Furthermore, the circulating levels of IGF-I-BP, a binding protein that regulates the availability and activity of IGF-I, are more than four times higher in PV patients than in normal controls [27]. Thus, the increased sensitivity of PV erythroid progenitors to IGF-I provide an attractive mechanism to account for the EPO-independent survival of these cells.

9.2.1
Expression of Bcl-xL Is Deregulated in PV Erythroid Progenitors

That erythroid colonies from PV patients can survive and undergo maturation in vitro in the absence of EPO suggests that the antiapoptotic pathways usually activated via binding of EPO to its cognate receptor may be either constitutively active or induced by other growth factors. Interestingly, transfection of the human *bcl-2* gene into an IL-3-dependent, multipotent hematopoietic cell line allows these cells to survive in the absence of IL-3, both in serum-containing and serum-deprived conditions, and this survival is accompanied by multilineage differentiation [28], which suggests that a deregulated expression of an antiapoptotic protein could give rise to aberrant growth factor-independent hematopoietic progenitors.

Unlike normal erythroid colony-forming units (CFU-E), which require EPO to survive, a population of CFU-E in patients with PV can grow in the absence of EPO. These EPO-independent cells become the dominant population of erythroid progenitors as the disease progresses. But how do the CFU-E from PV patients escape apoptosis? This question has been partly answered with the finding that the EPO-independent erythroid cells express high levels of Bcl-xL when cultured in the absence of EPO (see Fig. 9.1), and that the expression of Bcl-xL in bone marrow erythroid cells is significantly higher in patients with untreated PV than in those with other myeloproliferative disorders or secondary erythrocytosis [29]. These findings are consistent with those obtained in a mouse erythroblast cell line in which the constitutive expression of Bcl-xL maintained cell survival in the absence of EPO [4].

If a deregulated expression of Bcl-xL may contribute to the EPO-independent survival of erythroid-lineage cells in PV, it is likely that an upstream mediator of the pathway that leads to the transcription of *bcl-xL* may be altered in PV progenitors. Since Stat5 transactivates the *bcl-x* gene in erythroid progenitors, a constitutively active Stat5 could be an attractive candidate to account for the EPO-independent expression of Bcl-xL. Although this hypothesis still awaits experimental confirmation, recent data obtained in platelets from PV patients show that neither Jak2 nor Stat5 are constitutively active in platelets [30]. Furthermore, it has been found that platelets do not express the thrombopoietin receptor, which explains the lack of Stat5

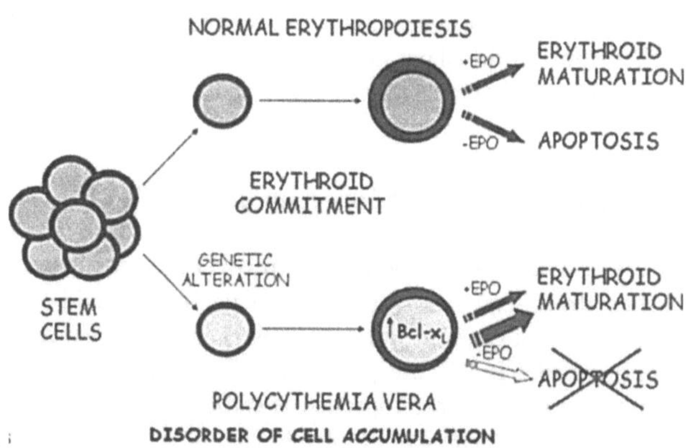

Fig. 9.1. Deregulated expression of Bcl-xL in erythroid cells from PV patients

activation in response to thrombopoietin. However, it is likely that an increased sensitivity of PV erythroid progenitors to a growth factor may account for the activation of Stat5 or other antiapoptotic signaling molecules.

As described above, IGF-I could be a likely candidate to explain how erythroid progenitors survive in the absence of EPO. To this end, although Stat5 does not seem to be activated by IGF-I, another member of the same family of transcription factors, Stat3 is activated by binding of IGF-I to its receptor, and this activation is mediated by Jak1 and Jak2 tyrosine kinases [31]. Consistent with this, Stat3 induces the expression of Bcl-xL and protects against apoptosis [32].

9.2.2 Other Pathways Likely to Be Involved in PV Erythroid Cell Survival

A number of growth factors, including IGF-I, trigger antiapoptotic pathways that are mediated by PI3K. An indirect target of PI3K is the serine-threonine Akt kinase that phosphorylates the proapoptotic protein Bad, preventing its binding to Bcl-xL and consequently enabling the cell to avoid apoptosis [33]. Thus, Bad phosphorylation by Akt in response to a growth factor or to a deregulated activation of this PI3K-dependent pathway could be a mechanism to deliver survival signals in PV erythroid cells. In addition, in platelet-derived growth factor (PDGF) signaling, NF-κB is a target of Akt [34]. NF-κB, which is known to inhibit apoptosis, is retained in the cytoplasm of unstimulated cells through an interaction with inhibitory proteins known as IκB. Following treatment with growth factors (epidermal growth factor, PDGF, and others), I-κB is phosphorylated by IKK (a kinase) and degraded by the proteasome, which causes the translocation of NF-κB to the nucleus and transcription of target genes.

It has been reported that upon PDGF stimulation, Akt transiently associates in vivo with IKK and induces IKK activation, causing the release of NF-κB to exert its antiapoptotic activity [34]. To this end, it has been recently established that NF-κB induces the expression of Bcl-xL through direct binding to a consensus sequence found in the bcl-x promoter [35]. Furthermore, an association of Akt, NF-κB and Bcl-xL has been provided in transgenic mice expressing a constitutively active form of Akt [36]. In this in vivo model, T lymphocytes overexpressing the transgene displayed elevated levels of Bcl-xL and enhanced NF-κB activation. Based on these findings, the growth factor-dependent activation of the PI3K-Akt-NF-κB pathway provides an attractive mechanism to account, either by itself or in combination with other transcriptional pathways (i.e., Jak2-Stats), for the EPO-independent expression of Bcl-xL in PV erythroid progenitor cells.

9.3 Future Research on the Molecular Basis of PV

More research needs to be done to uncover the genetic basis of PV. The recently published draft sequence of the human genome should help in achieving this goal. Sequencing of genomic libraries constructed from PV cells would detect the genetic abnormalities in PV, but given the effort and cost required to cover most of the genome, this technical approach is difficult to apply at present. In addition, other interesting strategies can be used to characterize the molecular defect leading to the development of PV. By using a subtractive hybridization technique to isolate cDNAs differentially expressed in PV patients versus normal controls, a new gene named PRV-1 that is highly expressed in PV granulocytes but undetectable in normal granulocytes, has been described [37], which opens a new line of investigation in the pathogenesis of PV. New large-scale screening strategies such as DNA microarray will also help establish a molecular fingerprint of PV cells and eventually identify differentially expressed genes able to explain the molecular basis of PV [38].

9.4 Summary

PV is a clonal disorder that arises from acquired genetic alterations in a hematopoietic stem cell. This disease is characterized by an increase in the number of erythroid cells, although elevated cell numbers in the myeloid and megakaryocyte lineages are also observed in PV patients. Furthermore, a significant number of patients develop acute myelogenous leukemia. In vitro studies have shown that PV progenitor cells are hypersensitive to a number of hematopoietic growth factors, and different alterations in signaling molecules have been reported. Among them, apoptosis inhibitors could contribute to the abnormal survival of progenitor cells and the acquisition of secondary genetic alterations that induce the leukemic transformation of PV progenitors. However, the molecular mechanisms leading to the transformation of a primitive stem cell and the multiple alterations shown in PV progenitor cells are still poorly understood.

References

1. Wu H, Liu X, Jaenisch R, Lodish HF (1995) Generation of committed erythroid BFU-E and CFU-E progenitors does not require erythropoietin or the erythropoietin receptor. Cell 83:59–67
2. Koury MJ, Bondurant MC (1990) Erythropoietin retards DNA breakdown and prevents programmed death in erythroid progenitor cells. Science 24:378–381
3. Koury MJ, Bondurant MC (1990) Control of red cell production: the roles of programmed cell death (apoptosis) and erythropoietin. Transfusion 30:673–674
4. Silva M, Grillot D, Benito A, Richard C, Nuñez G, Fernandez-Luna JL (1996) Erythropoietin can promote erythroid progenitor survival by repressing apoptosis through Bcl-xL and Bcl-2. Blood 88:1576–1582
5. Darnell JE, Kerr IM, Stark GM (1994) Jak-Stat pathways and transcriptional activation in response to IFNs and other extracellular signaling proteins. Science 264:1415–1421
6. Ihle JN (1996) Stats: signal transducers and activators of transcription. Cell 84:331–334
7. Zamorano J, Wang HY, Wang R, Shi Y, Longmore GD, Keegan AD (1998) Regulation of cell growth by IL-2: role of Stat5 in protection from apoptosis but not in cell cycle progression. J Immunol 160:3502–3512
8. Rui H, Xu J, Mehta S, Fang H, Williams J, Dong F, Grimley PM (1998) Activation of the Jak2-Stat5 signaling pathway in Nb2 lymphoma cells by an anti-apoptotic agent, aurintricarboxylic acid. J Biol Chem 273:28–32
9. Silva M, Benito A, Sanz C, Prosper F, Ekhterae D, Nuñez G, Fernandez-Luna JL (1999) Erythropoietin can induce the expression of Bcl-xL through Stat5 in erythropoietin-dependent progenitor cell lines. J Biol Chem 274:22165–22169
10. Dumon S, Santos SC, Debierre-grockiego F, Gouilleux-Gruart V, Cocault L, Boucheron C, Mollat P, Gisselbrecht S, Gouilleux F (1999) IL-3 dependent regulation of Bcl-xL gene expression by Stat5 in a bone marrow derived cell line. Oncogene 18:4191–4199
11. Socolovsky M, Fallon A, Wang S, Brugnara C, Lodish HF (1999) Fetal anemia and apoptosis of red cell progenitors in Stat5a-/-5b-/- mice: a direct role for Stat5 in Bcl-xL induction. Cell 98:181–191

12. Teglund S, McKay C, Schuetz E, van Deursen JM, Stravopodis D, Wang D, Brown M, Bodner S, Grosveld G, Ihle JN (1998) Stat5a and Stat5b proteins have essential and nonessential, or redundant, roles in cytokine response. Cell 93:841–850
13. Orkin SH (1992) GATA-binding transcription factors in hematopoietic cells. Blood 80:575–581
14. Weiss MJ, Orkin SH (1995) GATA transcription factors: key regulators of hematopoiesis. Exp Hematol 23:99–107
15. Weiss MJ, Orkin SH (1995) Transcription factor GATA-1 permits survival and maturation of erythroid precursors by preventing apoptosis. Proc Natl Acad Sci U S A 92:9623–9627
16. Gregory T, Yu C, Ma A, Orkin SH, Blobel GA, Weiss MJ (1999) GATA-1 and erythropoietin cooperate to promote erythroid cell survival by regulating bcl-xL expression. Blood 94:87–96
17. Bao H, Jacobs-Helber SM, Lawson AE, Penta K, Wickrema A, Sawyer ST (1999) Protein kinase B (c-Akt), phosphatidylinositol 3-kinase, and Stat5 are activated by erythropoietin (EPO) in HCD57 erythroid cells but are constitutively active in an EPO-independent, apoptosis-resistant subclone (HCD57-SREI cells). Blood 93:3757–3773
18. Kashii Y, Uchida M, Kirito K, Tanaka M, Nishijima K, Toshima M, Ando T, Koizumi K, Endoh T, Sawada K, Momoi M, Miura Y, Ozawa K, Komatsu N (2000) A member of forkhead family transcription factor, FKHRL1, is one of the downstream molecules of phosphatidylinositol 3-kinase-Akt activation pathway in erythropoietin signal transduction. Blood 96:941–949
19. Haseyama Y, Sawada K, Oda A, Koizumi K, Takano H, Tarumi T, Nishio M, Handa M, Ikeda Y, Koike T (1999) Phosphatidylinositol 3-kinase is involved in the protection of primary cultured human erythroid precursor cells from apoptosis. Blood 94:1568–1577
20. Chen Z, Notohamiprodjo M, Guan XY, Paietta E, Blackwell S, Stout K, Turner A, Richkind K, Trent JM, Lamb A, Sandberg AA (1998) Gain of 9p in the pathogenesis of polycythemia vera. Genes Chromosomes Cancer 22:321–324
21. Le Couedic JP, Mitjavila MT, Villeval JL (1996) Missense mutation of the erythropoietin receptor is a rare event in human erythroid malignancies. Blood 87:1502–1511
22. de Wolf JT, Beentjes JA, Esselink MT, Smit JW, Halie RH, Clark SC, Vellenga E (1989) In polycythemia vera human IL-3 and GM-CSF enhance erythroid colony growth in the absence of erythropoietin. Exp Hematol 17:981–983
23. Dai CH, Krantz SB, Dessypris EN, Means RT, Horn ST, Gilbert HS (1992) Polycythemia vera. II. Hypersensitivity of bone marrow erythroid, granulocyte-macrophage, and megakaryocyte progenitor cells to IL-3 and GM-CSF. Blood 80:891–899
24. Dai CH, Krantz SB, Green WF, Gilbert HS (1994) Polycythemia vera. III. Burst-forming units-erythroid (BFU-E) response to SCF and c-kit receptor expression. Br J Haematol 86:12–21
25. Correa PN, Eskinazi D, Axelrad AA (1994) Circulating erythroid progenitors in polycythemia vera are hypersensitive to insulin-like growth factor-I in vitro: studies in an improved serum-free medium. Blood 83:99–112
26. Mirza AM, Correa PN, Axelrad AA (1995) Increased basal and induced tyrosine phosphorylation of the insulin-like growth factor I receptor beta subunit in circulating mononuclear cells of patients with polycythemia vera. Blood 86:877–882
27. Mirza AM, Ezzat S, Axelrad AA (1997) Insulin-like growth factor binding protein-1 is elevated in patients with polycythemia vera and stimulates erythroid burst formation in vitro. Blood 89:1862–1869
28. Fairbairn LJ, Cowling GJ, Reipert BM, Dexter TM (1993) Suppression of apoptosis allows differentiation and development of a multipotent hematopoietic cell line in the absence of added growth factors. Cell 74:823–832
29. Silva M, Richard C, Benito A, Sanz C, Olalla I, Fernandez-Luna JL (1998) Expression of Bcl-x in erythroid precursors from patients with polycythemia vera. N Engl J Med 338:564–571
30. Moliterno AR, Hankins WD, Spivak JL (1998) Impaired expression of the thrombopoietin receptor by platelets from patients with polycythemia vera. N Engl J Med 338:572–580
31. Zong CS, Chan J, Levy DE, Horvath C, Sadowski HB, Wang LH (2000) Mechanism of Stat3 activation by insulin-like growth factor I receptor. J Biol Chem 275:15099–15105
32. Catlett-Falcone R, Landowski TH, Oshiro MM, Turkson J, Levitzki A, Savino R, Ciliberto G, Moscinski L, Fernandez-Luna JL, Nuñez G, Dalton WS, Jove R (1999) Constitutive activation of Stat3 signaling confers resistance to apoptosis in human U266 myeloma cells. Immunity 10:105–115
33. del Peso L, Gonzalez-Garcia M, Page C, Herrera R, Nuñez G (1997) Interleukin-3-induced phosphorylation of BAD through the protein kinase Akt. Science 278:687–689
34. Romashkova JA, Makarov SS (1999) NF-kappaB is a target of Akt in anti-apoptotic PDGF signalling. Nature 401:86–90
35. Chen C, Edelstein LC, Gelinas C (2000) The Rel/NF-kappaB family directly activates expression of the apoptosis inhibitor Bcl-xL. Mol Cell Biol 20:2687–2695

36. Jones RG, Parsons M, Bonnard M, Chan VS, Yeh WC, Woodgett JR, Ohashi PS (2000) Protein kinase B regulates T lymphocyte survival, nuclear factor kappaB activation, and Bcl-xL levels in vivo. J Exp Med 191:1721–1734
37. Temerinac S, Klippel S, Strunck E, Roder S, Lubbert M, Lange W, Azemar M, Meinhardt G, Schaefer HE, Pahl HL (2000) Cloning of PRV-1, a novel member of the uPAR receptor superfamily, which is overexpressed in polycythemia rubra vera. Blood 95:2569–2576
38. Pellagatti A, Vetrie D, Langford CF, Gama S, Eagleton H, Wainscoat JS, Boultwood J (2003) Gene expression profiling in polycythemia vera using cDNA microarray technology. Cancer Res 53: 3940–3944

Chapter 10

Involvement of Chromosome 9 and 11 in Familial and Sporadic Polycythemia Vera

Robert Kralovics

10.1 Introduction

Myeloproliferative disorders are acquired clonal diseases involving the pluripotent stem cell. The somatic mutations in myeloproliferative disorders lead to clonal expansion of the myeloid lineages with typically one lineage dominating in each type of myeloproliferative disorder. In polycythemia vera (PV), the expansion of the erythroid lineage results in a high erythrocyte mass, although thrombocythemia, high neutrophil counts, and splenomegaly are also present in a significant proportion of PV patients. The molecular lesion responsible for the PV disease phenotype is unknown. Clonality studies performed using G6PD isoenzyme expression demonstrated that PV is an acquired defect of the pluripotent stem cell [1]. The stem cell acquiring the PV mutation expands and subsequently, the terminally differentiated myeloid cells are all (or virtually all) derived from the PV stem cell clone. The contribution of the normal stem cell population to the production of circulating myeloid cells may in some patients become undetectable using sensitive clonality assays based on X chromosome inactivation. B lymphocytes are often derived from the PV stem cell clone but T lymphocytes are always polyclonal, i.e., derived from the non-PV clone, in all subjects studied [2]. Cytogenetic lesions are present in about 14% of PV patients at diagnosis but none of these lesions is specific for PV and all are shared among myeloproliferative disorders [3]. The most common cytogenetic abnormalities (present in about 8% of PV patients) are deletions involving chromosome 20q. Trisomies 1, 8, 9, and deletions on chromosomes 13q and 5q occur less frequently (0.5–3% of PV patients) [4].

Abnormal hematopoietic progenitor cell responses to cytokines have been consistently demonstrated in PV. The erythroid progenitors in PV exhibit colony formation independent of erythropoietin (EPO) in the absence of exogenous EPO in serum-containing cultures [5, 6]. In serum-free culture systems, hypersensitivity to other cytokines has also been reported. The abnormal responsiveness of PV progenitors to cytokines has promoted a number of studies focusing on cytokine receptor signaling and cytokine-dependent survival of PV progenitor cells. Quantitative abnormalities have been described in PV myeloid cells such as elevated phosphatase activity in erythroid progenitors [7], decreased SHP-1 phosphatase expression in PV erythroid cells [8], decreased thrombopoietin receptor expression in PV platelets [9], and increased expression of Bcl-xL in PV erythroid cells [10]. Changes in transcriptional regulation of the PRV-1 [11] and the CDKN2A [12] genes have also been observed in PV granulocytes, and cultured erythroid cells, respectively.

Our clinical and genetic studies of six families with PV have suggested that loss of heterozygosity (LOH) might play a role in PV pathogenesis [13]. To identify mutations of genes (or genomic regions) that cause the PV phenotype, we screened the whole genome for LOH without the bias of previously characterized cytogenetic lesions observed in myeloproliferative disorders. In this study, we identified two new genomic loci that undergo changes in the PV stem cells.

10.2 Results

10.2.1 Genome-wide Screening for LOH

To identify genomic regions with LOH, we compared DNA isolated from clonal granulocytes and polyclonal T cells or skin fibroblasts. Six subjects with PV had undergone the entire genome-wide LOH screening (two of these subjects had familial history of PV). We analyzed 382 autosomal microsatellite markers per DNA sample to cover the genome at 10 cM density. We identified LOH on the short arm of chromosome 9, and on the long arm of chromosome 11 (Fig. 10.1). The sizes of the LOH regions were about 40 cM on 9p, and about 70 cM on 11q. To estimate the frequency of LOH in these regions, we screened a total of 25 subjects with PV and 6 subjects with clonal essential thrombocythemia (ET). The 9pLOH was present in 3 of 10 sporadic subjects (33%) and 2 of 15 familial PV subjects and was not detected in any of the clonal ET subjects. The 11q LOH was observed only in one familial PV subject (the subject also had an LOH on chromosome 9p), and not in any clonal ET subject. The 11q LOH was found in a subject who also had a LOH on chromosome 9p.

10.2.2 Stem Cell Origin of LOH

Pluripotent stem cell defects are defined as acquired mutations occurring in a cell that gives rise to both myeloid and lymphoid progeny. To demonstrate that the LOH on chromosomes 9p, and 11q are stem cell lesions, we analyzed the presence of LOH

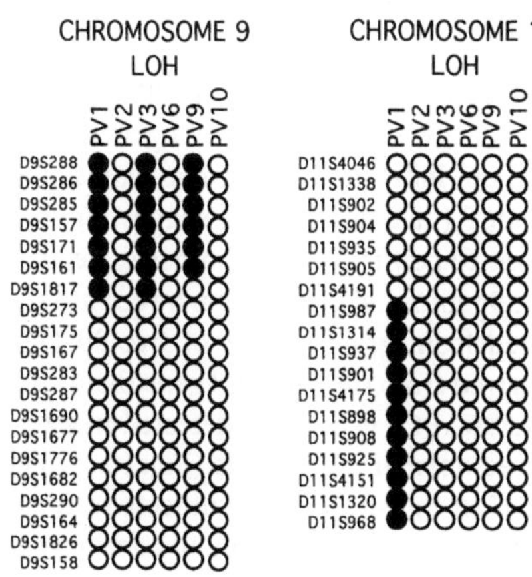

Fig. 10.1. Genome-wide screening for LOH in six PV subjects. The chromosomal regions involved in LOH were detected and are shown in *black* (uninformative markers are not shown)

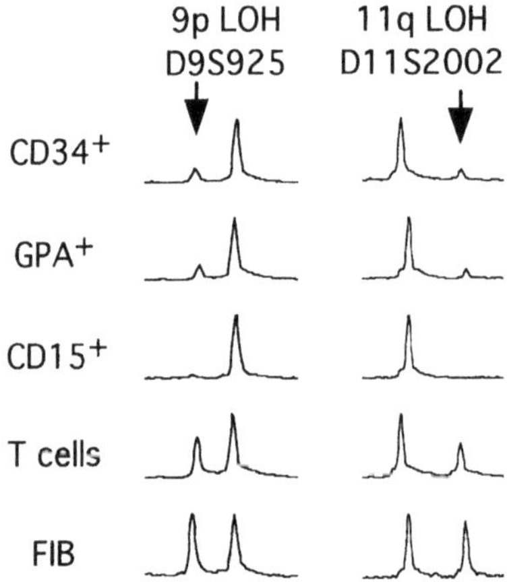

Fig. 10.2. Stem cell origin of LOH. The presence of the 9p and 11q LOH was studied in isolated populations of myeloid and lymphoid cells (*CD34+* early hematopoietic progenitors, *GPA+* glycophorin A+ erythroid cells, *CD15+* granulocytes, *T cells* T lymphocytes, *FIB* fibroblasts). The LOH is detectable in both myeloid cells and in a proportion of T lymphocytes, indicating that the LOH originated in the pluripotent stem cell. The allele involved in the LOH is indicated by *arrows*

in both myeloid and lymphoid cells of PV subjects. As shown in Fig. 10.2, the LOH is detectable in the myeloid lineages as well as in about 30% of T lymphocytes. This finding indicates that the LOH detected on 9p and 11q are clonal stem cell lesions. In addition to clonality analysis using LOH, we also analyzed the clonality of the same cell isolates using X-chromosome inactivation pattern assay. We found no significant differences between clonality data obtained by LOH analysis and by X-chromosome inactivation pattern analysis (data not shown). These data demonstrate that virtually all clonally derived cells are positive for the presence of LOH. Interestingly, in the subject positive for both 9p and 11q LOH we observed about 15% of CD34+ early hematopoietic progenitor cells that were not clonal (i.e., not derived from the PV stem cell clone) in either of the LOH assays or in the IDS clonality assay. This may be due to lymphoid contamination of the CD34+ cell isolate or due to a small population of normal polyclonal CD34+ cells without LOH in this subject. CD15+ granulocytes isolated to homogeneity were 100% clonal and all were positive for the LOH.

10.2.3
The LOH on Chromosome 9p Is Due to Mitotic Recombination

Since the 9p LOH occurred with highest frequency, we focused our studies primarily on this genomic region. Cytogenetic studies of the subjects with detectable 9p LOH did not indicate any terminal losses or deletions of the entire short arm of chromosome 9 (data not shown), suggesting that the LOH may be due to mitotic recombination. To confirm this hypothesis, we analyzed the copy number of genes mapping to the 9p minimal LOH region by quantitative genomic hybridization. DNA samples isolated from granulocytes of five 9p LOH+ subjects were hybridized with a probe derived from the SNAPC3 gene that is localized within the LOH region. Two copies of the SNAPC3 gene were detected in all five analyzed 9p LOH+ subjects as well as in three normal individuals (Fig. 10.3). These results indicate that the presence of 9p LOH in the studied PV subjects resulted from mitotic recombination events rather than interstitial or terminal deletions, in which case, only a single copy of the gene

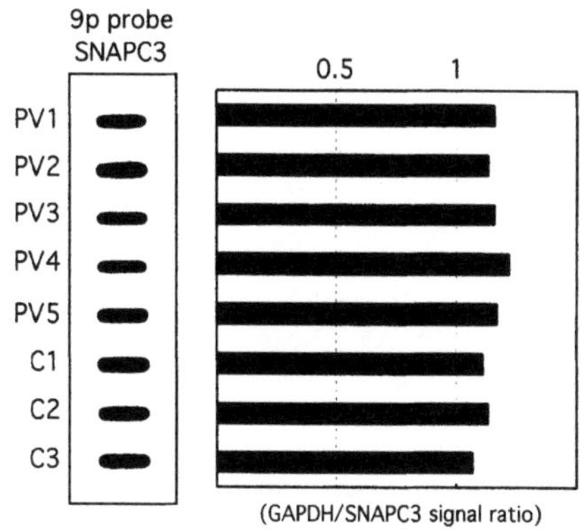

Fig. 10.3. Detection of mitotic recombination on chromosome 9p. Genomic hybridization of granulocyte DNA of five 9p LOH+ PV subjects and three normal controls with a probe derived from the 9p LOH region (SNAPC3 gene). The SNAPC3 hybridization signal was normalized against the hybridization signal obtained using the GAPDH control probe. The hybridization intensity of PV samples did not differ from the control DNA samples, suggesting that no loss of chromosomal material was present within the 9p LOH region. This finding indicates that LOH on chromosome 9p is due to mitotic recombination and is not a result of deletions

would be present. The LOH mechanism by mitotic recombination is further supported by the presence of LOH extending to the 9p telomere in all the analyzed subjects.

10.2.4 The PV Phenotype Is Not Linked to Any of the Previously Proposed Candidate PV Loci

We have previously described six families with PV (Fig. 10.4). The phenotype of all the affected family members was identical to sporadic PV including clonal hematopoiesis and EPO-independent erythroid colony formation. Four out of the six families (A–D) were used for linkage analysis since these consisted of at least two affected siblings. For these pedigrees, we calculated the power of linkage analysis using Monte-Carlo simulation assuming an autosomal dominant, rare, monogenic homo-

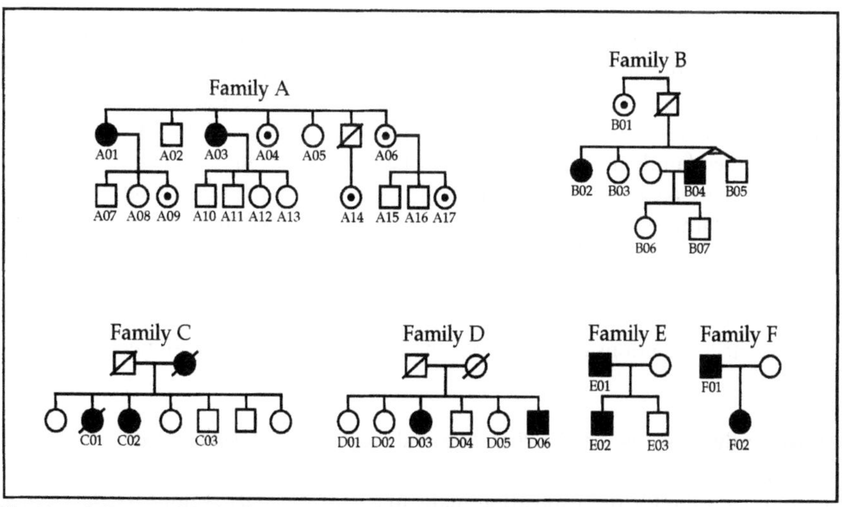

Fig. 10.4. Pedigrees of the PV families. Subjects with full PV phenotype are in *black*. Subjects with EPO-independent colony formation but otherwise normal phenotype are indicated with a *dot*

Table 10.1. Lod scores calculated for markers closely linked to the proposed candidate PV genes. Markers with a lod score below –2.0 exclude linkage (*CDR common deleted region*)

		0,001	0,01	0,05	0,1	0,2	0,3	0,4	Theta
Locus	Marker	0,1	1,0	5,0	10,0	21,0	34,0	55,0	Distance (cM)
EPO receptor		-3,16	-2,13	-1,30	-0,87	-0,41	-0,16	-0,04	
MPL		-2,24	-1,25	-0,57	-0,31	-0,10	-0,02	0,00	
20q CDR	D20S96	-2,03	-1,03	-0,36	-0,11	0,05	0,06	0,03	
20q CDR	D20S861	-4,40	-2,40	-1,03	-0,49	-0,10	0,01	0,01	
13q CDR	D13S153	-4,79	-2,78	-1,35	-0,75	-0,26	-0,08	-0,02	
5q CDR	D5S2077	-6,27	-4,20	-2,53	-1,67	-0,77	-0,30	-0,07	

zygous etiology with 70% penetrance. When only the subjects with the full PV phenotype were considered, the predicted lod scores were 2.43 ± 0.085 (max 4.4) at ζ (ζ the recombination value between simulated test locus and the gene)$=0$ and 159 ± 0.092 (max 3.7) at $\zeta=0$. When subjects positive for the EPO-independent erythroid colony assay were included as affected, the power of the analysis increased and the predicted lod scores were 2.98 ± 0.11 (max 5.2) at $\zeta=0$ and 1.97 ± 0.11 (max 4.7) at $\zeta=0.05$.

The involvement of the common deleted regions on chromosomes 20q, 13q, 5q and the c-mpl and EPO receptor genes have been proposed in the pathogenesis of myeloproliferative disorders including PV. We performed linkage analysis using microsatellite markers mapping to these loci. Only the affected subjects with the full PV phenotype were considered "affected" in the linkage analysis. Using lod scores below –2.0 to satisfy the criteria for exclusion of linkage, the linkage between the PV phenotype and the tested candidate PV loci were excluded (Table 10.1). When subjects positive for the EPO-independent erythroid colony assay were also considered as affected, the lod scores further decreased (data not shown).

10.2.5 Detailed Analysis of the Thrombopoietin Receptor Gene

The combined linkage analysis of families A, B, C and D (assuming genetic homogeneity) excluded the linkage between the PV phenotype and the c-mpl gene (lod score –2.24 and lod score –3.20 when subjects positive for the EPO-independent erythroid colony assay were included). Comparison of the segregation of the c-mpl gene alleles in the affected family members indicated that the affected subjects in families A and B did not share a common c-mpl gene allele (consistent with exclusion of linkage). However, in families C and D, the affected subjects shared a c-mpl gene allele that cannot conclusively exclude the c-mpl gene in these families. Therefore, we performed sequence analysis of the 12 c-mpl gene exons in the index subjects in families C and D and also in the families that were not included in the linkage studies (E and F). We did not detect mutations of the c-mpl gene in any of the analyzed subjects.

10.2.6 Linkage Analysis Between the PV Phenotype and the 9p and 11q LOH Regions

To examine if the PV predisposition maps to any of the LOH regions we performed linkage analysis using markers spanning the 9p and the 11q LOH. As shown in

Table 10.2. Lod scores calculated for markers spanning the 9p and 11q LOH regions. Markers with a lod score below -2.0 exclude linkage

Chromosome	Map position (cM)	Marker	0,001 0,1	0,01 1,0	0,05 5,0	0,1 10,0	0,2 21,0	0,3 34,0	0,4 55,0	Theta Distance (cM)
9	0	D9S288	-7,41	-4,40	-2,25	-1,34	-0,53	-0,19	-0,04	
	20,4	D9S285	-2,90	-1,80	-0,79	-0,36	-0,03	0,05	0,03	
	24,3	D9S157	-4,34	-2,35	-0,97	-0,42	0,01	0,12	0,07	
	33,4	D9S171	-3,68	-1,71	-0,46	-0,05	0,16	0,12	0,03	
	40,5	D9S161	-2,58	-1,55	-0,75	-0,41	-0,13	-0,04	-0,01	
	47,5	D9S1817	-4,83	-2,82	-1,40	-0,80	-0,29	-0,09	-0,02	
	54,7	D9S273	-4,83	-2,79	-1,20	-0,56	-0,09	0.04	0,04	
11	58	D11S41911	- 4,33	-2,32	-0,90	-0,34	0,07	0,13	0,05	
	64,3	D11S987	- 3,36	-2,31	-1,40	-0,91	-0,39	-0,14	-0,03	
	71,7	D11S1314	- 4,11	-2,13	-0,80	-0,31	0,01	0,05	0,01	
	78,6	D11S901	- 2,75	-1,74	-0,93	-0,51	-0,13	-0,01	0,00	
	90,5	D11S4175	- 1,46	-0,49	0,10	0,25	0,25	0,14	0,04	
	96,8	D11S898	- 1,68	-0,70	-0,05	0,17	0,25	0,17	0,05	
	106,3	D11S908	- 2,60	-1,55	-0.64	-0,23	0,08	0,13	0,08	
	112,2	D11S4195	- 8,56	-5,12	-2,41	-1,32	-0,41	-0,06	0,04	
	115,1	D11S4132	-10,76	-6,34	-3,00	-1,70	-0,62	-0,20	-0,04	
	117,3	D11S925	0,19	0,26	0,42	0,48	0,41	0,24	0,06	
	117,4	D11S4107	- 4,06	-2,98	-1,82	-1,11	-0,44	-0,16	-0,05	
	119,6	D11S1336	- 6,86	-3,89	-1,89	-1,11	-0,45	-0,17	-0,04	
	126,7	D11S4151	- 2,63	-1,62	-0,87	-0,53	-0,21	-0,08	-0,02	
	138,6	D11S1320	- 3,87	-2,33	-0,98	-0,44	-0,04	0,05	0,03	
	146,6	D11S968	- 4,31	-2,32	-0,96	-0,43	-0,04	0,04	0,02	

Table 10.2, the PV predisposition does not link to these loci. The calculated lod scores for most of the markers were below –2.0 that excludes linkage although some markers on chromosome 11 could not be excluded.

10.3 Conclusions

Excessive clonal expansion is the major phenotypic feature of the PV stem cell clone. To characterize genomic regions associated with this stem cell behavior, we screened the entire genome for LOH at high resolution using microsatellite analysis. We identified two genomic loci involved in LOH on chromosomes 9p and 11q. The LOH on chromosome 9p occurred with the highest frequency. We suspected mitotic recombination as the cause of LOH on chromosome 9p because (1) cytogenetic studies of the PV subjects with the 9p LOH did not reveal any losses of 9p, and (2) the chromosomal region involved in LOH extended to the 9p telomere. Therefore, we examined the number of 9p copies in five 9p LOH+ subjects and found no detectable losses of chromosomal material indicating that mitotic recombination is the mechanism of LOH in all the analyzed subjects. As a consequence, uniparental disomy is present in these subjects involving the entire short arm of chromosome 9. Unfortunately, none of the parents of the 9p LOH+ subjects were available for the analysis of parental origin of the disomic chromosomes. The 9p LOH due to mitotic recombination in PV is not detectable by cytogenetic analysis, fluorescent in-situ hybridization, or comparative genomic hybridization.

We characterized six families with multiple members diagnosed with PV. Four of these families were suitable for genetic linkage analysis. We examined the previously proposed PV locus candidates as well as the LOH regions identified in this study. None of the loci exhibited linkage with the familial PV predisposition. These data suggest that the genetic abnormalities including 20q, 13q and 5q deletions as well as LOH on chromosomes 9p and 11q are most likely secondary genetic changes. They might play a role in either providing clonal growth advantage to the PV stem cell clone or progression to leukemia. Our data also demonstrate the usefulness of genetic approaches to study myeloproliferative disorders.

10.4 Summary

Familial clustering of malignancies provides a unique opportunity to identify genetic determinants of cancer including hematological malignancies. PV is an acquired clonal myeloproliferative disorder. Although the vast majority of PV cases are sporadic, a few familial cases have been reported. We identified six families with multiple members affected with PV, all having clonal myelopoiesis. The predisposition to PV follows an autosomal dominant inheritance pattern with incomplete penetrance. Based on the clonality and genetic studies of these PV families, a model of the PV pathogenesis, in which LOH in the PV locus as the disease-initiating event, is discussed. Several previously proposed candidate PV loci (common deleted regions on 20q and 13q, c-mpl and EPO receptor genes) were excluded as the primary PV defect using linkage analysis. None of the familial PV subjects had cytogenetic abnormalities that would identify regions with LOH. Therefore, a genome-wide screening for LOH was performed in two familial subjects and one sporadic PV subject using microsatellite markers at 10 cM average spacing. Two loci with LOH were identified, one on chromosome 9p and the other on chromosome 11q. Further analysis of 10 sporadic and 15 familial PV subjects for the presence of both of these defects revealed that the 9p LOH was present in 3 of 10 sporadic subjects (33%) and 2 of 15 familial subjects (13%). We mapped the common LOH region on 9p to a location between D9S1813 and D9S1833 which spans about 40 cM. The 11q LOH was present in only 1 of 15 familial PV subjects (6%). The 11q LOH spans a 70 cM region between markers D11S2002 and 11qTER.

Linkage analysis performed with markers located within the two LOH loci excluded chromosome 9p as the locus implicated in the familial predisposition to PV. In addition, genetic linkage could also be excluded between PV and several loci previously implicated in the pathogenesis of PV. The LOH region on chromosome 11q could neither be excluded nor confirmed as the PV predisposition locus. The results of the genome-wide LOH and genetic linkage analyses demonstrate the complexity of genetic changes underlying the pathogenesis of PV.

References

1. Adamson JW, Fialkow PJ, Murphy S, Prchal JF, Steinmann L (1976) Polycythemia vera: stem-cell and probable clonal origin of the disease. N Engl J Med 295:913–916
2. Prchal JT, Prchal JF, Belickova M, Chen S, Guan Y, Gartland GL, Cooper MD (1996) Clonal stability of blood cell lineages indicated by X-chromosomal transcriptional polymorphism. J Exp Med 183:561–567
3. Diez-Martin JL, Graham DL, Petitt RM, Dewald GW (1991) Chromosome studies in 104 patients with polycythemia vera. Mayo Clin Proc 66:287–299
4. Bench AJ, Nacheva EP, Champion KM, Green AR (1998) Molecular genetics and cytogenetics of myeloproliferative disorders. Baillieres Clin Haematol 11:819–848
5. Prchal JF, Axelrad AA (1974) Bone-marrow responses in polycythemia vera (letter). N Engl J Med 290:1382
6. Prchal JF, Adamson JW, Murphy S, Steinmann L, Fialkow PJ (1978) Polycythemia vera. The in vitro response of normal and abnormal stem cell lines to erythropoietin. J Clin Invest 61:1044–1047
7. Sui X, Krantz SB, Zhao Z (1997) Identification of increased protein tyrosine phosphatase activity in polycythemia vera erythroid progenitor cells. Blood 90:651–657
8. Wickrema A, Chen F, Namin F, Yi T, Ahmad S, Uddin S, Chen YH, Feldman L, Stock W, Hoffman R, Platanias LC (1999) Defective expression of the SHP-1 phosphatase in polycythemia vera. Exp Hematol 27:1124–1132
9. Moliterno AR, Hankins WD, Spivak JL (1998) Impaired expression of the thrombopoietin receptor by platelets from patients with polycythemia vera [see comments]. N Engl J Med 338:572–580
10. Silva M, Richard C, Benito A, Sanz C, Olalla I, Fernandez-Luna JL (1998) Expression of Bcl-x in erythroid precursors from patients with polycythemia vera. N Engl J Med 338:564–571
11. Temerinac S, Klippel S, Strunck E, Roder S, Lubbert M, Lange W, Azemar M, Meinhardt G, Schaefer HE, Pahl HL (2000) Cloning of PRV-1, a novel member of the uPAR receptor superfamily, which is overexpressed in polycythemia rubra vera. Blood 95:2569–2576
12. Dai R, Krantz SB (2001) Increased expression of the INK4a/ARF locus in polycythemia vera. Blood 97:3424–3432
13. Kralovics R, Castilos FA, Prchal JT (1999) Familial polycythemia vera: mode of inheritance, clonality, and genetic analysis of candidate genes and chromosomal regions. Blood 94:113a

C Essential Thrombocythemia

Chapter 11

Essential Thrombocythemia: Regulation of Megakaryocytopoiesis

Sylvia Bellucci

11.1 Introduction

Essential thrombocythemia (ET) is characterized by an increased megakaryocyte (MK) proliferation, maturation and ploidy, leading to an increased number of circulating platelets. Although it now appears as a heterogeneous syndrome in particular in regard to the clinical manifestations and the prognosis [1], MK hyperproliferation and platelet hyperactivation can be considered as cardinal features of this disorder. There is no pathognomonic criterion for the diagnosis of ET. Thus ET must be first distinguished from the secondary thrombocytoses often due to iron depletion, an inflammatory state and/or splenectomy (see Chap. 1).

With that aim we recently reported that an increase in membrane and total platelet glycoprotein IV can be considered a common marker of chronic myeloproliferative disorders (cMPD) being observed in about 70% of patients; this increase is not observed in secondary thrombocytoses [2]. ET must also be distinguished from the other cMPDs [3]. In this disorder an autonomous MK colony formation and platelet hyperactivation have also been described. Taken together these data suggest a hyperreactivity to thrombopoietin (TPO) that is discussed in this chapter.

11.2 Evidence for the Existence of an Enhanced Megakaryocytopoiesis in ET

In vitro spontaneous MK colony formation (CFU-MK) in blood or bone marrow from ET patients has been noted in different culture media (methylcellulose, agar, plasma clot) used for MK progenitors cultures assays [4, 5]. This property is a particularly useful confirmative criterion for the diagnosis of ET [6]. The precise mechanism of the phenomenon remains to be elucidated. Thus, a recent study demonstrated that spontaneous MK growth involved only a fraction (about 20%) of the MK progenitors, from blood or bone marrow CD34+ cells. This property was not due to a paracrine stimulation since it was observed in limit dilutions [7]. Neither was it due to an autocrine stimulation by Mpl-ligand (or TPO), since neutralizing anti-Mpl-ligand antibody did not inhibit spontaneous growth. Furthermore, Mpl-ligand mRNA was either not detected by RT-PCR in CD34+ cells or only at extremely low levels, and finally it was shown that CD34+ cells do not secrete any detectable levels of biologically active Mpl ligand [7]. In addition, a c-mpl (TPO receptor) mutation/deletion by sequencing the entire coding region of the gene by PCR was not found [7, 8]. However, other authors have suggested that the Mpl ligand-Mpl loop might be involved in the phenomenon since it was abolished by antisense oligonucleotides against c-mpl

[9]. Soluble Mpl receptor was also able to markedly inhibit MK spontaneous growth [7]. Further studies are thus required to define the precise mechanism of this phenomenon, which can be inhibited by platelet factor 4 [10], a negative regulator of megakaryocytopoiesis [11].

Concerning the response to agonists, MK progenitor cells in ET have been shown to possess increased reactivity to interleukin 3. The sensitivity of MK precursors to TPO itself was then analyzed and hypersensitivity was recently demonstrated [12] (see Chap. 8). On the other hand, labeled ligand experiments showed after Scatchard analysis that platelets do not show an increase in the number of TPO receptors but on the contrary a marked decrease (about tenfold less) than the platelets from normal individuals [13]. This observation is controversial since it was not found in other ET [14], perhaps reflecting the heterogeneity of the disease. A more recent study confirmed the decrease in platelet TPO receptors observed in ET and showed no aberrant constitutive or TPO-induced tyrosine phosphorylation of this receptor or other proteins [15]. Therefore, an increased response of MK progenitors to TPO, after the step of binding to its receptor, via some different pathways of signal transduction possibly related to the hit of the malignant process, remains an attractive hypothesis which deserves to be tested.

Very interestingly, two recent studies have confirmed a decreased c-Mpl labeling of MKs in some subgroups of ET patients and found evidence of a correlation with thromboses and a more pessimistic prognosis, although the mechanisms involved remain to be elucidated [16, 17]. These cytoimmunological results contrast with those obtained in polycythemia vera (PV) or in idiopathic myelofibrosis where a very drastic decrease in (even a lack of) platelet cMpl receptors occurs in parallel with a defective TPO-induced protein tyrosine phosphorylation [14, 18].

Last, the possibility that the primary abnormality in ET was an increase in synthesis of TPO was ruled out. Thus, in ET, plasma TPO concentrations were found to be within the normal range and serum TPO either normal or only slightly raised [19]. This normal plasma concentration correlates well with its normal mRNA expression by bone marrow stromal cells, suggesting a normal synthesis by these cells [20]. In PV, since erythropoietin concentrations are regulated at the level of plasma production, erythropoietin levels are decreased. By contrast, in ET a marked decrease in TPO receptors leads to a defective binding of TPO [13] and since TPO concentrations are largely regulated by binding to platelets [21], plasma TPO is normal or subnormal and not as decreased as expected because of the elevated platelet count.

In a familial thrombocythemia with clinical features marked by erythromelalgia or atypical transient ischemic attacks simulating the phenotype of acquired ET, Wiestner et al. [22] recently described an activating donor splice site mutation in the TPO gene causing increased TPO production. This TPO gene mutation in hereditary ET leads to an abnormal processing of mRNA with normal coding sequences. This aberrant TPO mRNA has a much longer half-life and leads to increased levels of TPO in the affected family members, which can readily explain a phenotype characterized by an increase of clustered enlarged MKs in the bone marrow, spontaneous MK growth, platelet hyperreactivity and microvascular circulation disturbances very similar to that of acquired ET. Similar mutations have been reported in other familial thrombocythemias. However, formal proof that these familial hematopoietic disorders are polyclonal, which would establish the non-MPD nature of this disease, has not been reported yet. On the other hand, ET has been shown to be clonal or polyclonal [1], but such a mutation in the TPO gene was not found in 51 patients with either clonal or polyclonal acquired ET [23].

11.3 Evidence for "Hypersensitive" Platelets in ET

Indeed, the reproducible evidence of platelet activation in vivo in subjects with ET, as well as evidence of the beneficial effect of particular platelet cyclooxygenase inhibiting drugs such as aspirin and indomethacin and of cytoreduction of the platelet count, are all in support of in vivo hyperfunction of platelets playing a pivotal role in the pathophysiology of thrombotic complications in ET (for review see reference 24). Different biological techniques suggest the existence of an in vivo platelet hyperactivation in ET.

First, the presence of an excess of platelet clumps and aggregates in peripheral blood smears from ET patients. Ultrastructural studies confirm the appearance of activated platelets, since numerous pseudopodes and centralized granules are visualized. In vitro aggregation tests may show a spontaneous aggregation. After stimulation by ADP or collagen, aggregation is often decreased and may reflect a secondary storage pool defect.

Second, an increase in ET patients of plasma β-thromboglobulin (β-TG), a constituent normally present in alpha granules, reflects an increased release in vivo concomitantly with platelet hyperactivation. The concentration of β-TG in the MKs is within the normal range, ruling out a defect in synthesis. Recently, we have showed that this increase in ET of plasma β-TG persists even if the platelet count is normalized by chemotherapy [25]. Other constituents of alpha granules, such as endogenous thrombospondin are also expressed spontaneously at the platelet membrane, suggesting an in vivo platelet activation in ET [26].

Third, several authors have provided unequivocal evidence for platelet activation in vivo by measuring platelet-specific proteins or stable degradation products of platelet-derived thromboxane in urine, thereby avoiding artifacts from ex vivo platelet activation. The endogenous synthesis of thromboxane A2 by platelets was estimated by the measurement of their main stable metabolites in urine and was found to be increased. Particularly in symptomatic patients with arterial thrombosis, a spontaneous platelet activation with thromboxane B2 synthesis was found [27]. However, the physiopathogenesis of this in vivo platelet hyperactivation remains to be defined.

Finally, the role of TPO may be hypothesized. In vitro, TPO is able to enhance the platelet aggregation induced by the agonists ADP, thrombin and collagen [28]. Ex vivo, ET platelets show a variable response to exogenous TPO which is inversely proportional to the level of endogenous TPO, possibly indicating a role of TPO in the regulation of platelet function [29]. Furthermore, in some ET patients, TPO by itself leads to platelet aggregation, which is never observed in normal subjects. Thus endogenous TPO, the concentration of which is higher than expected according to the platelet count, may be considered as a positive modulator favoring the platelet hyperactivation observed in ET.

11.4 Conclusions

In ET there are several lines of evidence indicating hyperreactivity of MKs and of platelets to TPO, the plasma level of which is normal or slightly elevated. An increase in platelet glycoprotein IV has been observed in 70% of patients, the physiological relevance of which deserves to be analyzed. Overall, further studies are required to define the genetic abnormality(ies) responsible for this heterogeneous disorder and to enable a better knowledge and classification.

11.5 Summary

ET is one of the less-rare variants of cMPDs. This chapter discusses the possible link between spontaneous megakaryocytopoiesis, platelet hyperreactivity and hyperreactivity to TPO, the main growth factor for the MK lineage. Thus in ET there is an increased proliferation of MK progenitors, even under culture conditions without any known MK colony-stimulating factors. An increased reactivity of MK progenitors to TPO has been recently demonstrated. A defective clearance of TPO by MKs and platelets because of a reduced number of TPO receptors is possible. A point mutation in the TPO gene as the cause of increased TPO production in hereditary ET can readily explain both spontaneous megakaryocytopoiesis and platelet-mediated microvascular manifestations simulating the phenotype of acquired ET. Neverthe-

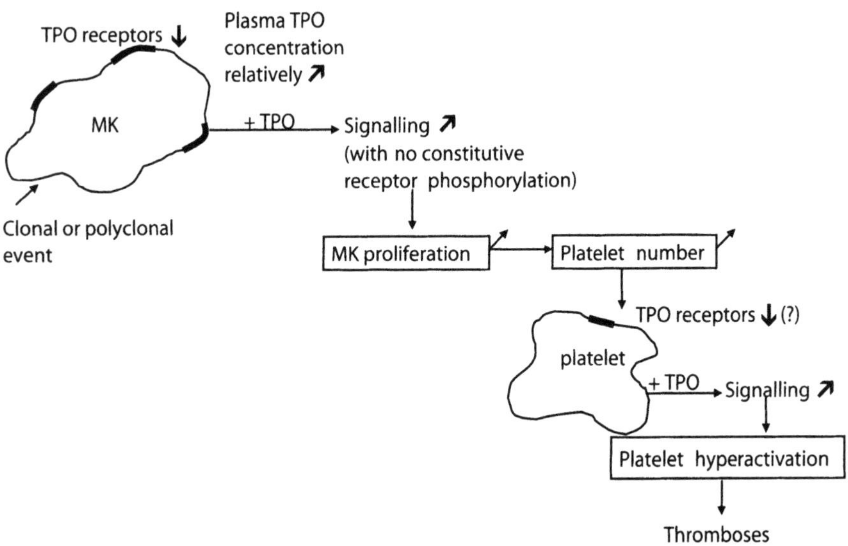

Fig. 11.1. Some unknown clonal or polyclonal event(s) lead to a malignant process responsible for the development of abnormal MKs with hypersensitivity to TPO accounting for an increase in MK precursors proliferation, platelet number and platelet reactivity. This MK and platelet hyperreactivity occur although the numbers of MK TPO receptors and possibly platelet TPO receptors are decreased, suggesting an exacerbation of cellular signaling by the involvement of new and/or abnormal pathways in relation to the malignant process

less, until now no mutation of the TPO structural gene, as shown in families with hereditary ET, and no mutations in the TPO receptor have been found in patients with acquired ET. On the other hand, TPO is able to enhance platelet aggregation induced by ADP, thrombin and collagen. Thus hyperreactivity of ET platelets to TPO has been suggested to explain platelet hyperactivation in vivo. MK and platelet hyperreactivity to TPO in ET is illustrated schematically in Fig. 11.1.

No specific abnormality has been found in this disorder. Thus, the evidence of the precise genetic abnormalities responsible for this very heterogeneous syndrome requires further investigation.

References

1. Nimer SD (1999) Essential thrombocythemia: another "heterogeneous disease" better understood? Blood 93:415–416
2. Thibert V, Bellucci S, Cristofari M, Gluckman E, Legrand C (1995) Increased platelet CD36 constitutes a common marker in myeloproliferative disorders. Br J Haematol 91:618–624
3. Thiele J, Kvasnicka HM, Werden C, Zankovich R, Diehl V, Fischer R (1996) Idiopathic primary osteomyelofibrosis: a clinicopathological study on 208 patients with special emphasis on evolution of disease features, differentiation from essential thrombocythemia and variables of prognosis impact. Leuk Lymphoma 22:303–317
4. Han ZC, Briere J, Abgrall JF, Sensebe L, Nedellec G, Parent D, Guern G (1987) Spontaneous formation of megakaryocyte progenitors (CFU-MK) in primary thrombocythemia. Acta Haematol 78:51–53
5. Juvonen E, Ikkala E, Oksanen K, Ruutu T (1993) Megakaryocyte and erythroid colony formation in essential thrombocythemia and reactive thrombocytosis: diagnostic value and correlation to complications. Br J Haematol 83:192–197
6. Michiels JJ, Juvonen E (1997) Proposal for revised diagnostic criteria of essential thrombocythemia and polycythemia vera by the Thrombocythemia Vera Study Group. Semin Thromb Hemost 23:339–347
7. Taksin AL, Le Couedic JP, Dusanter-Fourt I, Masse A, Giraudier S, Katz A, Wendling F, Vainchenker W, Casadevall N, Debili N (1999) Autonomous megakaryocyte growth in essential thrombocythemia and idiopathic myelofibrosis is not related to a c-mpl mutation or to an autocrine stimulation by Mpl-L. Blood 93:125–139
8. Kiladjian JJ, Elkassar N, Hetet G, Briere J, Grandchamp B, Gardin C (1997) Study of the thrombopoietin receptor in essential thrombocythemia. Leukemia 11:1821–1826
9. Li Y, Hetet G, Kiladjian JJ, Gardin C, Grandchamp B, Briere J (1996) Protooncogene c-mpl is involved in spontaneous megakaryocytopoiesis in myeloproliferative disorders. Br J Haematol 92:60–66
10. Han ZC, Bellucci S, Tenza D And Caen JP (1990) Negative regulation of human megakaryocytopoiesis by human platelet factor 4 and betathromboglobulin: comparative analysis in bone marrow cultures from normal individuals and patients with essential thrombocythemia and immune thrombocytopenic purpura. Br J Haematol 74:395–401
11. Han ZC, Sensebe L, Abgrall JF, Briere J (1990) Platelet factor 4 inhibits human megakaryocytopoiesis in vitro. Blood 75:1234–1239
12. Axelrad AA, Eskinazi D, Correa PN, Amato D (2000) Hypersensitivity of circulating progenitor cells to megakaryocyte growth and development factor (PEGrHU-MGDF) in essential thrombocythemia. Blood 96:3310–3321
13. Li J, Xia Y, Kuter DJ (1999) Interaction of thrombopoietin with the platelet c-mpl receptor in plasma: binding, internalization, stability and pharmacokinetics. Br J Haematol 106:345–356
14. Moliterno AR, Hankis D, Spivak JL (1998) Impaired expression of the thrombopoietin receptor by platelets from patients with polycythemia vera. N Engl J Med 338:572–580
15. Horikawa Y, Matsumura I, Hashimoto K, Shiraga M, Kosugi S, Tadokoro S, Kato T, Miyazaki H, Tomiyama Y, Kurata Y, Matsuzawa Y, Kanakura Y (1997) Markedly reduced expression of platelet c-mpl receptor in essential thrombocythemia. Blood 90:4031–4038
16. Teofili L, Pierconti F, Di Febo A, Maggiano N, Vianelli N, Ascani S, Rossi E, Pileri S, Leone G, Larocca LM, De Stefano V (2002) The expression pattern of c-mpl in megakaryocytes correlates with thrombotic risk in essential thrombocythemia. Blood 100:714–717
17. Mesa RA, Hanson CA, Li C-Y, Yoon S-Y, Rajkumar V, Schroeder G, Tefferi A (2002) Diagnostic and prognostic value of bone marrow angiogenesis and megakaryocyte c-Mpl expression in essential thrombocythemia. Blood 99:4131–4137

18. Moliterno AR, Spivak JL (1999) Posttranslational processing of the thrombopoietin receptor is impaired in polycythemia vera. Blood 94:2555–2561
19. von dem Borne AE, Folman C, Linthorst GE, Porcelijn L, van den Ouderijn S, van der Schoot CE, de Haas M (1998) Thrombopoietin and its receptor: structure, function and role in the regulation of platelet production. Baillieres Clin Haematol 11:409–426
20. Hirayama Y, Sakamaki S, Matsunaga T, Kuga T, Kuroda H, Kusakabe T, Sasaki K, Fujikawa K, Kato J, Kogawa K, Koyama R, Niitsu Y (1998) Concentrations of thrombopoietin in bone marrow in normal subjects and in patients with idiopathic thrombocytopenic purpura, aplastic anemia, and essential thrombocythemia correlate with its mRNA expression of bone marrow stromal cells. Blood 92:46–52
21. Fielder PJ, Gurney AL, Stefanich E, Marian M, Moore MW, Carver-Moore K, De Sauvage FJ (1996) Regulation of thrombopoietin levels by c-mpl mediated binding to platelets. Blood 87:2154–2161
22. Wiestner A, Schlemper RJ, Van Der Maas Apc, Skoda RC (1998) An activating splice donor mutation in the thrombopoietin gene causes hereditary thrombocythaemia. Nat Genet 18:49–52
23. Harrison CN, Gale RE, Wiestner AC, Skoda RC, Linch DC (1998) The activating splice mutation in intron 3 of the thrombopoietin gene is not found in patients with nonfamilial essential thrombocythaemia. Br J Haematol 102:1341–1343
24. Bellucci S, Michiels JJ (2000) Spontaneous proliferative megakaryocytopoiesis and platelet hyperreactivity in essential thrombocythemia: is thrombopoietin the link? Ann Hematol 79:51–58
25. Bellucci S, Ignatova E, Jaillet N, Boffa MC (1993) Platelet hyperactivation in patients with essential thrombocythemia is not associated with vascular endothelial cell damage as judged by the level of plasma thrombomodulin, protein S, PAI-1, t-PA and vWF. Thromb Haemost 70:736–742
26. Legrand C, Bellucci S, Disdier M, Edelman L, Tobelem G (1991) Platelet thrombospondin and glycoprotein IV abnormalities in patients with essential thrombocythemia: effect of alpha interferon treatment. Am J Hematol 38:307–313
27. Rocca B, Ciabattoni G, Tartaglione R, Cortelazzo S, Barbui T, Patrono C, Landolfi R (1995) Increased thromboxane biosynthesis in essential thrombocythemia. Thromb Haemost 74:1225–1230
28. Chen J, Herceg-Harjacek L, Groopman JE, Grabarek J (1995) Regulation of platelet activation in vitro by the c-mpl ligand, thrombopoietin. Blood 86:4054–4062
29. Usuki K, Iki S, Endo M, Izutsu K, Inoue K, Nishimura T, Urabe A (1997) Influence of thrombopoietin on platelet activation in myeloproliferative disorders. Br J Haematol 97:530–537

Chapter 12

Hereditary Thrombocythemia

Radek C. Skoda, Adrian Wiestner, Nico Ghilardi, Stephan Padosch

12.1 Thrombocythemia Caused by Mutations in the TPO Gene

Thrombopoietin (TPO) is the most potent humoral regulator of platelet formation [1] and was therefore an obvious candidate gene for hereditary thrombocythemia (HT). Physiologically, TPO serum concentrations are very low, ranging between 0.25 and 1 p*M* (15–60 pg/ml). Circulating TPO is mainly produced by the liver and the kidneys and TPO mRNA levels in these organs remain unchanged during thrombocytopenia. Familial occurrence of syndromes resembling myeloproliferative disorders (MPDs) offers the possibility of applying genetic linkage analysis to identify the chromosomal localization and ultimately of finding the mutated gene(s). This approach led to the identification of mutations in the TPO gene as the cause in four families with HT (Table 12.1). Here we discuss our current understanding of how these TPO mutations lead to thrombocytosis.

Table 12.1. Summary of TPO mutations causing hereditary thrombocythemia

Initial case report	Inheritance	Platelet count ($\times 10^9$/l)	Complications	Gene mutation	Molecular mechanism	Remarks
[2]	Autosomal dominant, 11 affected, 4 generations	533–1516	Vasoocclusive	TPO, G→C in intervening sequence 3 position +1 [5]	Loss of uORF-mediated repression [5]	Leukemoid reaction in one child [3]
[7]	Autosomal dominant	700–1000	Vasoocclusive	TPO, A→G in intervening sequence 3 +5 [7]	Not determined	Polyclonal hematopoiesis
[8]	Autosomal dominant, 5 affected, 3 generations	847–1600		TPO, ΔG in 5'-UTR [8]	Loss of uORF-mediated repression [9]	
[10]	Autosomal dominant, 4 affected, 3 generations	833–1986		TPO, G→T in 5'-UTR [11]	Loss of uORF-mediated repression [9]	

12.1.1 A Splice Donor Mutation in TPO Causes Hereditary Thrombocythemia in a Dutch Family

A large pedigree with 11 affected individuals in four generations (Fig. 12.1) and clinical features resembling ET was described [2]. Three HT patients had both vasoocclusive and hemorrhagic symptoms, three patients only vasoocclusive symptoms and

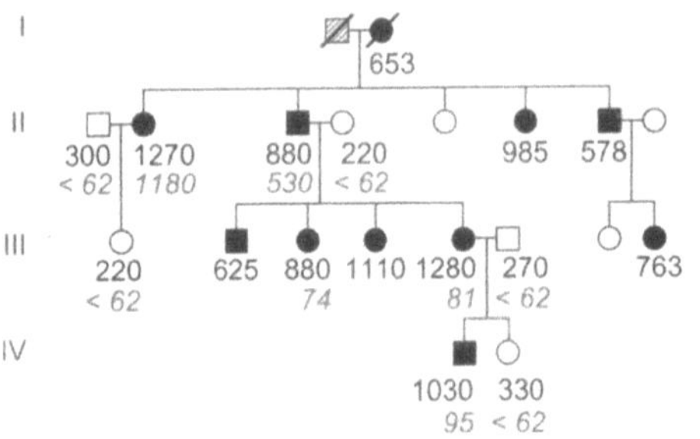

Fig. 12.1. Pedigree of the Dutch family (*filled symbols* affected individuals, *open symbols* normal individuals, *crossed symbols* deceased). Numbers below the symbols represent platelet counts $\times 10^9$/l; numbers in italics indicate TPO serum concentrations in pg/ml [5]

five patients were asymptomatic. Symptoms correlated with age but not with platelet count. ADP-induced platelet aggregation was abnormal in all affected individuals. No chromosomal abnormalities were found. Interestingly, at the age of 6 weeks, the youngest affected family member (IV/1) displayed hepatosplenomegaly and a leukemoid reaction, which lasted for several months [3, 4]. At the age of 5 years, he had thrombocytosis, but was otherwise healthy and without medication.

In this family, genetic analysis revealed linkage for the TPO locus (lod score of 3.5) and allowed the first gene mutation, which causes HT, to be defined [5]. Sequencing of the TPO gene showed that affected family members carry a point mutation in the +1 position of the splice donor of intron 3. This G→C transversion preferentially causes exon skipping and results in loss of exon 3 (Fig. 12.2). Exon 3 normally encodes a large part of the 5'-untranslated region (5'-UTR), which contains several upstream AUG (uAUG) codons. RNA that contains such uAUGs is poorly translated, because these uAUGs force the ribosome to initiate translation and to synthesize short peptides defined by the corresponding upstream open reading frames (uORFs). Thus, the presence of uAUGs prevents the ribosome from reaching the physiological start site (Fig. 12.3). The normal TPO mRNA was shown to be strongly inhibited by such uAUGs (Fig. 12.4). Directed mutagenesis of all uAUGs in the TPO mRNA restored full translational efficiency, demonstrating that translational inhibition of TPO biosynthesis is entirely mediated by uORFs [6]. The uORF defined by the seventh uAUG was shown to exert the strongest negative effect on translation [6]. This uAUG is in a good Kozak consensus and the uORF extends beyond the physiological start site, thus pre-

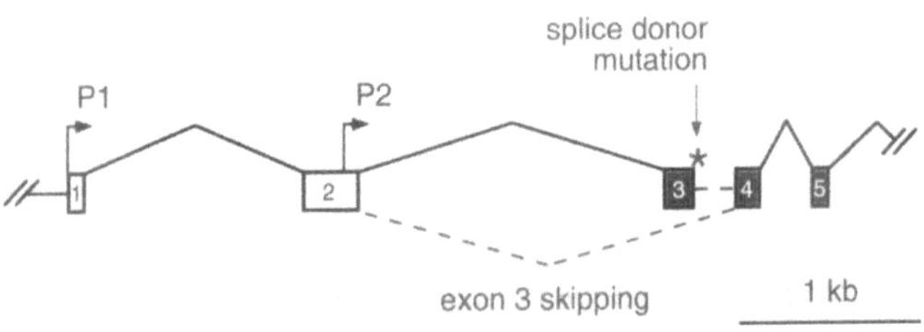

Fig. 12.2. The TPO splice donor mutation causes exon 3 skipping. The region between exons 1 and 5 is drawn. *Open boxes* represent non-coding exons, *filled boxes* exons encoding TPO protein. *Arrows* indicate transcription start sites for the P1 and P2 promoter and the *asterisk* marks the position of the G→C splice donor mutation. Transcripts from P2 are more abundant than from P1. Exons connected by *solid lines* represent normal splicing and the *dashed lines* indicate the consequences of the TPO mutation on splicing

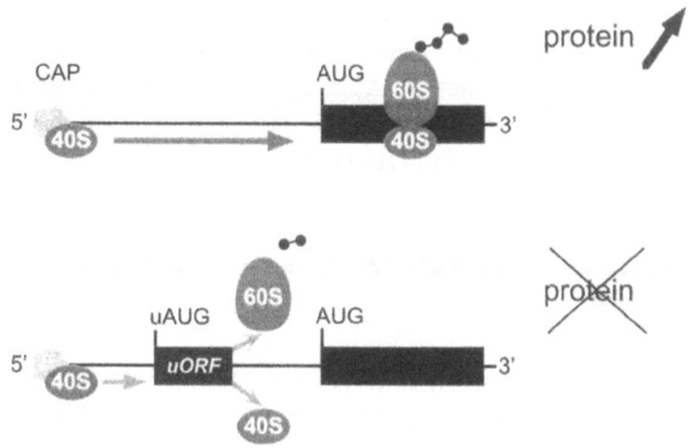

Fig. 12.3. *Top* The ribosomal 40S subunit binds the 5' cap structure of mRNA (cap-dependent mechanism of initiation) and migrates along the 5'-UTR in search for an appropriate initiator AUG codon (scanning process). Recognition of the physiological start AUG leads to assembly of the 60S ribosomal subunit and initiation of protein synthesis. *Bottom* A 5'-UTR containing an uAUG codon causes premature initiation leading to synthesis of a short peptide encoded by the uORF. The uAUG inhibits translation of the physiological protein by preventing the ribosome from reaching the start codon

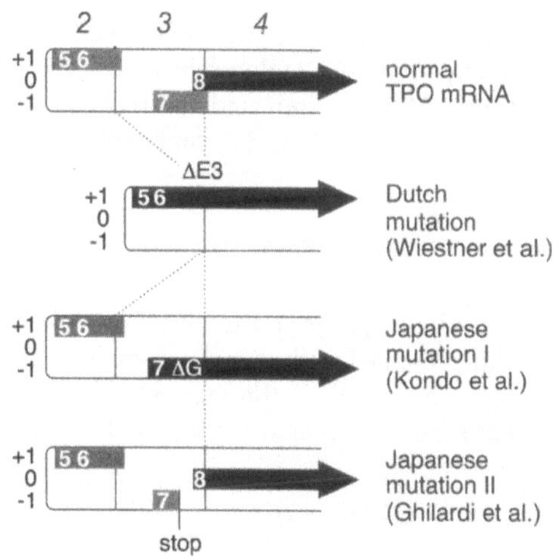

Fig. 12.4. TPO transcripts starting from the main promoter in exon 2 are shown. Boxes numbered in italic represent exons. The uORFs are drawn as thick lines and are placed into one of the three reading frames (+1, 0, −1). The TPO coding region is shown as a *thick arrow*. Numbers indicate the order in which the uAUGs appear in the full length TPO mRNA (therefore uAUGs 1–4 are not shown). The eighth AUG is the physiological initiation codon. Translation of normal TPO mRNA is physiologically almost completely inhibited by the presence of uORFs in the 5'-UTR. In particular, uORF7 is a potent inhibitor of translation, most likely because of its extension beyond the physiological start site. A splice donor mutation in the Dutch HT family at position +1 of the splice donor causes exon 3 skipping (ΔE3) that deletes uORF7 and shifts the TPO coding sequence into reading frame +1. TPO translation now initiates from the fifth and sixth AUG. A mutation located at position +5 of the same splice donor downstream [7] is expected to result in the same alterations. The Japanese mutation I consists of a single G nucleotide deletion (ΔG) that shifts the TPO coding sequence into reading frame −1. TPO translation now initiates from the seventh AUG. Note that both the Dutch and the Japanese mutation I create altered TPO signal peptides, but do not alter the sequence of the mature TPO protein. Both signal peptides remain functionally active and promote secretion of a biologically active TPO protein. The Japanese mutation II creates a premature stop codon in uORF7. This allows reinitiation of translation at the physiological start site (the eighth AUG) [13]

venting reinitiation (Fig. 12.4). Because of exon 3 skipping, the mutant TPO mRNA lacks uORF7 and uORF5 is placed in-frame with the TPO coding sequence (Fig. 12.4). The resulting new N-terminus affects the TPO signal peptide, but not the mature TPO protein. Importantly, the new signal peptide was shown to be a functionally active [5]. Thus, the mutated allele causes overproduction of TPO protein through the loss of physiological repression of translation.

Interestingly, an A→G substitution located four bases downstream of the Dutch mutation in the splice donor of TPO intron 3 has been reported for another HT family in a meeting abstract [7]. Although this mutation does not affect the most conserved residues of the splice donor, it is expected to cause the same aberrant splicing as the Dutch mutation. A full report on this family has not been published to date.

12.1.2 Deletion of a Single Nucleotide in the 5′-UTR Causes a Frame Shift in uORF7 in a Japanese HT Family

In a Japanese family with HT, affected family members displayed elevated TPO serum levels (Fig. 12.5) and carried a single G nucleotide deletion (ΔG) in uORF7 of the TPO gene [8]. No information on the clinical course of affected individuals was available. The ΔG caused a frameshift, which places uORF7 in frame with the TPO coding sequence (Fig. 12.4). This eliminates the strong inhibitory effect of uORF7 and again creates a novel N-terminus for the TPO signal peptide [9]. Similar to the Dutch mutation, this novel N-terminus still functioned as a signal peptide that ensured secretion of correctly processed, biologically active TPO protein [9]. Thus, through a different mutation, uORF7 is eliminated and translational repression is lost, resulting in elevated TPO serum levels and thrombocytosis.

12.1.3 A Nonsense Mutation in the 5′-UTR Causes Shortening of uORF7 in a Japanese HT Family

In an unrelated Japanese HT family, thrombocytosis was first detected in a 4-year-old boy who presented with cutaneous malignant lymphoma [10]. Subsequent family investigation revealed thrombocytosis in three additional family members (Fig. 12.6). No vasoocclusive or hemorrhagic symptoms were reported for any of the

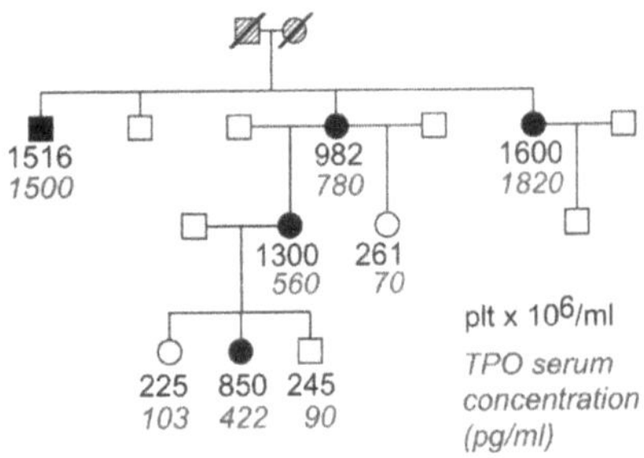

Fig. 12.5. Pedigree of the Japanese family I. For explanation of symbols, see Fig. 12.1 [8]

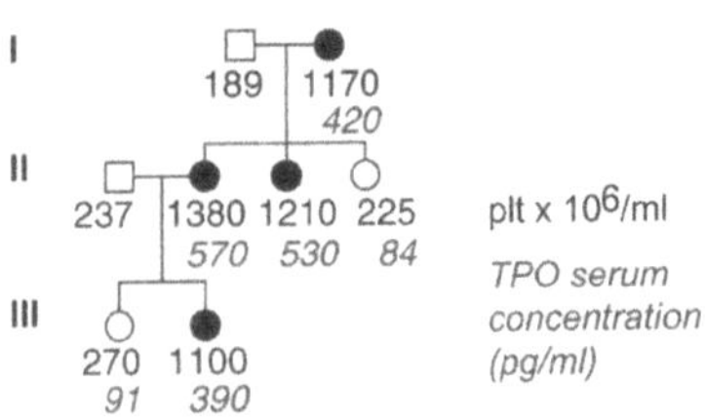

Fig. 12.6. Pedigree of the Japanese family II. For explanation of symbols, see Fig. 12.1 [8]

family members. Serum TPO concentrations were elevated in all affected individuals and a point mutation in the TPO 5'-UTR was found [11]. This G→T mutation creates a novel stop codon, which shortens uORF7 by 42 nucleotides (Fig. 12.4). Thereby a gap of 31 nucleotides is generated between uORF7 and the physiological TPO start codon, which allows translational reinitiation resulting in enhanced translational efficiency and overproduction of TPO [11].

12.1.4 Summary

Mutations of the TPO gene are very rare causes of thrombocytosis. To date, fewer than 20 familial syndromes have been described in the literature. Within these hereditary syndromes, TPO mutations account for about one-quarter of HT. It is remarkable, that all four known TPO alleles change or inactivate the inhibitory effect of uORF7 on translation [12]. Thus, uORF7 seems to be physiologically important for maintaining a normal platelet count. This also suggests that there is no platelet-sensing mechanism able to detect thrombocytosis and downregulate TPO production in patients carrying the mutations.

12.2 Hereditary Thrombocythemia Caused by Genes Other Than TPO

In other HT families, genetic analysis TPO has allowed TPO to be excluded as the candidate gene, indicating that HT is a syndrome of heterogeneous disorders [13, 14]. The ongoing search for the mutated gene(s) in these pedigrees will likely increase our understanding of the regulation of thrombopoiesis and may yield important new clues for acquired ET. Particularly interesting is a Spanish family with variable manifestations of clinical pictures resembling the three forms of MPDs [15]. Three patients had ET, two polycythemia vera (PV) and one osteomyelofibrosis (Fig. 12.7). The penetrance appeared to be considerably less than 100%.

Two models can be postulated. One is the classical loss of heterozygosity (LOH) paradigm, where somatic mutation inactivates the second allele (Fig. 12.8a). Alternatively, an autosomal dominant predisposition is inherited that increases the likelihood of acquiring a mutation at a second locus (Fig. 12.8b). At present, we cannot dis-

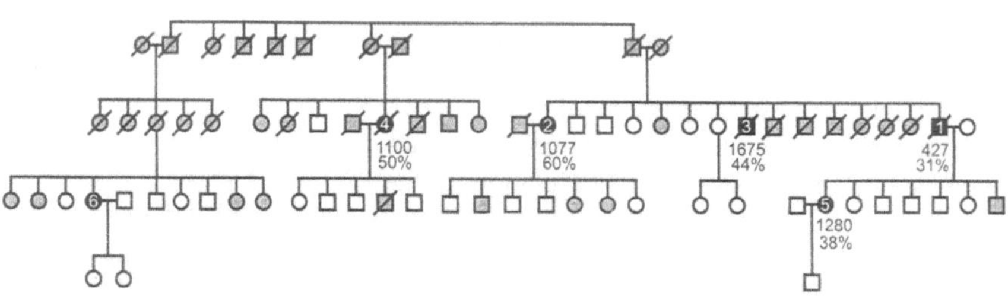

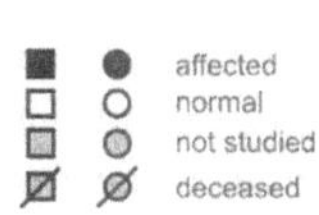

Fig. 12.7. Pedigree of the Spanish family. For explanation of symbols, see Fig. 12.1. The numbers below the symbols represent platelet counts × 10^9/l; numbers with % indicate the hematocrit

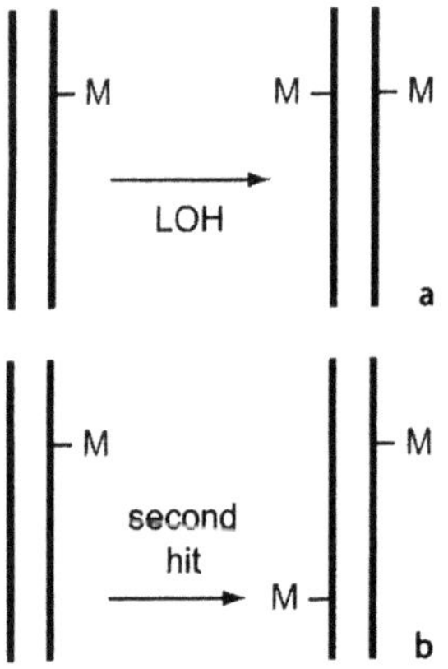

Fig. 12.8a, b. Model to explain low penetrance and variable expressivity of MPD in the Spanish family. **a** LOH results in two mutated alleles at the same chromosomal locus. **b** The germ line mutation at the first locus predisposes to the acquisition of additional mutations at the second

tinguish between these alternative models. We excluded the TPO gene by negative linkage (R.C.S., unpublished results) and obtained preliminary data suggesting cosegregation with the MPL (TPO receptor) locus. The calculated lod score for the allele segregation was 1.8, which is suggestive of, but not yet sufficient to prove, linkage. However, sequencing of the MPL exons and intron boundaries did not reveal a mutation (S.P. and R.C.S., unpublished results). Further analysis including more members of the family will be necessary to clarify these issues. Given the size of this pedigree, genetic analysis will likely allow us to define the chromosomal locus responsible for the disease yielding new hypotheses. The study of inherited forms of MPD continues to provide a powerful approach for gaining new insights into the pathophysiology of megakaryopoiesis and MPD.

Recently, in a Japanese pedigree of HT a unique point mutation (Ser505Asn) was identified in the transmembrane domain of the c-mpl protein. This mutation was identified in all of the eight members with thrombocythemia, but in none of the other eight unaffected members of this family. Ba/F3 cells expressing the mutant Asn505 acquired interleukin-3-independent survival capacity, whereas those expressing wild-type Ser505 did not [16].

12.2.1 Summary

Patients with HT (sometimes also called familial essential thrombocythemia or familial thrombocytosis) display constantly elevated platelet counts and clinical features resembling essential thrombocythemia (ET). Several families with HT have been described and in all these pedigrees, the pattern of inheritance is compatible with an autosomal dominant trait. Mutations in the TPO gene have been discovered in four HT families. In each of them a different mutation was found, defining four different mutant TPO alleles. Interestingly, all four alleles cause thrombocytosis through a translational mechanism, which increases production of TPO protein and results in elevated TPO serum concentrations. In other HT families, genetic analysis allowed TPO to be excluded as the candidate gene, indicating that HT is a syndrome of heterogeneous disorders. Recently, an activating point mutation in the c-mpl gene was described. The ongoing search for the mutated gene(s) in these pedigrees will likely increase our understanding of the regulation of thrombopoiesis and may yield important new clues for acquired ET.

References

1. Kaushinsky K (2003) Thrombopoietin: a tool for understanding thrombopoiesis. J Thromb Haemost 1: 1587–1592
2. Schlemper RJ, van der Maas APC, Eikenboom JCJ (1994) Familial essential thrombocythemia: clinical characteristics of 11 cases in one family. Ann Hematol 68:153–158
3. van Dijken PJ, Woldendorp KH, van Wouwe JP (1996) Familial thrombocytosis in infancy presenting with a leukaemoid reaction. Acta Paediatr 85:1132–1134
4. van Dijken PJ (1997) Essential thrombocythemia in a 5-month-old infant [letter; comment]. J Pediatr Hematol Oncol 19:354
5. Wiestner A, Schlemper RJ, van der Maas AP, Skoda RC (1998) An activating splice donor mutation in the thrombopoietin gene causes hereditary thrombocythaemia. Nat Genet 18:49–52
6. Ghilardi N, Wiestner A, Skoda RC (1998) Thrombopoietin production is inhibited by a translational mechanism. Blood 92:4023–4030
7. Jorgensen MJ, Raskind WH, Wolff JF, Bachrach HR, Kaushansky K (1998) Familial thrombocytosis associated with overproduction of thrombopoietin due to a novel splice donor site mutation (abstract). Blood 92 [Suppl 1]:205a
8. Kondo T, Okabe M, Sanada M, Kurosawa M, Suzuki S, Kobayashi M, Hosokawa M, Asaka M (1998) Familial essential thrombocythemia associated with one-base deletion in the 5'-untranslated region of the thrombopoietin gene. Blood 92:1091–1096
9. Ghilardi N, Skoda RC (1999) A single-base deletion in the thrombopoietin (TPO) gene causes familial essential thrombocytosis through a mechanism of more efficient translation of TPO mRNA (letter). Blood 94:1480–1482
10. Kikuchi M, Tayama T, Hayakawa H, Takahashi I, Hoshino H, Ohsaka A (1995) Familial thrombocytosis. Br J Haematol 89:900–902
11. Ghilardi N, Wiestner A, Kikuchi M, Oshaka A, Skoda RC (1999) Hereditary thrombocythemia in a Japanese family is caused by a novel point mutation in the thrombopoietin gene. Br J Haematol 107:310–316
12. Cazzola M, Skoda RC (2000) Translational pathophysiology: a novel molecular mechanism of human disease. Blood 95:3280–3288
13. Kunishima S, Mizuno S, Naoe T, Saito H, Kamiya T (1998) Genes for thrombopoietin and c-mpl are not responsible for familial thrombocythaemia: a case study. Br J Haematol 100:383–386
14. Wiestner A, Padosch SA, Ghilardi N, Cesar JM, Odriozola J, Shapiro A, Skoda RC (2000) Hereditary thrombocythaemia is a genetically heterogeneous disorder: exclusion of TPO and MPL in two families with hereditary thrombocythaemia. Br J Haematol 110:104–109
15. Perez-Encinas M, Bello JL, Perez-Crespo S, De Miguel R, Tome S (1994) Familial myeloproliferative syndrome. Am J Hematol 46:225–229
16. Ding J, Komatsu H, Wakita A, Kato-Uranishi M, Ito M, et al (2004) Familial essential thrombocythemia associated with a dominant-positive activating mutation of the c-MPL gene, which encodes the receptor for thrombopoietin. Blood 103:4198–4200

Thromboembolic Complications in Essential Thrombocythemia: the Role of the Analysis of the Platelet Proteome

Petro E. Petrides, Britta Seidemann, Brigitte Wittmann-Liebold

13.1 Introduction

Essential thrombocythemia (ET) is associated with both an increased risk of thromboembolic and bleeding complications [1]. The efficacy of aspirin and cytoreductive therapy supports the concept that platelets are functionally altered in individuals with ET and contribute to the complications. However, there is no linear relationship between platelet count and risk of thromboses since the complications can occur even at low platelet counts [2] and do not necessarily occur at high platelet counts. This maybe due to a patient-specific potential to aggregate and/or the individual modulation of the activity of platelets by nonthrombocytic factors such as plasma proteins or other cellular elements.

In 1856 Virchow described the triad "blood vessels, constituents of the blood and blood flow (viscosity)" as the important factors for the development of a thrombosis [3, 4]. The endothelium could be altered in individuals with ET because endothelial cells are also derived from bone marrow stem cells. The endothelium is also a target organ since it is influenced by circulating cells (platelets, granulocytes, monocytes) and soluble factors such as cholesterol and coagulation proteins. Therefore, in order to understand what determines the development of thromboses in ET, soluble factors, other cellular elements (granulocytes and monocytes) as well as platelets and their products have to be studied.

13.2 Role of Coagulation Factors

Several attempts have been made to delineate a potential contribution of coagulation factors (Factor V Leiden, prothrombin gene polymorphism, homocysteine, antithrombin 3 and others) to the development of thromboses in patients with ET. No conclusive results have been obtained yet, however [5–10] (Table 13.1).

13.3 Role of Granulocyte Activation and Leukocyte/Platelet Aggregates

Granulocytes and monocytes express molecules with pro- or anticoagulatory activity. Therefore they are able to cause functional alterations in endothelial cells, platelets or other leukocytes. This cellular interaction is mediated either by direct contact (aggregation) or soluble factors.

Granulocytes are activated in patients with ET (as determined by activation mark-

Table 13.1. Possible role of thrombophilic factors in ET

Parameter investigated	Conclusions	Reference
Factor V Leiden, prothrombin gene polymorphism	Association of prothrombin gene polymorphism with vasomotor symptoms; no correlation with thrombotic complications	[5]
Factor V Leiden	Possibly considered to identify patients with higher risk	[6]
Prothrombin gene polymorphism	Associated with increased occurrence of thrombotic complications	[7]
Factor V Leiden, protein S, protein C, antithrombin 3, prothrombin gene polymorphism, anticardiolipin antibodies	Higher prevalence of Factor V Leiden in patients; possible contribution	[8]
Homocysteine	70% have elevated homocysteine, but no correlation with thrombosis	[9]
Homocysteine	Homocysteine elevated, but not regarded as an additional risk factor	[10]

ers such as CD11b, elastase and myeloperoxidase), but no correlation with a history of thrombosis has been proven so far [11]. However, overexpression of PRV-1 (= CD177, see Chap. 6 and [12]) in granulocytes of ET patients seems to be associated with a higher risk of thrombosis [13].

Platelets and monocytes can form aggregates by way of surface-expressed P-selectin (CD62P) to P-selectin ligand 1, a leukocyte receptor [14]. In ET patients with increased platelet counts circulating platelet/monocyte or platelet/granulocyte/monocyte aggregates are elevated; in addition upon stimulation with ADP there is a further increase in the formation of aggregates. Patients with a previous history of microvascular complications or thromboses show an increase in the number of spontaneously formed aggregates [15–17].

13.4 Platelet Factors

Platelets are anucleated cellular constituents that adhere at sites of endothelial damage. They are critical effectors of hemostasis and thrombosis and regulators of inflammation, tissue repair and immune responses. In ET platelets play a major role in the development of thromboembolic complications. That the functional disturbances which are acquired with this disease are heterogeneous is concluded from HUMARA studies (see Chap. 14), clinical presentation and response to anagrelide (Chap. 15).

Platelets produce a variety of factors which can be analyzed. Although elevations of platelet products such as vascular endothelial growth factor (vEGF) or bFGF, selectins or thrombomodulin have been described indicating platelet and endothelial activation, no role for these parameters in the prediction of thromboembolic complications has been established yet [18, 19].

Inborn polymorphisms of several surface glycoprotein molecules that play a key role in platelet adhesion, activation and aggregation may also contribute to an increased aggregability of platelets. One of these (the P1 allele of GPIIIa) seems to be associated with an increased risk of arterial thrombosis in patients in polycythemia vera [5]. Other heritable factors such as the response to platelet stimuli, as shown in the Framingham heart study in which participants and family members were assayed for epinephrine, ADP and collagen-induced aggregation, may also play an important role [20]. In some individuals with arterial thrombotic complications hypersensitivity to ADP and epinephrine or only to epinephrine (sticky platelet syndrome) has been observed [21].

Instead of screening platelets for quantitative and qualitative alterations in certain proteins a more global approach would target the whole platelet for proteins affecting aggregability. This can be achieved by analysis of the proteome.

13.5 Analysis of the Platelet Proteome

13.5.1 Principles of Proteome Analysis

Proteome analysis is based on a combination of protein separation by two- dimensional gel electrophoresis (2-DE) and mass spectrometric (MS) analysis in connection with protein and gene databases. In 2-DE proteins are separated according to their isoelectric points and subsequently according to their molecular masses. The separation results in a characteristic spot pattern for each cell type which can vary depending upon the physiological state of the cell (resting or activated). The spot patterns are compared using imaging software packages (such as Phoretics or Melanie). For characterization the protein spots are excised from the gel and digested by trypsin, a sequence-specific protease, prior to their elution and analysis by MS.

Figure 13.1. shows a two-dimensional gel (32×24 cm, pI range 4.0–10.0, MW range 10,000 to 100,000 Da) of a proteome of platelets obtained from a healthy individual after obtaining informed consent. Several hundred protein spots are visible. For identification the spots are excised from the gel and subjected to trypsin digestion for 20 h at pH 7.8, desalting by ZipTips (Millipore) and subsequent application to MALDI (matrix-assisted laser-desorption ionization) MS. As matrices dihydrobenzoic acid or alpha-cyano-4-hydroxycinnamic acid are used. The addition of these organic acids is necessary to obtain good crystals with embedded peptide for ionization. The mixture is applied to the target of the Bruker Daltonik Reflex III mass instrument. The mass analysis is done by the time-of-flight (TOF) method calibrated with standard peptides and by internal tryptic fragments. The mass spectrum yields the tryptic masses of the protein which are then compared with all tryptic masses of the proteins collected in the protein database (SwissProt) in order to search for the identity of the investigated protein. Since the tryptic masses are characteristic for each individual protein the tryptic mass spectrum can be regarded as a mass fingerprint characteristic of this protein (PMF, peptide mass fingerprint). For the identification of the protein the software packages Mascot

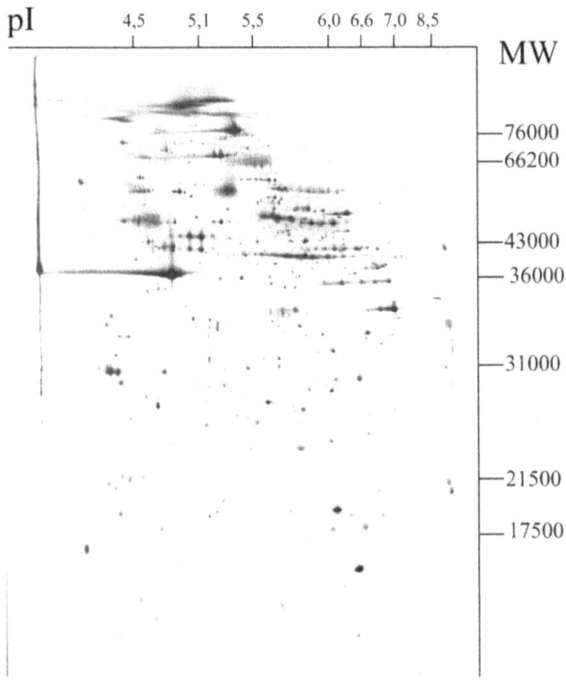

Fig. 13.1. Proteome of human platelets: 10 µg of whole platelet extract (diluted 1:1) was separated by 2-DE (15% PAGE in the second dimension) and stained with silver nitrate. Several hundred protein spots are visible [26]

(www.matrixscience.com) and Biotools (Bruker Daltonik) are used. In Fig. 13.2, two examples of the identification of platelet proteins utilizing this approach are shown.

MALDI-MS is the method of choice for the identification of proteins. If proteins are not present in any of the databases or cannot be identified unambiguously, further analysis can be performed by LC-MS (liquid chromatography linked to an electrospray-ionization MS, ESI-MS). With this method more peptide masses can be detected. After further fragmentation of selected peptide ions in the collision cell of this mass spectrometer additional information of partial sequences can be gained. This makes the identification of the protein in question more safe.

13.5.2 The Platelet Proteome in ET

Early studies in the pre-MS era applied 2DE to the study of the platelet cytoskeleton [22–24]. The results are available at www.expasy.ch/ch2d/ or http://ca.expasy.org/Ch2d/. After the introduction of MS, proteins translocating to the cytoskeleton after stimulation with thrombin were analyzed [25].

At that time we started to investigate the proteomes of individuals with ET. After obtaining informed consent, the platelets isolated from several adult patients with ET and a child with thrombocythemia due to chronic myeloid leukemia (CML) were analyzed [26]. Figure 13.3 shows the 2-DE of the cytosolic extract of purified platelets of

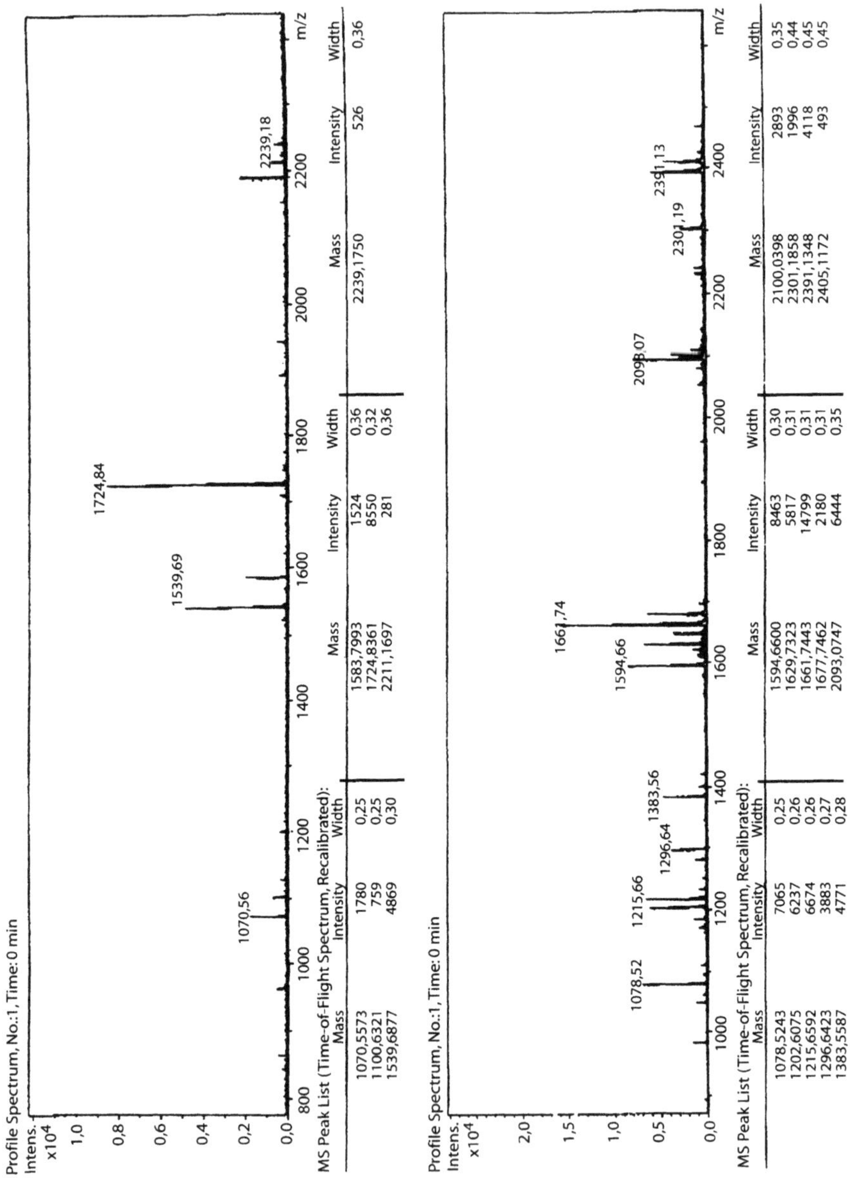

MS Peak List (Time-of-Flight Spectrum, Recalibrated):

Mass	Intensity	Width
1070,5573	1780	0,25
1100,6321	759	0,25
1539,6877	4869	0,30
1583,7993	1524	0,36
1724,8361	8550	0,32
2211,1697	281	0,36
2239,1750	526	0,36

MS Peak List (Time-of-Flight Spectrum, Recalibrated):

Mass	Intensity	Width
1078,5243	7065	0,25
1202,6075	6237	0,26
1215,6592	6674	0,26
1296,6423	3883	0,27
1383,5587	4771	0,28
1594,6600	8463	0,30
1629,7323	5817	0,31
1661,7443	14799	0,31
1677,7462	2180	0,31
2093,0747	6444	0,35
2100,0398	2893	0,35
2301,1858	1996	0,44
2391,1348	4118	0,45
2405,1172	493	0,45

Fig. 13.2. Peptide mass fingerprint of two platelet proteins. *Upper panel* Platelet basic protein precursor; *lower panel* transgelin 2 [26]

a patient with ET, and Fig. 13.4 illustrates the gel of another patient in comparison with controls and other ET patients. The differences are listed in Table 13.2. The most marked differences became apparent when the platelet proteome of a child with thrombocythemia (which turned out to be due to CML due to the presence of the BCR-ABL transcript) was compared with those of adult ET patients (Fig. 13.5). Several differences were revealed (Table 13.3.).

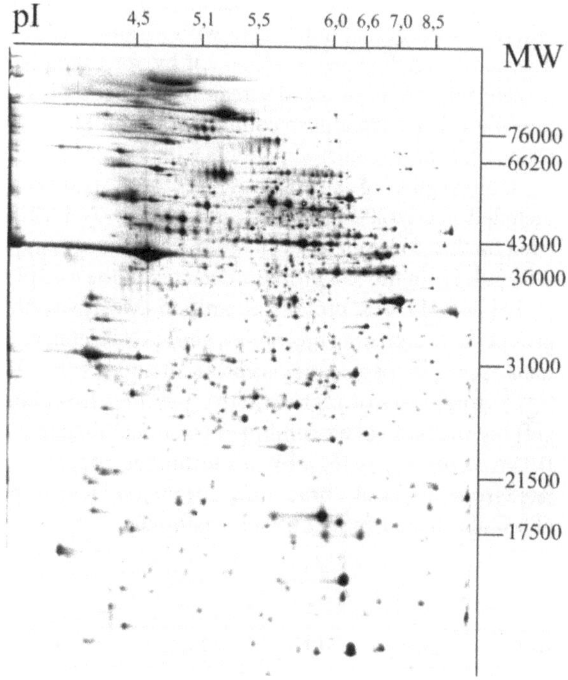

Fig. 13.3. 2-DE of platelet extract from an adult patient with ET [26]

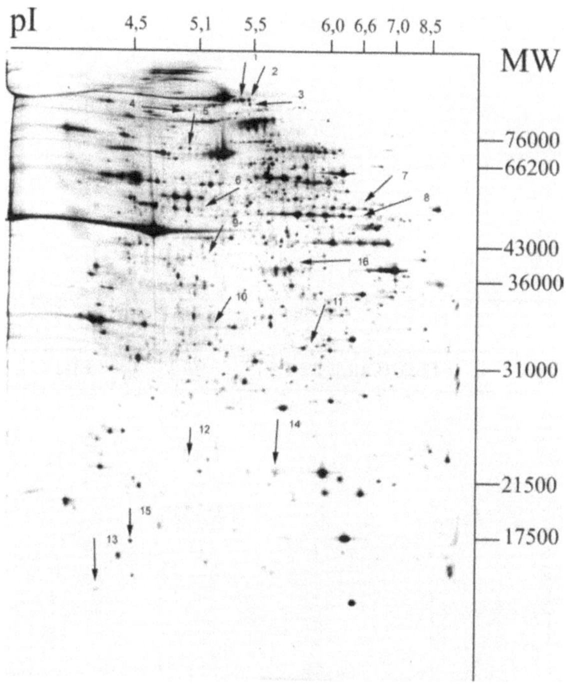

Fig. 13.4. 2-DE of platelet extract of a patient in comparison with control and two other ET patients (*spots 1–16*, see Table 13.2) [26]

These data show that by using this technique, differences in cytosolic platelet proteins among different individuals with ET and in CML with thrombocythemia can be detected. After further development by, for example, fractionation of the complex protein mixture in order to screen for proteins with low abundance or by selecting phosphorylated proteins in combination with ESI-MS, the method is currently being tested on a large cohort of patients with ET [26].

At the beginning of the century a cytosolic platelet proteome was generated which included nearly 200 proteins using MALDI-TOF [27]. Meanwhile the analysis has been further developed to expand the proteome to approximately 2300 protein spots [28–30]. From the 536 proteins detected in the 4–5 pI range, 284 could be identified by ESI-MS/MS. The proteins identified (see at www.bioch.ox.ac.uk/glycob/) can be grouped into signaling molecules, and cytoskeletal, vesicular and mitochondrial proteins as well as membrane receptors and others (Fig. 13.6).

To isolate sets of representative peptides from complex mixtures, a chromatographic method called combined fractional diagonal chromatography (or COFRADIC) was developed [31]. By this technique cysteine-containing peptides can be isolated from the platelet proteome. The method may be particularly useful for peptides of low abundance or hydrophobic peptides.

Table 13.2. Spot differences in 2-DE in three adult patients with ET [26]

Spot	Control	ET-1	ET-2	ET-3
1	–	+	+	+
2	–	+	+	+
3	–	+	–	–
4	–	–	+	–
5	+	+	–	+
6	–	–	–	+
7	+	–	+	+
8	+	–	+	+
9	–	–	–	+
10	–	–	–	+
11	–	–	+	–
12	+	–	+	+
13	+	–	+	+
14	+	–	+	+
15	–	+	+	+
16	+	–	–	–

Table 13.3. 2-DE in one child with thrombocythemia caused by CML versus three adults with ET [26]

Spot	Child (CML)	ET-1	ET-2	ET-3
A	+	–	–	–
B	–	+	+	+
C	+	–	–	–
D	+	–	–	–
E	+	–	–	–
F	+	–	–	–
G	–	+	+	+
H	+	–	–	–
I	+	–	–	–
J	+	–	–	–
K	+	–	–	–
L	+	–	–	–

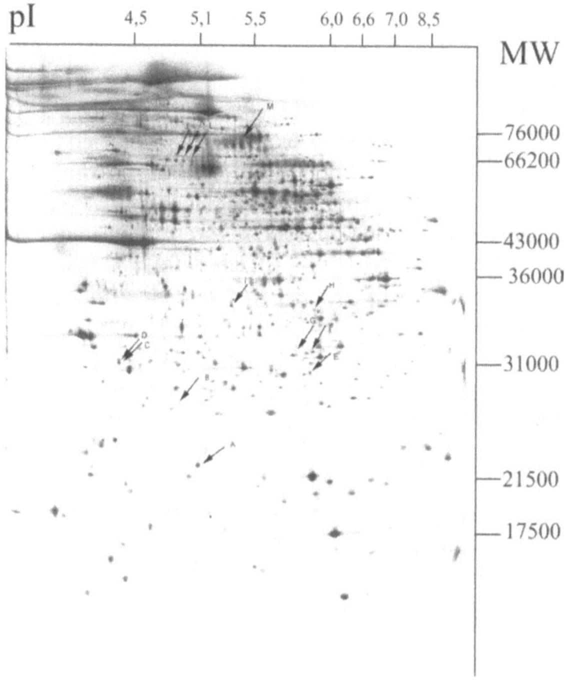

Fig. 13.5. 2-DE of platelet extract of a child with CML and thrombocythemia as compared to three adult ET patients (*spots A to L*, see Table 13.3) [26]

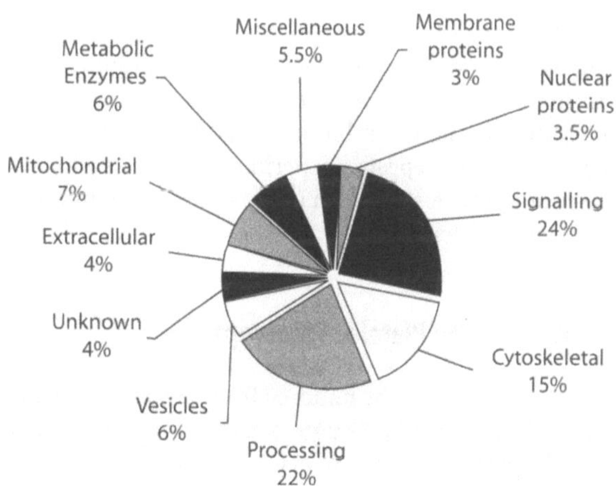

Fig. 13.6. Pie chart representing categories of protein function found in the platelet proteome (4–11 pI range) following 2-DE separation [29]

13.5.3 The Platelet Phosphoproteome

Signaling in platelets is regulated through tyrosine phosphorylation and dephosphorylation which is triggered by the various stages of platelet activation. By proteomic analysis these events can be further dissected. Either by prelabeling with 32P-orthophosphate or by the use of phosphotyrosine antibodies [27, 32], phosphorylation of specific proteins can be studied.

In addition, the phosphorylation events which take place during platelet activation (or possibly constitutively in ET) can be subjected to analysis. Maguire et al. [33] have studied proteins phosphorylated on their tyrosine residues after stimulation of the platelets with thrombin. Tyrosine phosphorylated proteins from both quiescent and thrombin-activated platelets were prefractionated with a monoclonal phosphotyrosine antibody and then subjected to 2-DE analysis. When the gels from quiescent and activated platelets were compared, more than 60 additional spots became apparent in the platelet proteome after thrombin activation.

13.5.4 The Platelet Secreteome

Upon activation, platelets secrete a variety of different molecules which act upon other cells (paracrine regulation) or upon the platelet itself (autocrine regulation). These molecules are stored in α-granules (cationic proteins, coagulation factors, glycoproteins, PDGF, TGF-β), dense granules (ADP, ATP, serotonin) and lysosomes (acid hydrolases). Upon activation granules move to the cell membrane, fuse and release their contents in the external space.

To study the proteins released by the platelet after activation (the secreteome) platelets can be stimulated with thrombin [34, 35] or thrombin receptor activated peptide (TRAP) [36]. The supernatant can either be subjected to 2-DE or after digestion with trypsin the resulting peptides may be separated by cation exchange chromatography and reverse-phase chromatography and subsequently introduced into an ion trap mass spectrometer. Using this approach more than 300 proteins were identified in the thrombin-activated platelet secreteome. Of these, 82 were consistently found in repeated experiments, 40% of which were already known and 60% were not previously known (such as secretogranin III, cyclophilin, calumenin) to be present in platelets.

13.6 Analysis of the Platelet Transcriptome

Platelets are formed by budding from megakaryocytes from which they take over the cytosolic contents. Although platelets do not have a nucleus they still contain mRNA and the protein translation machinery which can be turned on upon activation of the platelet. When RNA is isolated from platelet preparations and hybridized to Affimetrix oligonucleotide arrays, nearly 3000 distinct messages can be identified [37, 38]. When the platelet transcriptome is compared with the proteome there is a good correlation: about two-thirds of secreted proteins are detectable at the mRNA level. In addition, messages for proteins not previously reported can be detected. Some may represent residual megakaryocyte messages (and therefore reveal some information on this precursor cell), but many of the previously unreported genes are expressed in platelets. Despite the absence of gene transcription the platelet proteome is mirrored in the transcriptome.

13.7 Gene Expression Profiling in CD34 Derived Megakaryocytes

In addition, first gene expression profiling studies have been performed with CD34 derived megakaryocytes from normal individuals and patients with ET: proapoptotic genes such as BAX, BNIP3 and BNIP3L are down regulated in ET megakaryocytes together with genes which are components of the mitochondrial pereability transition pore complex which is pivotal for apoptosis. On the other hand antiapoptotic genes such as the IGF-I receptor, CFLAR or the SDF1-gene are upregulated [39].

13.8 Summary

Recent advances in proteomics and genomics have paved the ground for a more holistic analysis of the platelet biology under normal and pathological conditions. The ability to analyze the protein composition inside and outside the platelet (secreteome) under quiescent and activated conditions and to combine these data with the transcriptome will allow, in the future, disease-relevant proteins and genes (contributing to thromboembolic complications or marking the disease) also to be identified in ET. The technical advances outlined here have meanwhile also been applied to other fields in hematology [40, 41].

References

1. Schafer AI (1984) Bleeding and thrombosis in the myeloproliferative disorders. Blood 64:1–12
2. Regev A, Stark P, Blickstein D, Lahav M (1997) Thrombotic complications in ET with relatively low platelet counts. Am J Hematol 56:168–172
3. Virchow R (1856) Gesammelte Abhandlungen zur wissenschaftlichen Medizin. Meringer, Frankfurt, p.219
4. Blann AD, Lip GYH (2001) Virchow's triad revisited; the importance of soluble coagulation factors, the endothelium and platelets. Thromb Res 101:321–327
5. Afshar-Kharghan V, Lopez JA, Gray LA, et al (2004) Hemostatic gene polymorphisms and the prevalence of thrombotic complications in PV and ET. Blood Coagul Fibrinolysis 15:21–24
6. Ruggeri M, Gisslinger H, Tosetto A, et al (2002) Factor V Leiden mutation carriership and venous thromboembolism in PV and ET. Am J Hematol 71:1–6
7. Gisslinger H (2003) personal communication
8. Jensen MK, deNully Brown P, Thorsen S, Hasselbalch HC (2002) Frequent occurrence of anticardiolipin antibodies, factor V Leiden mutation and perturbed endothelial function in chronic myeloproliferative disorders. Am J Hematol 69:185–191
9. Faurschou, M, Nielsen, OJ, Jensen MK, Hasselbalch HC (2000) High prevalence of hyperhomocysteinemia due to marginal deficiency of cobalamin or folate in chronic myeloproliferative disorders. Am J Hematol 65:136–140
10. Gisslinger H, Rodeghiero F, Ruggeri M, et al (1999) Homocysteine levels in polycythemia vera and essential thrombocythemia. Br J Haematol 105:551–555
11. Falanga A, Marchetti M, Evangelista V, et al (2000) Polymorphonuclear leukocyte activation and hemostasis in patients with ET and PV. Blood 96:4261–4266
12. Stroncek DF, Caruccio L, Bettinotti M (2004) CD 177: a member of the Ly-6 gene superfamily involved with neutrophil proliferation and polycythemia vera. J Translational Med 2:8–18
13. Griesshammer M, Klippel S, Strunck E, et al (2004) PRV-1 mRNA expression discriminates two types of essential thrombocythemia. Ann Hematol 83:364–370
14. Freedman JE, Loscalzo J (2002) Platelet-monocyte aggregates: bridging thrombosis and inflammation. Circulation 105:2130–2132

15. Jensen MK, deNully Brown, Lund BV, et al (2001) Increased circulating platelet-leukocyte aggregates in myeloproliferative disorders is correlated to previous thrombosis, platelet activation and platelet count. Eur J Hematol 66:143–151
16. Kaplar M, Kappelmayr J, Kiss A, Szabo K, Udvardy M (2000) Increased leukocyte platelet adhesion in chronic myeloproliferative disorders with high platelet counts. Platelets 11:183–184
17. Villmow, T, Kemkes-Matthes B, Matzdorff AC (2003) Markers of platelet activation and platelet-leukocyte interaction in patients with myeloproliferative syndromes. Thromb Res 108:139–145
18. Musolino C, Calabro L, Bellomo G, et al (2002) Soluble angiogenic factors: implications for chronic myeloproliferative disorders. Am J Hematol 69:159–163
19. Musolino C, Alonci A, Bellomo G, et al (2000) Markers of endothelial and platelet status in patients with ET and PV. Hematology 4:397–402
20. O'Donnell CJ, Larson MG, Fen D, et al (2001) Genetic and environmental contributions to platelet aggregation: the Framingham heart study. Circulation 103:3051–3056
21. Frenkel, EP, Mammen EF (2003) Sticky platelet syndrome and thrombocythemia. Hematol Oncol Clin N Am 17:63–83
22. Giometti CS, Anderson NG (1984) Protein changes in activated human platelets. Clin Chem 30:2078–2083
23. Hanash SM, Neel JV, Baier LJ, et al (1986) Genetic analysis of 33 platelet polypeptides: detection in two dimensional polyacrylamide gels. Am J Hum Genet 38:352–360
24. Gravel P, Sanchez JC, Walzer C, et al (1995) Human blood platelet protein map established by two dimensional polyacrylamide gel electrophoresis. Electrophoresis 16:1152–1159
25. Gevaert K, Eggermont L, Demol H, Vandekerckhove J (2000) A fast and convenient MALDI-MS based proteomic approach: identification of components scaffolded by the actin cytoskeleton of activated human thrombocytes. J Biotechnol 78:259–269
26. Petrides PE, Seidemann B, Wittmann-Liebold B (unpublished) Platelet proteomics in patients with primary thrombocythemia
27. Marcus K, Immler D, Sternberger J, Meyer HE (2000) Identification of platelet proteins separated by two dimensional gel electrophoresis and analyzed by matrix assisted laser desorption/ionisation time of flight mass spectrometry and detection of tyrosine phosphorylated proteins. Electrophoresis 21:2622–2636
28. Bruschi M, Musante L, Candiano G, et al (2003) Soft immobilized pH gradient gels in proteome analysis: a follow up. Proteomics 3:821–825
29. O'Neill EE, Brock CJ, von Kriegsheim AF, et al (2002) Towards complete analysis of the platelet proteome. Proteomics 2:288–305
30. Garcia A, Prabhakar S, Brock CJ, et al (2004) Extensive analysis of the human platelet proteome by two dimensional gel electrophoresis and mass spectroscopy. Proteomics 4:656–668
31. Gevaert K, Ghesquire B, Staes A, et al (2004) Reversible labeling of cysteine containing peptides allows their specific chromatographic isolation for non gel proteomic studies. Proteomics 4:897–908
32. Immler D, Gremm D, Kirsch D, et al (1998) Identification of phosphorylated proteins from thrombin-activated human platelets by two-dimensional gel electrophoresis by electrospray ionization-tandem mass spectrometry (ESI-MS/MS) and liquid chromatography electrospray ionization mass spectrometry (LC-ESI-MS). Electrophoresis 19:1015–1023
33. Maguire PB, Wynne KJ, Harney DF, et al (2002) Identification of the phosphotyrosine proteome from thrombin activated platelets. Proteomics 2:642–648
34. Maguire PB, Fitzgerald DJ (2003) Platelet proteomics. J Thromb Haemost 1:1593–1601
35. Coppinger JA, Cagney G, Toomey S, et al (2004) Characterization of the proteins released from activated platelets leads to localization of novel platelet proteins in human atherosclerotic lesions. Blood 103:2096–2104
36. Garcia A, Pradbhakar S, Hughan S, et al (2004) Differential proteome analysis of TRAP-activated platelets: involvement of DOK-2 and phosphorylation of RGS proteins. Blood 103:2088–2095
37. Gnatenko DV, Dunn JJ, McCorkle SR, et al (2003) Transcript profiling of human platelets using microarray and serial analysis of gene expression. Blood 101:2285–2293
38. McRedmond JP, Park SD, Reilly DF, et al (2004) Integration of proteomics and genomics in platelets: a profile of platelet proteins and platelet specific genes. Mol Cell Proteomics 3:133–144
39. Tenedini E, Fagioli ME, Vianelli N, Tazzari PL, Ricci F, Tagliafico E, Ricci P, Gugliotta L, Martinelli G, Tura S, Baccarini M, Ferrari S, Catani L (2004) Gene expression profiling of normal and malignant CD34-derived megakaryocytic cells. Blood, in press
40. Seshi B (2004) Proteomics knocks on hematology's door. Blood 103:3607
41. Cristea IM, Gaskell SJ, Whetton AD (2004) Proteomics techniques and their application to haematology. Blood 103:3624–3634

Chapter 14

Clonality Studies in Essential Thrombocythemia

Rosemary E. Gale

14.1 Introduction

Essential thrombocythemia (ET) is a chronic myeloproliferative disorder (cMPD) in which the predominant feature is megakaryocytic hyperplasia with a sustained elevation of the platelet count. Patients may have a prolonged and relatively benign clinical course, with the major complication being thrombotic and hemorrhagic events, but in some patients the disease is progressive, either to one of the other cMPDs (polycythemia vera or myelofibrosis) or to acute leukemia [1]. The Polycythemia Vera Study Group (PVSG) has introduced criteria to discriminate ET from other cMPDs, but there are no specific markers for ET and the diagnosis remains one of exclusion (see Chap. 1). In practice this presents a diagnostic dilemma, in particular as the introduction of automated full blood counting in routine clinical practice has led to the detection of an increasing number of individuals with a thrombocytosis. In addition, with current estimates suggesting that 10% to 25% of the patients may be less than 40 years of age, it is no longer considered to be a disease just of the elderly, and this has important implications for long-term therapy with potentially leukemogenic agents.

ET is traditionally considered to be a clonal disorder originating in a single pluripotent stem cell, and this was thought to be one of the major ways in which it could be discriminated from a secondary or reactive thrombocytosis (RT) which should arise from a polyclonal expansion of many cells. Under ideal circumstances an assay for a clonal population should identify a disease-specific marker such as the t(9;22) chromosomal translocation in chronic myeloid leukemia (CML) which gives rise to the *bcr-abl* fusion transcript. However, karyotypic abnormalities are rare in ET and where found may be a consequence of therapy. For example, one study has shown that many patients with chromosome 17p deletion have been treated with hydroxyurea [2]. Other cancer-associated markers include activation of oncogenes, inactivation of tumor suppressor genes, and microsatellite instability, but none of these has been shown to be a consistent feature of ET. In order to study clonality in ET it has therefore been necessary to use the indirect approach of analyzing X-chromosome inactivation patterns (XCIPs).

14.2 XCIPs: Methods and Interpretation

The principle of random X-chromosome inactivation of one X-chromosome in every mammalian female cell as the mechanism to compensate for the gene dosage from two X-chromosomes was hypothesized by Lyon and exploited by Fialkow as a tool to determine clonality [3]. The method relies on both the ability to distinguish between the two X-chromosome alleles using polymorphic markers, and to determine the relative proportion of inactivation for each allele in a population of cells. This can be achieved at the protein level using phenotypic expression of isoenzymes of glucose-6-phosphate dehydrogenase (G6PD), at the DNA level using differential methylation patterns of X-linked markers such as the restriction enzyme polymorphism in the phosphoglycerate kinase gene or the trinucleotide repeat sequence in the human androgen receptor gene (HUMARA), and at the RNA level using expression of transcripts from polymorphic loci such as the iduronate sulfatase, p55 palmitoylated membrane protein and G6PD genes [4]. Each method has a number of advantages and disadvantages, and both DNA and RNA analyses should be carried out wherever possible. RNA methods are particularly useful in ET to study XCIPs in platelets, but the latter are by nature very sticky and can contaminate (and therefore confound results in) other cell types such as T lymphocytes.

In recent years a number of factors influencing XCIPs have been demonstrated and it is important that they are taken into account when interpreting what the patterns might mean [4]. The first criterion established in earlier studies for defining a clonal population was that it should have >75% expression of one allele [5]. This was an arbitrary rather than an absolute value, and was presumed to indicate divergence from the normal polyclonal pattern which was expected to show approximately 50% expression of each allele, consistent with a random process. However, study of blood cells from hematologically normal females has shown that approximately one-quarter have a pattern which is apparently 'clonal' by this definition. Mathematical modeling of the observed distribution of XCIPs indicates that there are probably six to eight stem cells committed to hematopoiesis at the time of X-chromosome inactivation. Therefore, a skewed or imbalanced XCIP does not always signify a clonal population and it is necessary to use a control tissue from the same individual to determine their constitutive XCIP. This must come from the same embryological origin as the tissue under analysis as XCIPs are tissue-specific, and skin or fibroblasts are not suitable as a control for hematopoietic cells [6]. For ET, T-lymphocytes can be used as the control as they are not thought to be involved in the pathological process, they originate from the same stem cell as myeloid cells, and their XCIPs correlate well with those from neutrophils. We therefore include the requirement that to be clonal a patient must have >20% difference between their neutrophil and T-cell XCIPs, which accommodates technical differences both between and within sample analyses.

A further factor of especial importance to the cMPDs is that a skewed XCIP of myeloid cells can be acquired with increasing age, and extreme skewing with >90% expression of one allele is common in elderly females (33%) compared to younger females (3%) [4]. The effect on XCIPs is not generally apparent until the seventh decade, but longitudinal analyses in cats and studies of women aged 73 to 101 years have suggested that the process is progressive [7, 8]. Furthermore, there may be a genetic component which causes gradual selection of stem cells expressing one X-chromosome [8, 9]. To exclude age-related skewing we have therefore introduced a third specification that, to be classified as having clonal myelopoiesis, a patient must be 65 years or less.

14.3 Clonality Results in ET Patients

Several studies of XCIP analysis in ET patients have been reported but only recent studies can be adequately evaluated with respect to constitutive and age-related skewing. If the criteria defined above are applied, then results of neutrophil XCIPs from four such studies suggest that ET is a heterogeneous disorder [10–13] (Table 14.1). Many patients do have a clonal disorder as expected, but approximately one-half of the patients evidently have polyclonal myelopoiesis, even though they fulfill all the current PVSG criteria for a diagnosis of ET. Typical XCIPs from our patients are shown in Fig. 14.1 and results from 31 patients in Fig. 14.2. These results raise a number of issues, in particular whether the underlying pathologies and clinical courses of the two groups of patients are different, and whether they represent a varying spectrum of the same disease or are different diseases.

14.4 Issues Raised by Clonality Results

Lineage Restriction. Some patients may appear to have polyclonal myelopoiesis because their clonality is restricted to the megakaryocytic lineage. This can be studied using platelet RNA and megakaryocytic DNA, and results to date suggest that it is an infrequent event. In one study of ten patients with polyclonal granulocytes, three had clonal platelets [10]; in two other studies no such patients were found out of 17 analyzed [11, 12]. This issue requires further examination in larger studies.

Table 14.1. XCIP studies of neutrophils in ET patients, excluding all patients with constitutive and age-related skewing

Reference	No. of patients	Clonal hematopoiesis	Polyclonal hematopoiesis
[10]	31	17 (55%)	14 (45%)
[11]	23	10 (43%)	13 (57%)
[12]	32	17 (53%)	15 (47%)
[13]	48	33 (69%)	15 (31%)
Total	134	77 (57%)	57 (43%)

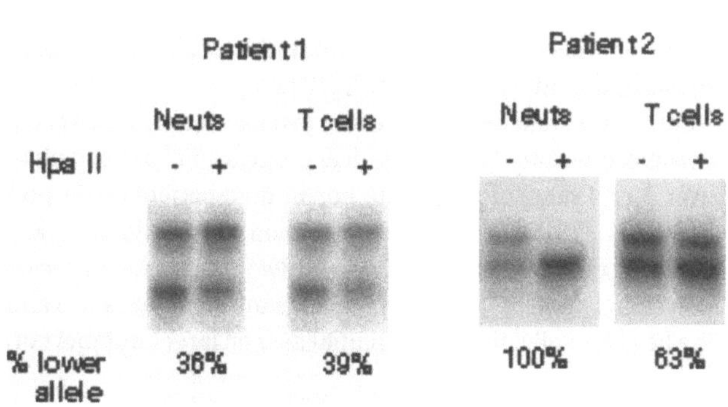

Fig. 14.1. Representative XCIPs using the HUMARA assay on DNA from neutrophils (*Neuts*) and T cells of patients with polyclonal (*patient 1*) and clonal (*patient 2*) myelopoiesis. Digests in the absence of *HpaII* (–) show the size of the two X-chromosome alleles, and in the presence of *HpaII* (+) show the relative expression of the two alleles

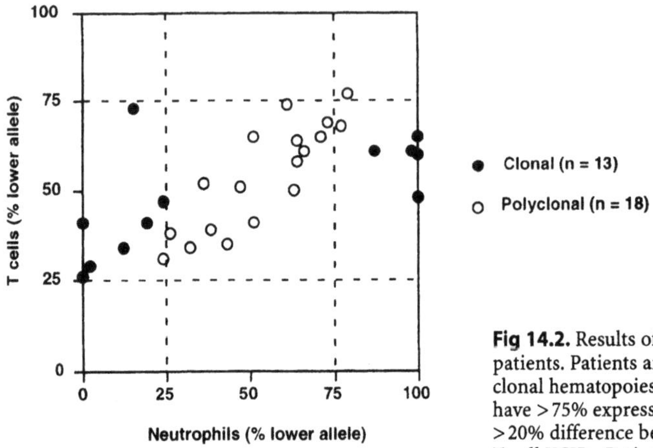

Fig 14.2. Results of XCIPs in 31 ET patients. Patients are defined as having clonal hematopoiesis (*closed circles*) if they have >75% expression of one allele and >20% difference between neutrophil and T-cell XCIPs. Patients with polyclonal hematopoiesis (*open circles*) have 75% expression of one allele in at least one sample and <20% difference between the two samples. One patient had >75% expression in both samples but RNA results indicated she had polyclonal hematopoiesis

Disease Progression. It is possible that polyclonal myelopoiesis represents the preliminary disease phase which only progresses to clonal disease with the acquisition of a pathogenic alteration providing the cell with a growth or survival advantage. For example, in the mouse model of polycythemia, infection with the spleen focus forming virus causes a polyclonal erythrocytosis which requires a further 'hit' to transform to leukemia [14]. XCIP analysis is not a sensitive technique, and a balanced, apparently polyclonal pattern could obscure the presence of a minor clone of cells. If the growth advantage is small it might be many years before such a clone becomes evident. At present there is only anecdotal evidence in small numbers of patients to examine these issues. It is probable that at least some patients present with clonal myelopoiesis as a significant number have been reported with a clonal XCIP within 1 year of diagnosis [10–12], although this does not exclude the possibility of an asymptomatic polyclonal disease phase. Furthermore, many of the patients reported with a polyclonal pattern were tested more than 3 years after diagnosis, suggesting that they are unlikely to have a slowly emerging clone [10–13].

A related issue is whether it is patients with clonal disease who are more likely to progress to myelofibrosis or acute leukemia. Again, information on this is limited and is confounded by the possibility of therapy-induced transformation from potentially leukemogenic agents. Two patients we studied with monoclonal myelopoiesis had myelofibrosis at the time of their first XCIP analysis, one of these acquired a trisomy chromosome 9 and transformed to acute myeloid leukemia (AML), and the other developed chromosome 20q- [11]. No clinical progression has been observed in six clonal patients over 3 or 4 years of follow-up, nor in nine patients with polyclonal disease. Similarly, Shih et al. [13] observed transformation to AML in one patient treated with busulfan, and progression to myelofibrosis in two patients with a clonal XCIP but none with a polyclonal pattern. These numbers are too small to draw valid conclusions and indicate the need for collection of sequential data on larger numbers of patients over many years.

Presence of Polyclonal Progenitors in Clonal Disease. It is unclear whether normal polyclonal progenitor cells remain in patients with clonal disease but are suppressed within the marrow environment. For example, in CML the presence of polyclonal CD34+ cells can be demonstrated, at least in the early stages of chronic disease, and can be used for autologous transplantation [15]. To date, XCIP studies of purified progenitor cells from ET patients have suggested that neutrophil XCIPs reflect the pattern in the earliest detectable stem cells [11, 12]. In addition, infusion of CD34+ cells from four ET patients into NOD/SCID mice reproduced the same XCIP in the mice as in the patient [16]. There is also no evidence to date that treatment restores polyclonal hematopoiesis in clonal ET patients. A number of the patients reported with a clonal XCIP had been treated with interferon or hydroxyurea at the time of testing [10–12], and Sacchi et al. [17] studied 11 patients before and after 6 months of interferon and observed no change in XCIPs.

Clinical Implications of Clonality. Comparison of clinical characteristics between clonal and polyclonal patients have shown that they do not differ with respect to age, platelet count, splenomegaly or incidence of hemorrhage. However, patients with polyclonal disease may have a decreased risk of thrombosis. In three different studies, thrombotic events were observed in 2/13 (15%), 1/15 (7%) and 1/15 (7%) polyclonal patients, respectively, compared to 6/10 (60%), 7/17 (41%) and 11/33 (33%) clonal patients [11–13]. These results are preliminary but have important implications for the stratification of patients and prospective use of therapy. For example, in one retrospective analysis, polyclonal patients were found to have received less cytoreductive therapy [18].

14.5 Analysis of Mutations in Candidate Cytokine/Cytokine Receptor Genes

Thrombopoietin (TPO). The primary regulator of megakaryocyte/platelet production is now known to be TPO [19]. It is constitutively synthesized, and circulating levels are thought to be controlled by megakaryocyte/platelet mass. However, in ET patients TPO levels are generally normal or even increased. Recent studies have shown that normal TPO production is suppressed at the level of translation, and four different point mutations in the 5′ regulatory region of the TPO gene have been described in families with hereditary thrombocytosis [20]. They lead to increased TPO levels and thrombocytosis by reducing the suppression of translation. The acquisition of such mutations could therefore cause or contribute to the thrombocytosis in ET, particularly in patients with polyclonal myelopoiesis. Until recently, no such mutations had been detected [21,22]. In 2004, however, Moliterno and colleagues described a thrombopoietin receptor polymorphism (G1283T or K39N, resp.) which is restricted to African Americans and designated Mpl Baltimore. The polymorphism appears to conform to a pattern of autosomal dominance with incomplete penetrance in that some heterozygotes have normal platelet counts whereas others have elevations of platelet counts that satisfy cMPD diagnostic criteria [23].

Transforming Growth Factor β (TGFβ). Several lines of evidence have indicated that TGFβ is involved in the regulation of megakaryopoiesis and may contribute to the pathogenesis of ET. Megakaryocytic progenitors in ET patients show a reduced in vitro sensitivity to the inhibitory effect of TGFβ [24], and potentially pathogenic mutations of the TGFβ receptor type II (TGFβRII) gene have been reported in a few patients [25]. Since abnormalities in this gene are a feature of solid tumors [26], it is a suitable candidate for a tumor marker in ET patients with clonal disease. We therefore screened neutrophil DNA from ET patients for mutations in the TGFβRII kinase domain using SSCP analysis [27]. One heterozygous amino acid substitution, Ser553Thr, was detected in 3/60 patients (5%) which might influence kinase activity as the receptor is known to autophosphorylate on several serine residues. However, the same heterozygous substitution was identified in 3/146 normal controls (2%), and the hematologically normal daughter of one ET patient was homozygous for the alteration, indicating that it is unlikely to be of pathological significance.

14.6 Conclusions

The use of XCIP analysis to study hematopoiesis in ET patients has demonstrated that this is a biologically heterogeneous disorder. The usefulness of this approach is limited, as in general it can only be applied to younger females, but the ability to detect potentially different subgroups of patients may serve as a tool to identify more specific disease markers which can then be extended to all patients.

References

1. Murphy S (1999) Diagnostic criteria and prognosis in polycythemia vera and essential thrombocythemia. Semin Hematol 36 [Suppl 2]:9–13
2. Sterkers Y, Preudhomme C, Lai J-L, Demory J-L, Caulier M-T, Wattel E, Bordessoule D, Bauters F, Fenaux P (1998) Acute myeloid leukemia and myelodysplastic syndromes following essential thrombocythemia treated with hydroxyurea: high proportion of cases with 17p deletion. Blood 91:616–622
3. Fialkow PJ (1972) Use of genetic markers to study cellular origin of development of tumors in human females. Adv Cancer Res 15:191–226
4. Gale RE (1999) Evaluation of clonality in myeloid stem-cell disorders. Semin Hematol 36:361–372
5. Vogelstein B, Fearon ER, Hamilton SR, Preisinger AC, Willard HF, Michelson AM, Riggs AD, Orkin SH (1987) Clonal analysis using recombinant DNA probes from the X-chromosome. Cancer Res 47:4806–4813
6. Gale RE, Wheadon H, Boulos P, Linch DC (1994) Tissue specificity of X-chromosome inactivation patterns. Blood 83:2899–2905
7. Abkowitz JL, Catlin SN, Guttorp P (1996) Evidence that hematopoiesis may be a stochastic process in vivo. Nat Med 2:190–197
8. Christensen K, Kristiansen M, Hagen-Larsen H, Skytthe A, Bathum L, Jeune B, Andersen-Ranberg K, Vaupel JW, Orstavik KH (2000) X-linked genetic factors regulate hematopoietic stem-cell kinetics in females. Blood 95:2449–2451
9. Abkowitz JL, Taboada M, Shelton GH, Catlin SN, Guttorp P, Kiklevich JV (1998) An X chromosome gene regulates hematopoietic stem cell kinetics. Proc Natl Acad Sci U S A 95:3862–3866
10. El-Kassar N, Hetet G, Briere J, Grandchamp B (1997) Clonality analysis of hematopoiesis in essential thrombocythaemia: advantages of studying T lymphocytes and platelets. Blood 89:128–134
11. Harrison CN, Gale RE, Machin SJ, Linch DC (1999) A large proportion of patients with a diagnosis of essential thrombocythemia do not have a clonal disorder and may be at lower risk of thrombotic complications. Blood 93:417–424
12. Chiusolo P, Ortu La Barbera E, Laurenti L, Piccirillo N, Sora F, Giordano G, Urbano R, Mazzucconi MG, De Stefano V, Leone G, Sica S (2001) Clonal hemopoiesis and risk of thrombosis in young female patients with essential thrombocythemia. Exp Hematol 29:670–676

13. Shih L-Y, Lin T-L, Lai C-L, Dunn P, Wu P-N, Kuo M-C, Lee L-C (2002) Predictive values of X-chromosome inactivation patterns and clinicohematologic parameters for vascular complications in female patients with essential thrombocythemia. Blood 100:1596–1601
14. Hankins WD, Troxler D (1980) Polycythemia- and anemia-inducing erythroleukemia viruses exhibit differential erythroid transforming effects in vitro. Cell 22:693–699
15. Delforge M, Boogaerts MA, McGlave PB, Verfaillie CM (1999) BCR/ABL–CD34+HLA-DR– progenitor cells in early chronic phase, but not in more advanced phases, of chronic myelogenous leukemia are polyclonal. Blood 93:284–292
16. Gale RE, Ings S, Harrison CN, Linch DC (unpublished observations)
17. Sacchi S, Gugliotta L, Papineschi F, Liberati AM, Rupoli S, Delfini C, Ruggeri M, Cavanna L, Bucalossi A, Benedetti E, Ferrandina C, Vinci G, Morselli M, Torelli G (1998) Alfa-interferon in the treatment of essential thrombocythemia: clinical results and evaluation of its biological effects on the hematopoietic neoplastic clone. Italian Cooperative Group on ET. Leukemia 12:289–294
18. Briere J, Guilmin F, Chait Y, Kiladjian JJ, Gardin C, Elkassar N, Grandchamp B (1999) Is clonality status of young females with essential thrombocythaemia (ET) a reliable parameter for indication of cytoreductive treatment. Blood 94 [Suppl 1]:111a
19. Kaushansky K, Drachman JG (2002) The molecular and cellular biology of thrombopoietin: the primary regulator of platelet production. Oncogene 21:3359–3367
20. Cazzola M, Skoda RC (2000) Translational pathophysiology: a novel molecular mechanism of human disease. Blood 95:3280–3288
21. Harrison CN, Gale RE, Wiestner AC, Skoda RC, Linch DC (1998) The activating splice mutation in intron 3 of the thrombopoietin gene is not found in patients with non-familial essential thrombocythaemia. Br J Haematol 102:1341–1343
22. Allen AJR, Gale RE, Harrison CN, Machin SJ, Linch DC (2001) Lack of pathogenic mutations in the 5′-untranslated region of the thrombopoietin gene in patients with non-familial essential thrombocythaemia. Eur J Hematol 67:232–237
23 Moliterno AR, Williams DM, Gutierrez-Alamillo LI, Salvatori R, Ingersoll RG, Spivak JL (2004) Mpl Baltimore: A thrombopoietin receptor polymorphism associated with thrombocytosis. Proc Natl Acad Sci 101: 11444–11447
24. Zauli G, Catani L, Gugliotta L, Gaggioli L, Vitale L, Belmonte MM, Aglietta M, Bagnara GP (1991) Essential thrombocythemia: impaired regulation of megakaryocyte progenitors. Int J Cell Cloning 9:43–56
25. Niitsu Y, Sakamaki S, Kuroda H, Matsunaga T, Hirayama Y, Kusakabe T, Akiyama T, Sasaki K (1998) Mutation of the type II TGF-b receptor gene in patients with essential thrombocythemia may cause an escape from suppression of megakaryopoiesis by TGF-β. Blood 92 [Suppl 1]:422a
26. Grady WM, Myeroff LL, Swinler SE, Rajput A, Thiagalingam S, Lutterbaugh JD, Neumann A, Brattain MG, Chang J, Kim SJ, Kinzler KW, Vogelstein B, Willson JK, Markowitz S (1999) Mutational inactivation of transforming growth factor beta receptor type II in microsatellite stable colon cancers. Cancer Res 59:320–324
27. Sud R, Gale RE, Harrison CN, Machin SJ, Linch DC (2000) Mutations in the TGFβRII gene are unlikely to be responsible for the reduced sensitivity to TGFβ in megakaryocytes from patients with essential thrombocythaemia. Blood 96 [Suppl 1]:743a

Chapter 15

Molecular and Preclinical Aspects of Anagrelide Action

Petro E. Petrides

15.1 Introduction

Anagrelide is the most important contribution to the therapeutic options in the Ph-negative cMPDs over the last decade. The substance belongs to the group of imidazole(2,1-b)chinazoline-2-compounds (Fig. 15.1). Anagrelide, which is orally bioavailable, has a relatively poor solubility in water.

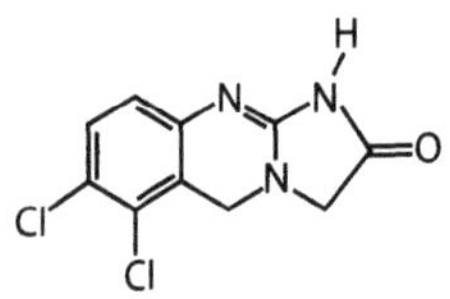

Fig. 15.1. Structural formula of anagrelide

Initially on the basis of in vitro investigations an antiaggregating activity on platelets was attributed to the substance. Thereafter, experiments in humans showed, however, that anagrelide under in vivo conditions has only limited influence on platelet function but rapidly lowers platelet counts. This caused the initiation of a series of clinical studies which led to the approval of the substance in the US and Canada under the name Agrylin (Shire Pharmaceuticals, USA), in Switzerland under the name Xagrid and in several countries of the European community under the name Thromboreductin (AOP Pharmaceuticals, Austria). A comprehensive review of its clinical efficacy has recently been published [1].

15.2 Platelet-Antiaggregating Properties in Animals and Humans

In 1979 an antiaggregating activity of anagrelide in experimental animals (Rhesus monkeys, rats, rabbits and dogs) was observed. Under in vitro conditions the substance inhibited in a dose-dependent manner the ADP and collagen-induced aggregation of platelets in platelet-rich plasma [2].

The same activity was also present in humans [3–5]. Under these experimental conditions the activity of anagrelide, and also that of its metabolites (see below) which can be generated under the influence of enzymes in plasma, platelets and other blood cells, can be tested. Biologically active metabolites, which are possibly produced in intestinal or hepatic metabolic pathways, are not recognized in this assay.

Platelet function can be regulated through the intracellular turnover of cyclic nucleotides which is determined by adenylcyclases and phosphodiesterases. Physio-

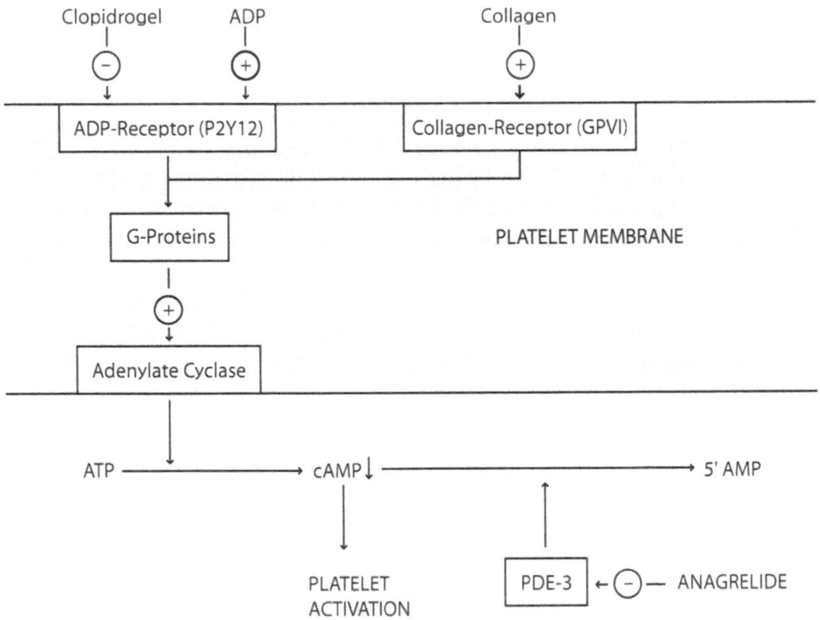

Fig. 15.2. Mechanism of anagrelide upon platelets

logical platelet antagonists as well as various vasodilators inhibit platelet function by activating adenyl and guanyl cyclases thereby increasing intraplatelet cAMP and cGMP levels. This elevation interferes with basically all known platelet-activating signal pathways and blocks intracellular signaling networks, cytoskeletal rearrangements and fibrinogen receptor activation [6–9]. Target molecules of cyclic nucleotides are cAMP- or cGMP-dependent protein kinases which mediate their effects through phosphorylation of specific substrates.

Anagrelide inhibits platelet function by inhibiting a type 3 phosphodiesterase [10, 11] with a subsequent increase in cAMP (Fig. 15.2).

The effects of anagrelide on the aggregation of platelets have also been observed with aggregometric measurements after the oral intake of daily total dosages of 6 or 8 mg in human volunteers [12]. Anagrelide also inhibits the release of arachidonic acid metabolites from human platelets after stimulation with thrombin [13].

When tested on whole blood or platelet-rich plasma of patients with myeloproliferative disorders anagrelide did not, however, change the spontaneous or induced platelet aggregation [14]. Moreover, in vivo platelet function is also not influenced since the bleeding time measured after 4 to 10 days treatment with anagrelide (daily dosage 4–6 mg) is not changed [14]. However, this observation does not rule out the possibility that the effects of anagrelide only become clinically visible when anagrelide is combined with other substances that affect platelets (e.g., aspirin, clopidogrel).

15.3 Platelet-Lowering Effects in Humans

In humans, but not in experimental animals, anagrelide causes a decrease in the platelet count [15–18]. In cell culture the action is also species-specific. Anagrelide inhibits the maturation and thereby the size and ploidy of megakaryocytes [19–21]. This activity is not mediated through the phosphodiesterase system; the underlying molecular mechanism is under investigation (see below). In a double-blind study in 15 healthy volunteers (5 probands on placebo, and 5 each on 1 and 2 mg anagrelide), besides the platelet count decrease, a slight shortening of the platelet survival time was observed (from 8.4 to 7.8 days). Effects on prothrombin time, partial thromboplastin time, bleeding time, hemoglobin, reticulocytes, leukocytes and differential were not seen [14].

Because of the short half-life of anagrelide an increase in the platelet count with an overshoot is observed about 4 to 8 days after discontinuation of the drug.

15.4 In Vivo Activities of Anagrelide in Patients with Thrombocythemias

Bellucci et al. [22] observed an increase in the platelet volume in three patients with primary thrombocythemia. Such an effect cannot be observed upon treatment with hydroxyurea or interferon-α. Membrane protein glycoprotein IV (CD36) which was elevated in the platelets of the patients remained elevated after normalization of their platelet count. In addition, the absence of aggregation induced by epinephrine or the presence of an abnormal thrombospondin band were not eliminated upon anagrelide treatment. From these observations the authors concluded that anagrelide effectively lowers the platelet count but does not cause functional or biochemical alterations to the platelets. This could explain a residual risk for thromboembolic complications upon anagrelide therapy (see below).

Lev et al. [23] in 16 patients with primary thrombocythemia investigated the plasma concentration of various cytokines (TGFβ, PDGF, bFGF) before therapy and after normalization of the platelet count. The plasma levels of all three cytokines were elevated in all patients. After normalization of the platelet count, the plasma levels of TGFβ and bFGF remained elevated, which indicates a participation of these cytokines in the development of primary thrombocythemia. The concentrations of these mediators within the platelets were normal (TGFβ), elevated (bFGF) or diminished (PDGF).

Laguna et al. [24] analyzed the plasma levels of thromboxane B2 and PDGF in 17 patients with primary thrombocythemia. The levels of thromboxane were elevated and normalized under therapy. PDGF levels, however, were diminished but not influenced by therapy with anagrelide.

Tomer [25] investigated in vivo megakaryocytopoiesis in patients with primary thrombocythemia under therapy with anagrelide. Megakaryocytopoiesis in the bone marrow was quantified by flow cytometry. During therapy the number of megakaryocytes [identified through the lineage marker CD41 (GPIIb)] diminished in the bone marrow, and their diameter decreased from 46 to 40 μm, their volume from 48 to 34×10^3 μm^3, and their ploidy from 32 N (with some 64 and 128 forms) to the nor-

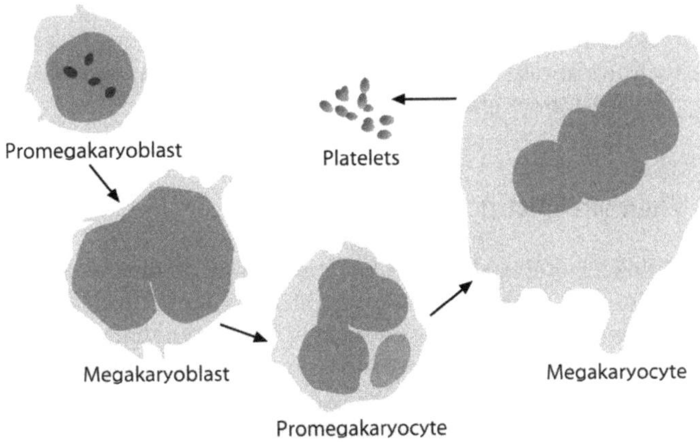

Fig. 15.3. The promegakaryoblast is the first morphologically recognizable megakaryocyte precursor in the bone marrow. Megakaryoblasts have a diameter of 15–50 μm and large oval nuclei (with two sets of chromosomes = 4N) and a basophil cytoplasm without granules. Promegakaryocytes are 20–80 μm in diameter and possess developing granules. Megakaryocytes are up to 150 μm in diameter, undergo endomitosis and become polyploid through repetitive DNA replications without cell division. Most megakaryocytes have eight sets of chromosomes (= 16N). Cytokines such as interleukin-3 and thrombopoietin participate in the development of the megakaryocytes

mal 16N ploidy. Thereby the total megakaryocyte mass was reduced by 66% which correlated with the decrease in platelet count. These results confirmed the observations in cell culture (see above) in which anagrelide decreased the platelet level by inhibition of the hyperproliferation and differentiation of megakaryocytes.

Thiele and coworkers [26, 27] investigated megakaryocytopoiesis in ten patients with idiopathic myelofibrosis (IMF) and five patients with primary thrombocythemia using immunohistochemical and morphometric methods (using the differentiation marker CD61a). According to these authors the reduction in megakaryocytopoiesis by anagrelide was due to a specific arrest in the development of megakaryopoiesis with the production of more mature platelet-secreting cellular forms. This led to a significant left shift with an increased presence of diploid 2N-promegakaryoblasts and megakaryoblasts (Fig. 15.3). The total number of all CD61a-positive megakaryocytes was not altered. An effect of anagrelide on the formation of connective tissue fibers in primary thrombocythemia or IMF was not found.

Yoon et al. [28] in a prospective study investigated possible alterations of the bone marrow in patients with IMF under treatment with anagrelide through sequential biopsies. They observed an increase in the megakaryocyte number (identified through the determination of so-called UEA-1 antigens) and a left shift. The concentrations of PDGF and TGFβ were not affected which possibly also explained the missing (inhibiting) influence on fibrosis of the bone marrow (duration of observation up to 4 years).

15.5 Nonhematological Effects

In experimental animals anagrelide has a positive inotropic and vasodilatory effect [29]. This effect is possibly again mediated through a phosphodiesterase 3 which is present in vascular smooth muscle cells. In humans (e.g., patients with myeloproliferative syndromes), the initiation of therapy with anagrelide can cause a decrease in systolic and diastolic blood pressures which under maintenance therapy increase to their initial values. Some of the adverse effects of anagrelide are due to these inotropic/vasodilatory effects [1].

15.6 Pharmacokinetics

Following oral intake of a radioactive (100 µCi of the 14C-labeled substance) test dosage of 1 mg in fasted healthy volunteers, a rapid increase in the anagrelide plasma level was seen with a maximum after 1 hour (3 ng/ml), followed by a relatively rapid decrease within 6 to 8 hours and a slow decrease to about 10% of the maximum value within 24 hours [30]. The estimated terminal elimination half-life was about 3 days. The intake of food slows the resorption of anagrelide with a subsequent prolongation of the plasma half-life. Clinical experience with anagrelide in therapeutic dosages in patients shows, however, that its efficacy is not influenced by food intake.

The excretion of the radioactivity occurred primarily through the kidneys, i.e., within 6 days about 75% of the radioactivity was secreted in the urine and about 10% from the liver through the bile into the feces. At least four different metabolites (two "major" metabolites, 44% and 24% respectively, and two "minor" metabolites, 7% and 2% respectively) were detectable in urine by reverse-phase HPLC (in the original publication, however, no chromatograms were shown), and anagrelide itself represented only 1% of the whole activity excreted in the urine.

There are marked differences between this distribution of urine metabolites and that found in dogs, monkeys and rats. Whereas the total activity in monkeys is similar (64%), it is much lower in dogs and rats (35% and 42% respectively). Moreover, the quantitative distribution is quite different from species to species, which could explain the lack of platelet-reducing activity of anagrelide in animals. It is unknown which of the metabolites still possesses biological activity.

Lane et al. [31] have identified a water-soluble metabolite designated FL603 which does not possess the imidazole side chain and which is much more soluble in water than anagrelide (Fig. 15.4). The report, however, does not contain any information as to whether the metabolite is one of the substances in urine or how the metabolite was isolated. The intraperitoneal injection of FL603 in Balb/c mice caused a dose-dependent decrease of the circulating platelet counts. If the metabolite is active in mice it should normally not be produced in these animals. Under in vitro conditions the metabolite inhibited the replication and maturation of megakaryocytes (with a 50 times higher potency than anagrelide) without influencing the ADP-induced aggregation of platelets.

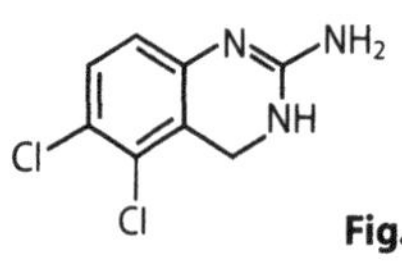

Fig. 15.4. Anagrelide metabolite FL603

Erusalimski et al. [32, 33] questioned the mechanism of action of anagrelide via a human-specific metabolite. These authors were not able to confirm the activity of the substance on megakaryocytes and in mice and showed that FL603 is also present in rats, dogs and rabbits in significant amounts. Hence they favored the hypothesis developed by McCarty which relates the species specificity of anagrelide to the c-mpl, the TPO-receptor which shows only 10% homology between humans and mice. In in vitro experiments anagrelide inhibited the thrombopoietin-stimulated proliferation of megakaryocytes which had been transfected with the human c-mpl receptor but not in those transfected with the mouse gene [34]. Rafil and Lane [35], however, do not accept this argument.

15.7 Summary

Anagrelide is a drug which reduces platelets in a species-specific manner. Despite its clinical efficacy, much has to be learned about its molecular mechanism of action in humans. The understanding of its activity is hampered by the fact that multiple metabolites are produced within the human body. Thus, it is still unclear whether its action on megakaryocytes is mediated through one of these metabolites (FL 603), another metabolite or anagrelide itself. The same is true for side effects observed during treatment (activity on type 3 phosphodiesterases in smooth muscle cells present in peripheral, central or intestinal arteries?). A potential influence on phosphodiesterases in human platelets can also not be ruled out. In view of the remarkable accumulation of knowledge on the signal transduction pathways in platelets, some of the old studies on platelets should be redone with anagrelide and its metabolites.

Since anagrelide and its metabolites can be identified by HPLC [36] and characterized by chromatography/mass spectrometry [37], anagrelide and derivatives have to be determined to provide a better understanding of important questions such as the development of primary resistance to the drug, individual dosage requirements, the metabolism of the drug, and which adverse effects are due to which metabolites.

References

1. Petrides PE (2004) Anagrelide: a decade of clinical experience with its use for the treatment of primary thrombocythemia. Expert Opin Pharmacother 5:1781–1798
2. Fleming JS, Buyniski JP (1979) A new potent inhibitor of platelet aggregation and experimental thrombosis, anagrelide (BL-4162A). Thromb Res 15:373–388
3. Tang SS, Frojmovic MM (1980) Inhibition of platelet function by antithrombotic agents which selectively inhibit low km cyclic AMP phosphodiesterase. J Lab Clin Med 95:241–257
4. Clark WF, Reid BD, Tevaarwerk GJM (1981) Anagrelide: inhibitor of collagen and immune complex induced platelet aggregation and release. Thromb Res 21:215–219
5. Smith JB (1992) Effect of thromboxane synthetase inhibitors on platelet function: enhancement by inhibition of phosphodiesterase. Thromb Res 28:477–485
6. Haslam RJ, Dickinson NT, Jang EK (1999) Cyclic nucleotides and phosphodiesterases. Thromb Haemost 82:412–423
7. Schwarz UR, Walter U, Eigenthaler M (2001) Taming platelets with cyclic nucleotides. Biochem Pharmacol 62:1153–1161
8. Feijge MA, Ansink K, Vanschoonveek K, Heemskerk JW (2004) Control of platelet activation by cyclic AMP turnover and cyclic nucleotide phosphodiesterase type-3. Biochem Pharmacol 67:1559–1567
9. Sim DS, Merrill-Skoloff G, Furie BC, Furie B, Flaumenhaft R (2004) Initial accumulation of platelets during arterial thrombus formation in vivo is inhibited by elevation of basal cAMP levels. Blood 103:2127–2134

10. Seiler S, Arnold AJ, Grove RI, et al (1987) Effects of anagrelide on platelet cAMP levels, cAMP dependent protein kinase and thrombin induced calcium fluxes. J Pharmacol Exp Ther 243:767–774
11. Gillespie E (1988) Anagrelide: a potent and selective inhibitor of platelet cyclic AMP phosphodiesterase enzyme activity. Biochem Pharmacol 37:2866–2868
12. Courtwright WE, Buchanon JO, Fleming JS, Taylor R (1983) The effect of multiple oral doses of anagrelide on ADP and collagen-induced platelet aggregation in normal male subjects. Clin Pharmacol Ther 220
13. Colton DG, Paige JB, Fleming JS, Buyniski JP (1982) Effect of the antithrombotic agent anagrelide (AL) on thrombin-stimulated human platelet arachidonic acid (AA) metabolism. Fed Am Soc Exp Biol (abstract 7557)
14. Balduini CL, Bertolino G., Noris P, Ascari E (1992) Effect of anagrelide on platelet count and function in patients with thrombocytosis and myeloproliferative disorders. Haematologica 77:40–43
15. Berger A, Arnold J, Dukstein W, et al (1983) 111Indium labelled autologous platelet survival during aggregation inhibition by anagrelide in normal volunteers. Clin Pharm Ther 33:219
16. Plapp F, Sinor L, Schmitz R, et al (1983) Effect of anagrelide on platelet counts and size. Abstract C52
17. Taylor R, Fleming S, Arnold J (1984) The effect on platelets of a stable orally active imidazoquinazoline. J Clin Pharmacol 24:423
18. Andes WA, Noveck RJ, Fleming JS (1984) Inhibition of platelet production induced by an antiplatelet drug, anagrelide, in normal volunteers. Thromb Hemost 52:325–328
19. Herron KJ, Fleming JS, Solberg LA (1986) Inhibition of megakaryocyte colonies in vitro by anagrelide. Clin Res 34:459
20. Solberg LA, Tefferi A, Oles KJ, Tarach JS, Petitt RM, Forstrom LA, Silverstein MN (1997) The effects of anagrelide on human megakaryocytopoiesis. Br J Haematol 99:174–180
21. Mazur EM, Rosmarin AG, Sohl PA, et al (1992) Analysis of the mechanism of anagrelide induced thrombocythemia in humans. Blood 79:1931–1937
22. Bellucci S, Legrand C, Boval B, Drouet L, Caen J (1999) Studies on platelet volume, chemistry and function in patients with essential thrombocythemia treated with anagrelide. Br J Haematol 104:886–892
23. Lev PR, Marta RF, Vassallu P, Molinas FC (2002) Variation of PDGF, TGF-β and bFGF levels in essential thrombocythemia patients treated with anagrelide. Am J Hematol 70:85–91
24. Laguna MS, Kornblihtt LI, Marta RF, Molinas FC (2000) Thromboxane B2 and platelet derived growth factor in essential thrombocythemia treated with anagrelide. Medicina (B Aires) 60:448–452
25. Tomer A (2002) Effects of anagrelide on in vivo megakaryocyte proliferation and maturation in essential thrombocythemia. Blood 99:1602–1609
26. Thiele J, Kvasnicka HM, Schmitt-Gräff A (2002) Anagrelide induzierte Veränderungen der Megakaryopoiese bei der Therapie thrombozythämischer chronischer myeloproliferativer Erkrankungen. Pathologe 23:426–432
27. Thiele J, Kvasnicka HM, Fuchs N, Brunnbauer K, Volkwein N, Schmitt-Graeff A (2003) Anagrelide induced bone marrow changes during therapy of chronic myeloproliferative disorders with thrombocytosis. An immunohistochemical and morphometric study of sequential trephine biopsies. Haematologica 88:1130–1138
28. Yoon S-Y, Li C-Y, Mesa RA, Tefferi A (1999) Bone marrow effects of anagrelide therapy in patients with myelofibrosis with myeloid metaplasia. Br J Haematol 106:682–688
29. Kastner PR, Fleming JS, Gillespie E, et al (1985) Inotropic and cardiovascular effects of anagrelide. Proc Fed Am Soc Exp Biol 44:716
30. Gaver RC, Deeb G, Pittman KA, Smyth RD (1981) Disposition of anagrelide, an inhibitor of platelet aggregation. Clin Pharmacol Ther 29:381–386
31. Lane WJ, Hattori K, Dias S, Peerschke EI, Moore MA, Blanset DL, Lang PC, Petrone M, Rafii S (2001) Anagrelide metabolite induces thrombocytopenia in mice by inhibiting megakaryocyte maturation without inducing platelet aggregation. Exp Hematol 29:1417–1424
32. Erusalimski JD, Hong Y, Franklin R (2002) Is the platelet lowering activity of anagrelide mediated by its major metabolite 2-amino-5,6-dichloro-3,4-dihydroquinazoline (RL603)? Exp Hematol 30:625–626
33. Erusalimski JD, Wang G, Hong Y (2002) The anagrelide metabolite 2-amino-5,6-dichloro-3,4-dihydroquinazoline (RL603) is a poor inhibitor of in vitro megakaryopoiesis (abstract 4950). Blood American Society of Hematology Annual Meeting
34. McCarty JM, Melone PM, Heisey C, Dessypris EN (2000) Differences in the species specific activity of anagrelide is mediated through the c-mpl receptor. Blood 96:743a
35. Rafil S, Lane W (2002) In response. Exp Hematol 30:626–627
36. Kerns EH (1987) Determination of anagrelide in plasma by capillary gas chromatography–mass spectrometry. J Chromatogr 416:357–364

D Chronic Idiopathic Myelofibrosis

Chapter 16

Prolactin-like Protein E and Megakaryocytopoiesis

Jiandie Lin, Daniel I.H. Linzer

16.1 Introduction

Pregnancy represents a unique stage of mammalian physiology. Concerted and dramatic changes take place in numerous physiological systems, and for the most part these changes are survivable and reversible. One of the systems which undergoes the most extensive alterations during gestation is the hematopoietic system: immune function is modified, preventing attack and rejection of a genetically distinct embryo; blood volume increases, enabling more efficient exchange of nutrients and wastes between the mother and fetus; erythrocyte mass increases, providing greater capacity for oxygen delivery and carbon dioxide removal; and platelet production accelerates, protecting the mother against vascular damage which might accompany the larger blood flow and the extensive remodeling of the vasculature near the implantation site. While these changes occur broadly throughout the mammalian class, rodents – especially mice and rats – offer the most convenient and widely used laboratory models for exploring the regulation of these changes.

16.2 Placental Hormones

The alterations which occur in the physiology of rodent pregnancy are coordinated by a number of hormones, some of which are present throughout adult life and some of which are pregnancy-specific. Among the pregnancy-specific hormones are a large group of proteins in the prolactin/growth hormone family. The timing and location of synthesis during gestation vary for these hormones, leading to a complex temporal and spatial pattern of hormone accumulation and corresponding bioactivity. Most of these hormones are produced by placental trophoblasts (extraembryonic cells which are derived from the fertilized egg), and some by uterine decidual cells. The placenta and associated decidual tissue thus combine to form a robust endocrine structure, with both embryo-derived and maternal components, which secretes many hormones only detected during gestation [1].

The first mouse and rat prolactin-related placental hormones discovered were placental lactogen I and II, hormones which bind to the prolactin receptor and functionally replace prolactin during pregnancy [2]. The next hormones identified were proliferin and proliferin-related protein [3, 4]. These two hormones represented the first "non-classical" hormones in this family – hormones which do not bind to the prolactin or growth hormone receptors. Proliferin and proliferin-related protein are positive and negative regulators of angiogenesis, respectively [5], and proliferin (also called mitogen-regulated protein) has been found to stimulate proliferation of mid-gestational uterine cells [6]. By regulating angiogenesis, proliferin and proliferin-related protein are predicted to act in establishing the appropriate vascular structure at the maternal-fetal interface [7].

As members of the cytokine superfamily, at least some of the prolactin-related hormones would be expected to target blood cells and regulate hematopoiesis. Thus, while increased levels of cytokines present in the nonpregnant state may occur during pregnancy and may account for much of the rise in erythrocyte and platelet production, it seems reasonable to predict that some of the unusual hematopoietic changes which occur during pregnancy might also depend on the actions of pregnancy-specific, placental hormones. If so, then these pregnancy-specific factors may provide unusual, and perhaps unique, ways to regulate cellular response. Our recent results with prolactin-like protein (PLP) E suggest that the approach of identifying novel placental hormones and then characterizing their activities does lead to potentially important new hematopoietic activities.

16.3 Prolactin-like Protein E

PLP-E is secreted as a glycoprotein of 236 amino acid residues, including six sites for N-linked glycosylation (Fig. 16.1). This hormone is synthesized exclusively by the trophoblast giant cells [8], highly polyploid cells which lie at the boundary of the extraembryonic compartment and which make direct contact with maternal decidual tissue and with maternal blood. Peak levels of PLP-E occur on days 10–12 of the 20-day mouse gestational period [8], with hormone concentrations in the maternal serum reaching in excess of 1 μg/ml [9]. The same hormone was also identified by Soares and co-workers, and was designated by them as PLP-G [10].

To determine which cells PLP-E might act upon, a modified hormone was generated as a fusion protein with alkaline phosphatase; this fusion protein enables the sensitive detection of hormone bound to cells, even when the hormone is in a crude protein preparation. Using this approach, specific binding of PLP-E was detected to megakaryocytes present in the mouse bone marrow and spleen [9]. Binding was seen to megakaryocytes from both pregnant and nonpregnant female mice, and from both female and male mice, demonstrating that while PLP-E is restricted to pregnancy, its receptor is not [9]. Moreover, the PLP-E receptor is also found to be expressed by rat megakaryocytes (Fig. 16.2), indicating that the PLP-E receptor is conserved among rodents. Despite the lack of a known homologue of PLP-E in humans, the mouse hormone also binds to human megakaryocytes [11], suggesting an even greater degree of

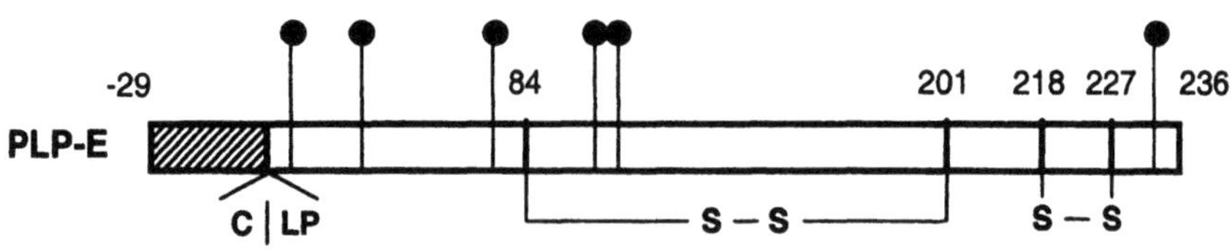

Fig. 16.1. Diagram of PLP-E. The PLP-E protein is depicted, showing the secretion signal sequence (*hatched box*), the cleavage site (between cysteine at –1 and leucine at +1), and the secreted protein (*open box*). The locations of consensus sites for N-linked glycosylation at residues 6, 28, 80, 119, 127 and 234 of the mature protein are represented by the *filled circles*, and the positions of the four cysteine residues are also indicated

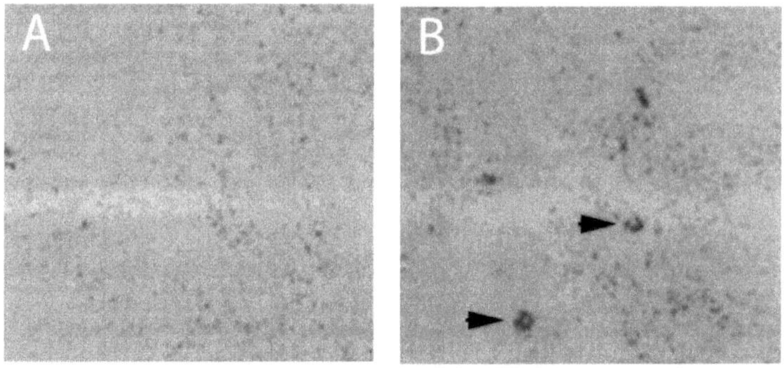

Fig. 16.2A, B. Binding of PLP-E to rat megakaryocytes. Alkaline phosphatase (**A**) or an alkaline phosphatase/PLP-E fusion protein (**B**) produced in transfected mammalian cells was incubated with sections from a rat spleen. Binding of the fusion protein, but not alkaline phosphatase, to megakaryocytes was detected (*arrows*)

conservation of the PLP-E receptor, and presumably of the PLP-E-induced signaling pathway and cellular effects, among mammals.

A number of megakaryocyte cell lines have been generated, and several of these were tested for PLP-E binding. If a cell line expressing the PLP-E receptor could be identified, then characterization of the receptor and of receptor-PLP-E binding kinetics would be relatively straightforward. Also, a megakaryocyte cell line which binds PLP-E would offer a system in which to explore the PLP-E signaling pathway and the biological effects of this hormone. Unfortunately, none of the cell lines examined to date display any PLP-E binding (Table 16.1), presumably because expression of the PLP-E receptor typically fails to be retained during the establishment of primary megakaryocyte precursor cells in culture and the formation of immortalized cell lines. This finding raises the possibility that continued activation of the PLP-E receptor in cell culture would act in opposition to immortalization and unlimited cell proliferation.

Thus, to test the effect of PLP-E on its target cells, it was necessary to utilize primary mouse bone marrow cultures. Megakaryocytes can be readily identified in these cultures, despite their low frequency, simply by size and morphology, or by staining for acetylcholinesterase or immunodetection of specific cell surface antigens. The effects of PLP-E, either alone or in combination with other cytokines, were

Table 16.1. PLP-E binding to hematopoietic cells

Species	Source of cells	Binding
Mouse	Bone marrow sections	+
	Spleen sections	+
	Fetal liver sections	+
	MEL (erythroleukemia) cell line [14]	–
	GM979 (erythroleukemia) cell line [15]	–
	L8057 (megakaryocyte) cell line [16]	–
	BaF3/mpl (thrombopoietin receptor-expressing) cell line [17]	–
Rat	Spleen sections	+
Human	Primary bone marrow cultures	+
	Meg-01 (megakaryocyte) cell line [18]	–
	Mo-7e (megakaryocyte) cell line [19]	–

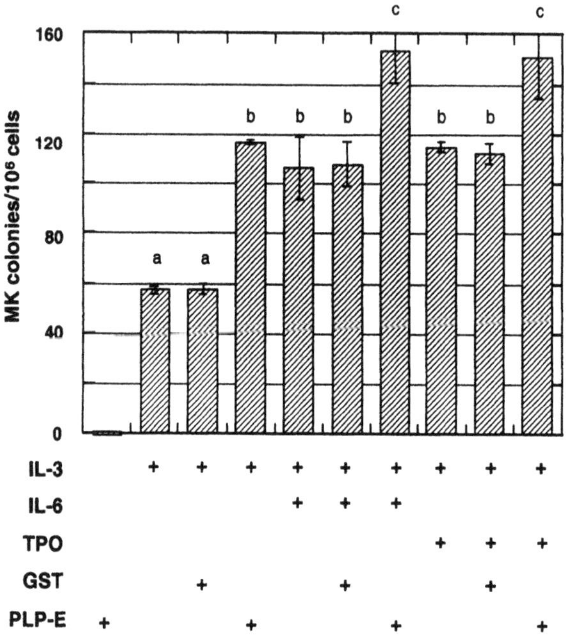

Fig. 16.3. Synergistic effects of PLP-E on megakaryocyte colony formation. One million bone marrow cells in semisolid medium were treated with a glutathione S-transferase/PLP-E fusion protein (*PLP-E*) or a glutathione S-transferase control (*GST*) in the absence or presence of interleukin 3 (*IL-3*), interleukin 6 (*IL-6*), and thrombopoietin (*TPO*). Statistical significance: *a* vs *b* $P<0.01$, *b* vs *c* $P<0.05$, *a* vs *c* $P<0.001$ (one-way ANOVA and a post-hoc Tukey's test). Reproduced with modification from [9]

scored by assessing changes in megakaryocyte size, ploidy, and colony numbers. PLP-E by itself stimulated increases in megakaryocyte size and DNA content, but did not cause any increase in the number of megakaryocyte colonies resulting from the survival and proliferation of CFU-MK in semisolid medium. The number of megakaryocyte colonies increased, as expected, upon addition of interleukin-3 (IL-3). Importantly, PLP-E in combination with IL-3, with IL-3 and IL-6, or with IL-3 and thrombopoietin (TPO), gave a synergistic increase in colony number (Fig. 16.3). Thus, PLP-E provides an activity that complements, rather than mimics, various other megakaryocytic factors. PLP-E may therefore account for some of the pregnancy-specific changes in platelet production by adding a novel activity to the mix of cytokines normally acting on the megakaryocyte lineage. PLP-E appears to act both on megakaryocyte progenitor cells and on megakaryocytes, and may influence cell survival or cell proliferation (based on the colony forming results) as well as cell differentiation.

Although readily detectable binding of PLP-E was observed primarily to megakaryocytes, effects of this hormone on other myeloid lineages have been observed. In the presence of PLP-E alone, primary mouse bone marrow cells do form some colonies in semisolid medium. These colonies do not stain for acetylcholinesterase and are negative for globin, indicating that the colonies are neither from CFU-MK or CFU-E, but instead develop from CFU-GM [12]. On human bone marrow cell cultures, in addition to its effects on megakaryocyte and granulocyte lineages, PLP-E has been found to act on erythroid progenitors [11]. Thus, PLP-E either targets common precursors for multiple myeloid lineages or expression and function of the PLP-E receptor continue after these precursors adopt restricted fates.

16.4 Conclusions

The discovery of PLP-E and its effects support the notion that investigations of hormones of pregnancy will lead to important new insights into physiological control. PLP-E represents only one of the numerous prolactin-like hormones produced in the mouse and rat placenta or decidua. Recently, another of these hormones, PLP-A, was found to inhibit the cytolytic activity of natural killer T cells [13]. Thus, the placental prolactin family includes hormones which target both myeloid and lymphoid lineages, and these hormones may prove to be of value in designing new strategies to regulate hematopoiesis both experimentally and clinically.

Acknowledgements. This work was supported by grant R01 HD24518 from the National Institutes of Health

References

1. Soares MJ, Müller H, Orwig KE, Peters TJ, Dai G (1998) The uteroplacental prolactin family and pregnancy. Biol Reprod 58:273–284
2. Kelly PA, Tsushima T, Shiu RPC, Friesen HG (1976) Lactogenic and growth hormone-like activities in pregnancy determined by radioreceptor assays. Endocrinology 99:765–774
3. Linzer DIH, Nathans D (1984) Nucleotide sequence of a growth-related member of the prolactin-growth hormone family. Proc Natl Acad Sci U S A 81:4255–4259
4. Linzer DIH, Nathans D (1985) A new member of the prolactin-growth hormone family expressed in mouse placenta. EMBO J 4:1419-1423
5. Jackson D, Volpert O, Bouck N, Linzer DIH (1994) Stimulation and inhibition of angiogenesis by placental proliferin and proliferin-related protein. Science 266:1581–1584
6. Nelson JT, Rosenzweig N, Nilsen-Hamilton M (1995) Characterization of the mitogen-regulated protein (proliferin) receptor. Endocrinology 136:283–288
7. Linzer DIH, Fisher SJ (1999) The placenta and the prolactin family of hormones – regulation of the physiology of pregnancy. Mol Endocrinol 13:837–840
8. Lin J, Poole J, Linzer DIH (1997) Two novel members of the PRL/GH family are expressed in the mouse placenta. Endocrinology 138:5535–5540
9. Lin J, Linzer DIH (1999) Induction of megakaryocyte differentiation by a novel pregnancy-specific hormone. J Biol Chem 274:21485–21489
10. Müller H, Orwig KE, Soares MJ (1998) Identification of two new members of the mouse prolactin gene family. Biochim Biophys Acta 1396:251–258
11. Lefebvre P, Lin J, Linzer DIH, Cohen I (2001) Murine Prolactin-like protein E synergizes with human thrombopoietin to stimulate expansion of human megakaryocytes and their precursors. Exp Hematol 29:51–58
12. Lin J, Toft DJ, Bengtson NW, Linzer DIH (2000) Placental prolactins and the physiology of pregnancy. Recent Prog Horm Res 55:37–52
13. Müller H, Liu B, Croy BA, Head JR, Hunt JS, Dai G, Soares MJ (1999) Uterine natural killer cells are targets for a trophoblast cell-specific cytokine, prolactin-like protein A. Endocrinology 140:2711–2720
14. Marks PA, Rifkind RA (1978). Erythroleukemia differentiation. Annu Rev Biochem 47:419–448
15. Zitnik G, Hines P, Stamatoyannopoulos G, Papayannopoulou T (1991) Murine erythroleukemia cell line GM979 contains factors that can activate silent chromosomal human gamma-globin genes. Proc Natl Acad Sci U S A 88:2530–2534
16. Hirabayashi Y, Inoue T, Yoshida K, Sasaki H, Kubo S, Kanisawa M, Seki M (1991) Murine acute leukemia cell line with megakaryocytic differentiation (MK-8057) induced by whole-body irradiation in C3H/He mice: cytological properties and kinetics of its leukemic stem cells. Int J Cell Cloning 9:24–42
17. Lok S, Kaushansky K, Holly RD, Kuijper JL, Lofton-Day CE, Oort PJ, Grant FJ, Heipel MD, Burkhead SK, Kramer JM, Bell LA, Sprecher CA, Blumberg H, Johnson R, Prunkard D, Ching AFT, Mathewes SL, Bailey MC, Forstrom JW, Buddle MM, Osborn SG, Evans SJ, Sheppard PO, Presnell SR, O'Hara PJ,

Hagen FS, Roth GJ, Foster DC (1994) Cloning and expression of murine thrombopoietin cDNA and stimulation of platelet production in vivo. Nature 369:565–568
18. Chen YZ, Gu XF, Caen JP, Han ZC (1994) Interleukin-3 is an autocrine growth factor of human megakaryoblasts, the DAMI and MEG-01 cells. Br J Haematol 88:481–487
19. Avanzi GC, Porcu P, Brizzi MF, Ghigo D, Bosia A, Pegoraro L (1991) Interleukin 3-dependent proliferation of the human Mo-7e cell line is supported by discrete activation of late G1 genes. Cancer Res 51:1741–1743

Chapter 17

Pathophysiology and Stem Cell Biology in Myelofibrosis with Myeloid Metaplasia

Marie-Caroline Le Bousse-Kerdilès, Marie-Claire Martyré

17.1 Introduction

Originally described by Heuck in 1879, myeloid metaplasia with myelofibrosis (MMM) was further classified by Dameshek [1] as a member of the chronic myeloproliferative disorders (cMPDs). Criteria for the diagnosis were first proposed by Laszlo [2]. They included splenomegaly, marrow fibrosis, leukoerythroblastosis with teardrop erythrocytes, extramedullary hematopoiesis, and absence of Philadelphia chromosome, a particular acquired genetic alteration (BCR-ABL) found in CML [3]. Actually, though karyotypic analyses have been crucial to flag oncogenes involved in the pathogenesis of hematological malignancies, data in MMM are still sparse and inconclusive. However, about 30% of the patients have cytogenetic abnormalities, with del(20q), del(13q) and partial trisomy 1q [4] accounting for 75% of all abnormalities at diagnosis. MMM is the rarest cMPD; its incidence was estimated to be 0.73 and 0.40 per 100,000 person years in males and in females respectively [5]. Its prognosis is poor with a median overall survival of 40 to 60 months. Treatments are still largely unsatisfactory since they do not significantly improve morbidity or mortality.

MMM is characterized by myeloproliferation, myelofibrosis, myelemia and progressive splenomegaly due to myeloid metaplasia; angiogenesis is also frequently observed. Although its pathogenesis has come to light during the last decade, it is not yet thoroughly elucidated. Several lines of evidence suggest that the disease arises from primitive stem cells, while the fibroblastic proliferation and activation resulting in marrow fibrosis is a secondary and reactive process. The hypothesis of a clonal expansion of a hematopoietic pluripotent stem/progenitor cell was first supported by genetic and enzyme studies [6–10]. Recent studies from the group of Praloran, within the framework of the French INSERM Research Network, have demonstrated that in MMM patients with cytogenetics abnormalities the clonality of the hematopoietic proliferation can be detected in CD34+ progenitors [11]. In contrast, the nonclonality of the fibroblast proliferation is supported by the findings of Castro-Malaspina et al. [12] and further confirmed by our group [11]. The reactive nature of the fibroblast proliferation in this disease was also documented by the report on resolution of bone marrow fibrosis following allogeneic bone marrow transplantation [13].

17.2 Promotion of Bone Marrow Fibrosis

In MMM, immunolocalization studies have demonstrated a marked neovascularization in the myelofibrotic bone marrow stroma together with an increased deposition of collagen types I, III, IV, V and VI, with type III being the predominant type. An increased deposition of interstitial and basement membrane proteins, fibronectin, laminin, tenascin and vitronectin has also been documented in the advanced stages of the disease [14].

A number of studies support the concept that the megakaryocytic lineage is pathogenically important in its generation [15–18]. Castro-Malaspina was the first to propose that the genesis of bone marrow fibrosis would result from the abnormal release of growth factor from megakaryocytes (MK) [19]. According to his hypothesis, the imbalance between the increased collagen production by a MK-derived growth factor, further identified as platelet-derived growth factor (PDGF) [20], and the decreased collagen degradation by platelet factor 4 (PF4), a collagenase inhibitor, would lead to the development of myelofibrosis. Based on this hypothesis, other groups have demonstrated quantitative abnormalities of PDGF in MMM platelets [21]. The release of PDGF, while undoubtedly participating in fibroblast proliferation, cannot account totally for the complexity of the myelofibrotic stroma. Therefore, the roles of two other fibrogenic factors, namely transforming growth factor-β (TGF-β) [22] and basic fibroblast growth factor (bFGF) [23], have received particular attention.

The involvement of TGF-β, synthesized in MKs and stocked in platelets, in marrow fibrosis was first supported by reports of elevated TGF-β levels in MKs and platelets from MMM patients [24–26] and was further strengthened by studies on myelofibrosis occurring in acute megakaryoblastic leukemia [27, 28]. Altogether, these findings strongly suggest that TGF-β and MKs are linked in the pathophysiology of MMM. Whereas myelofibrosis can also be observed in other chronic MPDs such as chronic myeloid leukemia (CML) and evolutive polycythemia vera (PV) [29], it is not commonly observed in essential thrombocythemia (ET) in which, though the MK/platelet population is expanded, TGF-β levels are within the normal range [21, 26].

Recent studies have demonstrated that bFGF is also highly expressed in circulating MKs and platelets from MMM patients [30]. Interestingly, while producing bFGF, MMM MKs do not export it, and cell lysis has been hypothesized for bFGF externalization. Given the dysplastic and necrotic appearance of MKs reported in MMM [31], this hypothesis is likely and could account for the elevated urinary [32] and serum [30] bFGF levels detected in MMM patients. Finally, additional factors could also be involved in the etiology of marrow fibrosis such as vascular endothelial growth factor (VEGF) [33, 34] and calmodulin [32], the levels of which are elevated in MMM patients.

17.3 Dysregulation of the Hematopoietic Progenitor Proliferation: Role of Growth Factors and Stroma

The myeloproliferation observed in MMM patients is characterized by an increased number, up to 2000-fold, of circulating CD34+ hematopoietic cells [35, 36]. This progenitor rise includes pluripotent, granulomacrophagic, erythroid, megakaryocytic and mastocytic progenitors [17, 37–39]. It probably results from cell flow from the fibrotic bone marrow into the circulation [40], since the increase of circulating progenitors contrasts with a relative reduction in the content of medullar progenitors. Spleen and liver also play a role in this progenitor augmentation [40]; our results showing a large number of CD34+ cells in the spleen pulp of splenectomized MMM patients support this assumption. Interestingly, the myeloproliferation is also associated with disturbances of the immune system. The lymphocytic compartment is altered [41, 42] and could be implicated in the induction and/or maintenance of the disease [43–45].

In MMM, scarce studies concern the pathogenesis of myeloproliferation. The hierarchical level, the primary mechanism, and the gene alteration responsible for emergence and expansion of the malignant clone are still unknown. When cultured at high concentrations in semisolid medium, unpurified hematopoietic progenitors from MMM patients give rise to spontaneous colonies of all myeloid lineages [35, 46, 47]. This autonomous growth disappears when purified CD34+ cells are plated [35], suggesting that growth factors, produced by accessory cells, are involved in the proliferation and/or differentiation of MMM hematopoietic progenitors; however, type, origin, and mechanisms of this growth factor production are not well understood.

Although CD34+ progenitors from MMM patients are not autonomous, they exhibit an impaired response to hematopoietic and fibrogenic growth factors that positively (SCF, IL-3, M-CSF, GM-CSF, bFGF) or negatively (TGF-β) control the proliferation and differentiation of their normal counterparts [35, 48]. This modified sensitivity is correlated with an altered expression of receptors to these growth factors [35, 48], suggesting alteration of hematopoietic progenitor response to regulatory growth factors as a possible mechanism for myeloproliferation in MMM. Such a role for fibrogenic cytokines in myeloproliferation, is particularly relevant with regard to MMM in which myeloproliferation and myelofibrosis are intimately associated.

The prominent proliferation of an abnormal MK population and its implications for the pathogenesis of MMM, via the release of numerous growth factors, caused a number of groups to search for the intimate mechanisms of this dysregulation. The potential implication of thrombopoietin (TPO) and its receptor c-Mpl was first investigated. Data from our group showed that c-Mpl is more highly expressed in circulating CD34+ progenitors from MMM patients than in CD34+ progenitors from normal bone marrow [49]. Given the role of c-Mpl in hematopoietic progenitor proliferation, it may be that overexpression in CD34+ cells is part of the mechanisms involved in their expansion in MMM. Interestingly, the in vitro autonomous growth observed in a small proportion of MK progenitors appears not to be due to a mutation of c-Mpl or to a autocrine/paracrine stimulation by TPO [50], but rather to result from the constitutive STAT5 activation via immunophilin FKBP51 overexpression [51]. Concerning c-Mpl expression in platelets, it has been reported to be decreased in MMM and PV patients [52]. Data are still controversial in ET, indicating either a reduced [53] or a normal [52] c-Mpl expression. Regarding the c-Mpl ligand, the increase in TPO is moderate, since we detected only a three- to fourfold increase in the serum from MMM patients [49]. These findings are in agreement with results reported by Wang et al. [54] and contrast with the high TPO levels detected in TPO-induced myelofibrosis models [55, 56], suggesting that the myelofibrosis observed in MMM and in these experimental models results from distinct processes.

Recently, results from our group have given prominence to the potential involvement of altered hematopoietic transcription factors in the dysregulation of the MK compartment in MMM patients. Actually, we demonstrated an increased level of GATA-1 expression in patients' peripheral blood mononuclear cells. Whereas such an increase in GATA-1 expression level was not observed in MMM CD34+ cells [57], the expression of its cofactor FOG1 (Friend of GATA-1) is significantly elevated in those cells as compared to CD34+ cells from healthy controls [57]. As GATA-1 also associates in a multiprotein complex with the stem cell leukemia gene (SCL) a crucial actor in early hematopoiesis, we sought for potential alteration in SCL expression. We demonstrated that SCL gene transcription is altered in patients' CD34+ progenitor cells since promoter 1b-initiated SCL transcription is restricted to primitive CD34+CD41− cells from patients while it is detectable in both primitive CD34+CD41− and megakaryocytic CD34+CD41+ progenitor subsets from healthy subjects. Interestingly, the SCL protein sublocalizations are different in MKs from patients and from healthy subjects [58]. Overall these findings highlight the possible contribution of hematopoietic transcription factors to the myeloproliferation process and to the MK compartment alteration that is a feature of MMM.

Beside MKs, several studies [35, 59, 60] have suggested that activated monocytes and/or macrophages also participate in the GF production detected in MMM patients. Actually, these cells are increased in number in bone marrow sections from MMM patients [31]. Furthermore, serum levels of M-CSF are increased in MMM and myelofibrosis post-PV and are significantly higher than in other cMPDs. Interestingly, in MMM, the M-CSF levels correlate with spleen size and myelemia [59]. Recent experiments from Praloran's group have shown an increased transcription of the M-CSF and of its c-fms receptor in circulating CD34+ cells from patients. Thus, it could be speculated that in MMM, M-CSF might activate macrophages to produce, together with MKs, cytokines/GF involved in both fibrosis and myeloproliferation. In addition to these cytokines, other GFs such as erythropoietin, stem cell factor and IL-6 [54] also are probably involved in the complex network leading to the development of MMM.

In addition to signals mediated by GFs through their cognate receptors, direct cell-cell interactions (between hematopoietic and stromal cells) or cell-matrix interactions also modulate genes involved in hematopoietic cell regulation. Interestingly, spleen fibroblasts from MMM patients display patterns in adhesion molecule expression, matrix component and hematopoietic GF production that are distinct from their normal counterparts [61]. Recent results from our group have shown that the in vitro growth of MMM CD34+ cells and their differentiation are dependent on their specific interaction with MMM fibroblasts, thus suggesting the interdependence of the progenitor/fibroblast couple in this disease [42, 62] and demonstrating the central role of stroma in hematopoiesis dysregulation in MMM.

17.4 Pathophysiological Hypothesis and Conclusion

Hematopoiesis is tightly regulated by cellular and matrix protein interactions occurring through specific cell surface adhesion structures, cell-derived cytokines and growth factors. Whereas the initial molecular defect leading to MMM is still

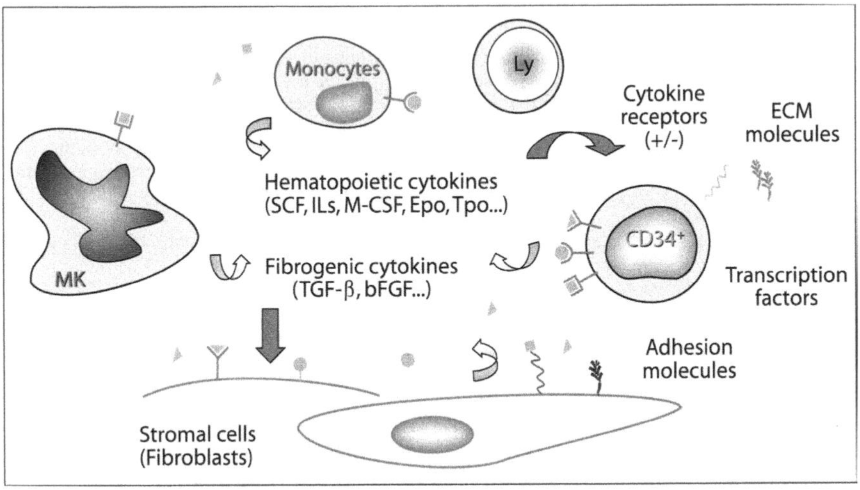

Fig. 17.1. Model of MMM pathogenesis

unknown, results from our group allowed us to propose a model of its pathogenesis (Fig. 17.1). In this model, it could be hypothesized that alteration of the dialog between CD34+ and stromal cells would result in the overproduction and release of several cytokines by cells from the hematopoietic clone (CD34+ cells, monocytes and MK). Among these molecules, cytokines/GF with fibrogenic and angiogenic activities (TGF-β, bFGF, PDGF, VEGF) would further activate stromal cells and subsequently make them produce extracellular matrix components as well as a number of cytokines/GF. These factors, alone or in synergy, would maintain the amplification of myeloid CD34+ progenitors potentially to the detriment of the lymphoid ones, the sensitivity of both toward positive and negative regulators and their signaling pathway being altered. Obviously, individually, each cytokine could not be considered as specific for the disease; the specificity of the pathological process more probably results from interactions within this cytokine network. Beside the crucial role of GF, the possible contribution of deregulated expression or activation of hematopoietic transcription factors in MMM pathogenesis is likely.

In conclusion, significant progress has been made in the understanding of the pathophysiological mechanisms involved in MMM. However, many questions remain to be answered to elucidate this puzzling process. Elaboration of new concepts in MMM pathogenesis could help establish germane biological markers of the disease and to set up more appropriate therapeutic approaches.

Acknowledgements. This work was financially supported by: INSERM Nos. 494016 and 4R006C, ANRB (Association Nouvelles Recherches Biomédicales), ARC No.1803, Fondation Contre La Leucémie No. 96003116, Ligue Nationale Contre Le Cancer No. 3D130C and Contrat Coopératif Institut Curie.

References

1. Dameshek W (1951) Some speculations on the myeloproliferative syndromes. Blood 6:372–376
2. Lazlo J (1975) Myeloproliferative myelosclerosis, extramedullary hematopoiesis, undifferentiated MPD and hemorrhagic thrombocythemia. Semin Hematol 12:409–432
3. Ward HP, Block MH (1971) The natural history of agnogenic myeloid metaplasia (AMM) and a critical evaluation of its relationship with the myeloproliferative syndrome. Medicine 50:357–420
4. Reilly JT, Snowden JA, Spearing RL, Fitzgerald PM, Jones N, Watmore A, Potter A (1997) Cytogenetic abnormalities and their prognostic significance in idiopathic myelofibrosis: a study of 106 cases. Br J Haematol 98:96–102
5. Reilly JT (1997) Idiopathic myelofibrosis: pathogenesis, natural history and management. Blood Rev 11:233–242
6. Kahn A, Bernard JF, Cottreau D, Marie J, Bovin P (1975) A G6PD variant with heterozygous expression in blood cells of a woman with primary myelofibrosis. Humangenetik 30:41–46
7. Jacobson RJ, Salo A, Fialkow PJ (1978) Agnogenic myeloid metaplasia: a clonal proliferation of hematopoietic stem cells with secondary myelofibrosis. Blood 51:189–194
8. Wang JC, Lang HD, Lichter S, Weinstein M, Benn P (1992) Cytogenetic studies of bone marrow fibroblasts cultured from patients with myelofibrosis and myeloid metaplasia. Br J Haematol 80:184–188
9. Kreipe H, Jacquet K, Feigner J, Radzun HJ, Parwaresch MR (1991) Clonal granulocytes and bone marrow cells in the cellular phase of agnogenic myeloid metaplasia. Blood 78:1814–1817
10. Buschle M, Janssen JWG, Drexler H, Lyons T, Anger B, Bartram CR (1988) Evidence for pluripotent stem cell origin of idiopathic myelofibrosis: clonal analysis of a case characterized by a N-ras gene mutation. Leukemia 2:658–660
11. Bilhou-Nabera C, Brigaudeau C, Clay D, Lai JL, Brouty-Boyé D, Vignon C, Gharbi MJ, Le Bousse-Kerdilès MC, Praloran V (2003) Does cytogenetic mosaicism in CD34+CD38low cells reflect the persistence of normal primitive hematopoietic progenitors in myeloid metaplasia with myelofibrosis? Blood 102:1551–1552
12. Castro-Malaspina H, Gay RE, Thanwar SL (1982) Characteristics of bone marrow fibroblast colony forming cells and their progeny in patients with myeloproliferative disorders. Blood 59:1046–1054
13. Dokal I, Jones L, Deenmamode M, Lewis SM, Goldman JM (1989) Allogenic bone marrow transplantation for primary myelofibrosis. Br J Haematol 71:158–160
14. Hasselbalch HC (1993) Idiopathic myelofibrosis. Clinical aspects and studies on extracellular matrix metabolism. Dan Med Bull 40:39–55
15. Thiele J, Kuemmel T, Sander C, Fisher R (1991) Ultrastructure of the bone marrow tissue in so-called primary (idiopathic) myelofibrosis-osteomyelosclerosis (agnogenic myeloid metaplasia). I. Abnormalities of megakaryopoiesis and thrombocytes. J Submicrosc Cytol Pathol 23:93–107
16. Burkhardt R, Frisch B, Bartl B (1982) Bone marrow biopsy in haematological disorders. J Clin Pathol 35:257–265
17. Hibbin JA, Njoku OS, Matutes E, Lewis SM, Goldman JM (1984) Myeloid progenitor cells in the circulation of patients with myelofibrosis and other myeloproliferative disorders. Br J Haematol 57:495–503
18. Marcus RE, Hibbin JA, Matutes E, Whittle N, Waterfield MD, Goldman JM (1986) Megakaryoblastic transformation of myelofibrosis with expression of c-sis oncogene. Scand J Haematol 36:186–193
19. Castro-Malaspina H (1984) Pathogenesis of myelofibrosis: role of ineffective megakaryopoiesis and megakaryocyte components. In: Berck P, Castro-Malaspina H, Wasserman LR (eds) Myelofibrosis and the biology of connective tissue. Alan R. Liss, New York, pp 427–454
20. Castro-Malaspina H, Rabbelino EM, Yen A, Nachman RL, Moore MA (1981) Human megakaryocyte stimulation of proliferation of bone marrow fibroblasts. Blood 57:781–787
21. Martyré MC (1995) TGF-beta and megakaryocytes in the pathogenesis of myelofibrosis in myeloproliferative disorders. Leuk Lymphoma 20:39–44
22. Ignotz R, Massague J (1986) Transforming growth factor-beta stimulates the expression of fibronectin and collagen and their incorporation into the extracellular matrix. J Biol Chem 261:4337–4345
23. Brunner G, Nguyen H, Gabrilove J, Rifkin DB, Wilson EL (1993) Basic fibroblast growth factor expression in human bone marrow and peripheral blood cells. Blood 81:631–638
24. Martyré MC, Magdelenat H, Bryckaert MC, Laine-Bidron C, Calvo F (1991) Increased intraplatelet levels of platelet-derived growth factor and transforming growth factor-β in patients with myelofibrosis with myeloid metaplasia. Br J Haematol 77:80–86
25. Martyré MC, Romquin N, Le Bousse-Kerdilès MC, Chevillard S, Benyahia B, Dupriez B, Demory JL, Bauters F (1994) Transforming growth factor-β and megakaryocytes in the pathogenesis of idiopathic myelofibrosis. Br J Haematol 88:9–16
26. Zauli G, Visani G, Catani L, Vianelli N, Gugliotta L, Capitani S (1993) Reduced responsiveness of bone marrow megakaryocyte progenitors to platelet-derived transforming growth factor β1, produced in normal amounts, in patients with essential thrombocythaemia. Br J Haematol 83:14–20

27. Terui T, Niitsu Y, Mahara K, Fujisaki Y, Urushizaki Y, Mogi Y, Kohgo Y, Watanabe N, Ogura M, Saito H (1990) The production of transforming growth factor-β in acute megakaryoblastic leukemia and its possible implication in myelofibrosis. Blood 75:1540–1548
28. Reilly JT, Barnett D, Dolan G, Forrest P, Eastham J, Smith A (1993) Characterisation of an acute micromegakaryocytic leukaemia: evidence for the pathogenesis of myelofibrosis. Br J Haematol 83:58–62
29. Buhr T, Georgii A, Choritz H (1993) Myelofibrosis in chronic myeloproliferative disorders. Incidence among subtypes according to the Hannover classification. Pathol Res Pract 189:121–127
30. Martyré MC, Le Bousse-Kerdilès C, Romquin N, Chevillard S, Praloran V, Demory JL, Dupriez B (1997) Elevated levels of basic growth factor in megakaryocytes and platelets from patients with idiopathic myelofibrosis. Br J Haematol 97:441–448
31. Thiele J, Braeckel C, Wagner S (1992) Macrophages in normal human bone marrow and in chronic myeloproliferative disorders: an immunohistochemical and morphometric study by a new monoclonal antibody (PG-M1) on trephine biopsies. Virchows Arch A Pathol Anat Histopathol 421:33–39
32. Dalley A, Smith JM, Reilly JT, MacNeil S (1996) Investigation of calmodulin and basic fibroblast growth factor (bFGF) in idiopathic myelofibrosis: evidence for a role of extracellular calmodulin in fibroblast proliferation. Br J Haematol 93:856–862
33. Di Raimondo F, Azzaro MP, Palumbo GA, Bagnato S, Stagno F, Giustolisi GM, Cacciola E, Sortino G, Guglielmo P, Giustolisi R (2001) Elevated vascular endothelial growth factor (VEGF) serum levels in idiopathic myelofibrosis. Leukemia 15:976–980
34. Chou JM, Li CY, Tefferi A (2003) Bone marrow immunohistochemical studies of angiogenic cytokines and their receptors in myelofibrosis with myeloid metaplasia. Leuk Res 27:499–504
35. Le Bousse-Kerdilès MC, Martyré MC, and the members of the French INSERM Research Network (2000) Pathogenesis of myelofibrosis with myeloid metaplasia. Springer Semin Immunopathol 21:491–508
36. Barosi G (1999) Myelofibrosis with myeloid metaplasia: diagnostic definition and prognostic classification for clinical studies and treatment guidelines. J Clin Oncol 17:2954–2970
37. Battegay EJ, Thomssen C, Nissen C, Gudat F, Speck B (1989) Endogenous megakaryocyte colonies from peripheral blood in precursor cell. Eur J Haematol 42:321–326
38. Chikkappa G, Carsten AL, Chanana AD, Chandra P, Cronkite EP (1978) Increased granulocytic, erythrocytic and megakaryocytic progenitors in myelofibrosis with myeloid metaplasia. Am J Hematol 4:121–131
39. Han ZC, Bellucci S, Wan HY, Caen JP (1992) New insights into the regulation of megakaryocytopoiesis by haemopoietic and fibroblastic growth factors and transforming growth factor beta-1. Br J Haematol 81:1–5
40. Wolf BC, Neiman RS (1987) Hypothesis: splenic filtration and the pathogenesis of extramedullary hematopoiesis in agnogenic myeloid metaplasia. Hum Pathol 1:77–80
41. Cervantes F, Hernandez-Boluda JC, Villamor N, Serra A, Montserrat E (2000) Assessment of peripheral blood lymphocyte subsets in idiopathic myelofibrosis. Eur J Haematol 65:104–108
42. Briard D, Brouty-Boyé D, Giron-Michel J, Azzarone B, Jasmin C, Le Bousse-Kerdilès MC (2003) Impaired NK cell differentiation of blood-derived CD34+ progenitors from patients with myeloid metaplasia with myelofibrosis. Clin Immunol 106:201–212
43. Reilly JT (1994) Pathogenesis of idiopathic myelofibrosis: present status and future directions. Br J Haematol 88:1–8
44. Caligaris Cappio F, Vigliani R, Novarino A, Camussi G, Campana D, Gavosto F (1981) Idiopathic myelofibrosis: a possible role for immune-complexes in the pathogenesis of bone marrow fibrosis. Br J Haematol 49:17–21
45. Hasselbach H, Jans H, Nielsen PL (1987) A distinct subtype of idiopathic myelofibrosis with bone marrow features mimicking hairy cell leukemia: evidence of an autoimmune pathogenesis. Am J Hematol 25:225–230
46. Han ZC, Brière J, Nedellec G, Algrall JF, Sensobe L, Parent D, Guern G (1988) Characteristics of circulating megakaryocyte progenitors (CFU-MK) in patients with primary myelofibrosis. Eur J Haematol 40:130–135
47. Kobayashi S, Teramura M, Hoshino S, Motoji T, Oshimi K, Mizoguchi H (1993) Circulating megakaryocyte progenitors in myeloproliferative disorders are hypersensitive to interleukin-3. Br J Haematol 83:539–544
48. Le Bousse-Kerdilès MC, Chevillard S, Charpentier A, Romquin N, Clay D, Smadja-Joffe F, Praloran V, Dupriez B, Demory JL, Jasmin C, Martyré MC (1996) Differential expression of transforming growth factor-β, basic fibroblast growth factor and their receptors in CD34+ hematopoietic progenitor cells from patients with myelofibrosis and myeloid metaplasia. Blood 88:4534–4546
49. Cocault L, Le Bousse-Kerdilès C, Flon M, Challier C, Clay D, Martyré MC, Souyri M (1998) TPO, c-mpl and megakaryocytes in idiopathic myelofibrosis (abstract). European Working Group on Myeloproliferative disorders of the European Haematology Association, Rotterdam, 12–14 March 1998

50. Taksin AL, Le Couedic JP, Dusanter-Fourt I, Massé A, Giraudier, Katz A, Wendling F, Vainchenker W, Casadevall N, Debili N (1998) Autonomous megakaryocyte growth in essential thrombocythemia and idiopathic myelofibrosis is not related to a c-mpl mutation or to an autocrine stimulation by Mpl-L. Blood 93:125–139
51. Giraudier S, Chagraoui H, Komura E, Barnache S, Blanchet B, LeCouedic JP, Smith DF, Larbret F, Taksin AL, Moreau-Gachelin F, Casadevall N, Tulliez M, Hulin A, Debili N, Vainchenker W (2002) Overexpression of FKBP51 in idiopathic myelofibrosis regulates the growth factor independence of megakaryocyte progenitors. Blood 100:2932–2940
52. Moliterno A, Hankins W, Spivak J (1998) Impaired expression of the thrombopoietin receptor by platelets from patients with polycythemia vera. New Engl J Med 338:572–580
53. Horikawa Y, Matsumura J, Hashimoto K, Shiraga M, Kosugi S, Tadokoro S, Kato T, Miyazaki H, Tomiyama Y, Kurata Y, Matsuzawa Y, Kanakura Y (1997) Markedly reduced expression of platelet c-mpl receptor in essential thrombocythemia. Blood 90:4031–4038
54. Wang JC, Chen C, Lou LH, Mora M (1997) Blood thrombopoietin, IL-6 and IL-11 levels in patients with agnogenic myeloid metaplasia. Leukemia 11:1827–1832
55. Villeval JL, Cohen-Solal K, Tulliez M, Giraudier S, Guichard J, Burstein SA, Cram EM, Vainchenker W, Wendling F (1997) High thrombopoietin production by hematopoietic cells induces a fatal myeloproliferative syndrome in mice. Blood 90:4369–4383
56. Yan XQ, Lacey D, Hill D, Chen Y, Fletcher F, Hawly RG, McNiece IK (1996) A model of myelofibrosis and osteomyelosclerosis in mice induced by overexpressing thrombopoietin (mpl ligand): reversal of disease by bone marrow transplantation. Blood 88:402–409
57. Martyré MC, Steunou V, Le Bousse-Kerdilès MC, Wietzerbin J (2003) Lack of alteration in GATA-1 expression in CD34+ hematopoietic progenitors from patients with idiopathic myelofibrosis. Blood 101:5087–5089
58. Steunou V, Le Bousse-Kerdilès MC, Colin-Micouin A, Clay D, Chevillard S, Martyré MC (2003) Altered transcription of the stem cell leukemia gene in myelofibrosis with myeloid metaplasia. Leukemia 10:1998–2006
59. Gilbert HS, Praloran V, Stanley ER (1989) Increased CSF-1 (M-CSF) in myeloproliferative disease: association with myeloid metaplasia and peripheral bone marrow extension. Blood 74:1231–1234
60. Rameshwar P, Denny TN, Stein D, Gascon P (1994) Monocyte adhesion in patients with bone marrow fibrosis is required for the production of fibrogenic cytokines: potential role for interleukin-1 and TGF-β. J Immunol 153:2819–2830
61. Brouty-Boyé D, Doucet C, Clay D, Le Bousse-Kerdilès MC, Lampilis TJ, Azzarone B (1998) Phenotypic diversity in human fibroblasts from myelometaplasic and non-myelometaplasic hematopoietic tissues. Int J Cancer 76:767–773
62. Brouty-Boyé D, Briard D, Le Bousse-Kerdilès MC, Clay D, Pottin-Clemenceau C, Azzarone B, Jasmin C (2001) Effect of human fibroblasts from myelometaplasic and non-myelometaplasic hematopoietic tissue on CD34+ stem cells. Int J Cancer 92:484–488

Chapter 18

Transforming Growth Factor β1 in Myelofibrosis

Pedro Gascon, Pranela Rameshwar

18.1 Introduction

Myelofibrosis is a chronic myeloproliferative disorder characterized by clonal expansion of hematopoiesis, fibrosis, hypercellularity, excessive deposits of extracellular matrix (ECM) proteins, and neoangiogenesis in the bone marrow (BM) [1]. Myelofibrosis could be idiopathic (IMF) or secondary to several diseases. In both cases its pathophysiology remains poorly defined. However, it is believed that the fibrosis, caused by excessive proliferation of polyclonal fibroblastic cells, is a reactive process secondary to dysfunctions caused by the clonal hematopoietic stem cell [2]. The experimental evidence indicates that the increased deposits of ECM proteins could be due to over-activation of the fibroblasts by soluble factors released from cells within the BM microenvironment. The candidate cells include monocytes, megakaryocytes and platelets [3, 4], and soluble factors include the fibrogenic cytokines: IL-1, TGF-β, PDGF and b-FGF [5]. More recently, a neurotransmitter with fibrogenic and neoangiogenic properties, substance P, has been implicated in patients with myelofibrosis [6]. In this review, we focus on the potential role of TGF-β1 in the development of BM fibrosis.

18.2 TGF-β1 in Hematopoiesis

Activated TGF-β1 exerts pleiotropic functions and its cellular sources include immune and non-immune cells [7–9]. The effects of TGF-β1 in a particular tissue could be different and this complex function could be demonstrated in the hematopoietic system. A positive, negative or blunting effect of TGF-β1 on the proliferation of hematopoietic progenitors depends on the degree of cell maturation [8, 9]. TGF-β1 also mediates terminal differentiation and apoptosis on hematopoietic progenitors [8, 9].

The effects of TGF-β1 on myeloid cell development appear to be more complex. Inhibitory effects have mainly been observed on the earlier myeloid progenitors [8–10]. However, as these same progenitors become more mature, the effects of TGF-β1 are slightly inhibitory or even stimulatory, depending on the presence of other soluble factors within the microenvironment. TGF-β1 synergizes with GM-CSF to stimulate the growth and terminal differentiation of murine granulocytic/monocytic progenitors. Consistent with this role on cell differentiation is the ability of TGF-β1 to upregulate the expression of receptors for GM-CSF and M-CSF in monocytic progenitors [8–10]. In this regard, the increased levels of TGF-β1 (Fig. 18.1) and M-CSF in

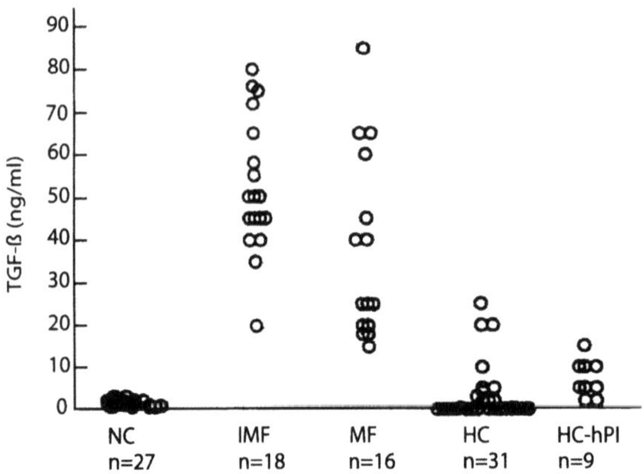

Fig. 18.1. Circulating levels of active TGF-β in patients with and without BM fibrosis. TGF-β was quantitated in serum from normal controls (NC) and patients using the CCL64 cell assay (from [11], with permission) (*IMF* idiopathic myelofibrosis, *MF* secondary myelofibrosis, *HC* hematological controls, *hPl* high platelet count)

myelofibrosis [3, 4, 11–13] might suggest a synergistic effect between the two factors contributing to myeloid expansion and an increase in monocytes/macrophages [14]. Since TGF-β1 is produced by myeloid cells, it could negatively and positively regulate myelopoiesis through autocrine and paracrine loops. These localized functions are plausible considering the anatomical structure of the BM.

18.3 Megakaryocytes in Myelofibrosis

Megakaryocytes and platelets are major sources of TGF-β1, which is stored in the intracytoplasmic α-granules and released at sites of injury upon stimulation by different cytokines such as IL-1, altered in myelofibrosis [3, 15]. TGF-β1 inhibits the early and late stages of megakaryopoiesis [8]. The literature overwhelmingly associates the megakaryocytic lineage with the pathophysiology of myelofibrosis. This link could be indirect through the production and release of fibrogenic cytokines, in particular PDGF, b-FGF and TGF-β1 (Table 18.1). Increased numbers of megakaryocytes, with dysplastic or necrotic features have been shown in the BM and circulation of patients with myelofibrosis [16, 17]. Although a cause–effect relationship has not been shown between megakaryocytes and the excessive deposits of ECM proteins and fibroblast proliferation, there is a high correlation between megakaryocytic

Table 18.1. Fibrogenic cytokines in patients with myelofibrosis

Growth factor	Bone marrow	Periphery	Reference(s)
TGF-β1	↑	↑ Serum	[11, 18]
		↑ PBMNs	[4]
		↑ Platelets	[12]
		↑ CD34+	[27]
b-FGF		↑ Serum	[11]
		↑ Megakaryocytes/platelets	[32]
		↑ CD34+	[27]
PDGF		↑ Platelets	[12]

hyperplasia and fibrosis (fibroblast proliferation and collagen deposition). Martyré et al. reported increased TGF-β levels in the platelets and in circulating mononuclear cells (characterized as cells of megakaryocytic lineage) of patients with myelofibrosis with myeloid metaplasia [4, 12]. Other studies have supported these findings by showing increased TGF-β in the BM and in the circulation of these patients [11, 18]. Earlier studies that showed stimulatory activity of megakaryocyte homogenates on fibroblasts [19] are consistent with megakaryocytes as sources of mitogen for fibroblasts: PDGF and TGF-β [19, 20].

18.4 TGF-β1: Relevance to Altered Gene Expression in Myelofibrosis

Perhaps the most relevant effect of TGF-β1 in myelofibrosis is its importance in the regulation of genes that encode ECM proteins [21]. The BM of patients with myelofibrosis has increased deposits of total collagen (interstitial and basement membrane) and includes types I, III, IV and V [22]. In advanced stages of myelofibrosis, there are increased deposits of laminin, fibronectin, vitronectin and tenascin [1]. The excessive deposits of these ECM proteins correlate with the increases in their biosynthesis, suggesting active molecular processes at the cellular level [23]. In fact, the goals of several research groups including our own are to dissect and understand these processes at the molecular level. Ultimately the pieces could be placed together for the design of effective therapies for the various aspects of the pathophysiology that are associated with myeloproliferative disorder.

A relevant function of TGF-β1 is its blunting effect on matrix degradation by inhibiting the expression of protease inhibitors [8]. This effect of TGF-β1 and its increase in myelofibrosis is consistent with the ubiquitous increase of ECM proteins in patients with myelofibrosis [1]. TGF-β1 appears to be central to the role of other fibrogenic cytokines in the development of myelofibrosis. For example, TGF-β1 regulates the mitogenic activity of EGF and PDGF on fibroblasts [20] and it supersedes other fibrogenic cytokines in the synthesis of ECM proteins [20, 23].

TGF-β1 modulates the expression of the integrins leading to altered adherence of cells to the matrix. A compelling role for TGF-β1 is that it mediates enhanced neoangiogenesis [8], a feature of the BM in myelofibrosis. Substance P, recently implicated in myelofibrosis [6], also exerts angiogenic properties [24]. Individually both substance P and TGF-β1 are mitogenic to fibroblasts [20, 25] and together they appear to exert enhanced and synergistic effects in the proliferation of BM fibroblasts (unpublished). However, the relationship between TGF-β1 and substance P in angiogenesis is yet to be determined.

18.5 Hematopoietic Progenitors in Myelofibrosis

Circulating hematopoietic stem cells in myelofibrosis [26] express elevated levels of stem cell factor, SCF [1], and mutation in the gene for its receptor, c-*kit*. This dysregulation of SCF–c-*kit* are thought to cause the high sensitivity of the myeloid progenitor cells to SCF, hence a proliferative advantage leading to the myeloid clone. Le Bousse-Kerdilès et al. studied the mechanism that could result from the abnormal proliferation of CD34+ hematopoietic progenitor cells in myelofibrosis and found that TGF-β1 expression is unaltered but the expression of the type II receptor is significantly decreased [27]. This finding might reconcile the inability of increased TGF-β1 in myelofibrosis patients to inhibit the proliferation of CD34+ cells. Contrasting results have been reported for b-FGF in which the ligand and receptors are consistently increased so as to allow expansion of the progenitors with concomitant increase in the proliferation of the fibroblastoid cells in the BM [27].

18.6 Monocytes/Macrophages in Myelofibrosis

Although there is a strong association between myelofibrosis and increases in the number of megakaryocytes, other cells could be involved in the pathophysiology of myelofibrosis. A role for monocytes in myelofibrosis is demonstrated in conditions with normal or low megakaryocytes. These include systemic lupus erythematosus, AIDS, acute myeloid leukemia, multiple myeloma, large granular lymphocytic leukemia and hairy cell leukemia [1, 28]. Despite the implication of other cells, TGF-β1 seems to be the constant parameter in the pathophysiology of myelofibrosis. Thus, it is tempting to speculate that TGF-β rather than the cells might be the key in understanding the pathophysiology of myeloproliferative disorders and the associated hematological abnormalities.

Monocytes/macrophages are ideal candidates: they are part of the BM stroma, are increased in myelofibrosis [14, 16, 29] and are major producers of relevant fibrogenic factors (IL-1, PDGF, TGF-β1, substance P) [5, 6]. Peripheral blood monocytes from idiopathic myelofibrosis (IMF) are activated [3, 15], which could lead to relevant immune-related processes. The circulating activated IMF monocytes contain increased intracellular TGF-β1 [3] and in the absence of cell stimulation, these monocytes produce aberrantly large amounts of IL-1 and TGF-β1 (Fig. 18.2) [3, 11, 15, 30]. The mechanism leading to the release of these two fibrogenic cytokines is unclear, although adhesion molecules might be involved [15]. Figure 18.3 summarizes the reports and describes a model to explain the activation of circulating monocytes in patients with myelofibrosis.

Other evidence of activation of the IMF monocytes includes CD25 upregulation and increased tyrosine phosphorylation in unstimulated IMF monocytes [3, 15]. A recent study in our laboratory showed that the transcriptional factor NF-κB is activated in IMF monocytes and could be central to their activation [30]. These studies were conducted with IMF monocytes in which RelA/p65, a subunit of NF-κB, had been transiently knocked out. Interestingly, exogenous IL-1 was able to restore the activation of the RelA/p65-depleted IMF monocytes, indicating an immune-mediated process in which other cells could be providing the 'pro-immune' signal. A summary of these findings is shown in Fig. 18.3. The results show that binding of the ubiquitous ECM proteins to the respective membrane proteins on IMF monocytes leads to NF-κB activation and translocation to the nucleus. This allows transcription and release IL-1, which stimulates the cells through an autocrine mechanism to produce TGF-β and possibly upregulation of adhesion molecules. As exogenous IL-1 induces the production of TGF-β1 despite the depletion of RelA, an alternate pathway is suggested and such a putative mechanism is shown in Fig. 18.4.

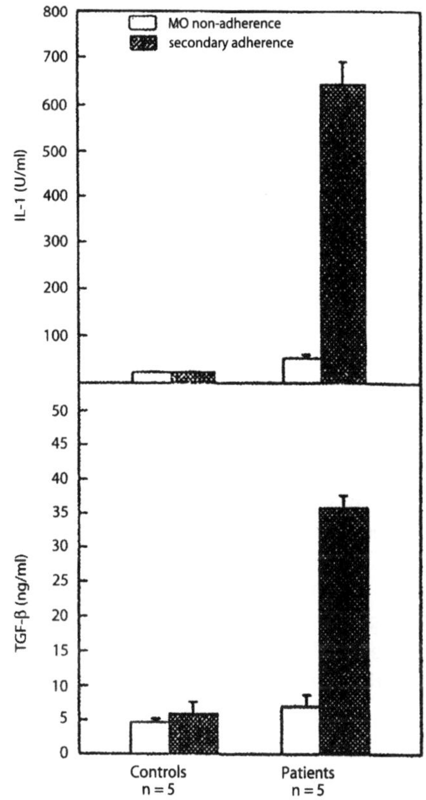

Fig. 18.2. Effect of adherence on the induction of IL-1 and TGF-β in IMF monocytes. IL-1 and TGF-β levels were quantified using the D10.G4.1 and CCL64 cell assays (from [3], with permission)

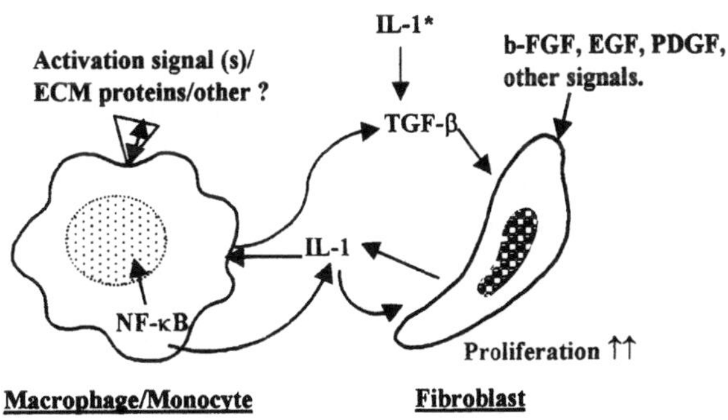

Fig. 18.3. Monocytes stimulated by ECM proteins and other putative 'factors'. NF-κB is activated and leads to the release of IL-1, which induces the production of TGF-β in an autocrine manner. IL-1, TGF-β and other putative ligands induce the proliferation of the fibroblasts
*Exogenous IL-1 induces TGF-β1

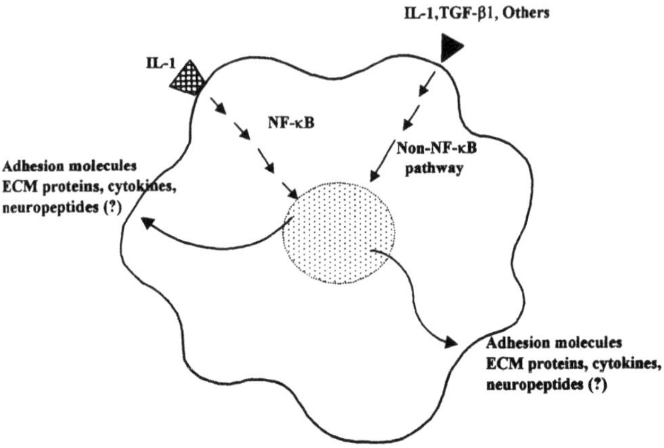

Fig. 18.4. In the absence of NF-κB, activation signals could utilize other putative intracellular pathways that converge on a common, but unidentified, signaling molecule(s) leading to the expression of the same genes that were induced through the activation of NF-κB. Multiple arrows represent a series of intracellular pathways

The increase in TGF-β1 in myelofibrosis is independent of the underlying cause of fibrosis [11], and this strongly favors a reactive process and suggests a common pathway, perhaps through TGF-β1, in the development of BM fibrosis and other associated pathophysiologies in the BM. The increase in TGF-β1 is not limited to the periphery but is also in the BM, as shown by several studies using BM biopsies from patients with myelofibrosis [9, 18]. If BM fibrosis could be extrapolated to lung fibrosis, then other TGF-β1-inducible genes might also be involved as recently reported [31]. Finally, the role of monocytes and macrophages in the development of BM fibrosis may also be inferred from an animal model of osteomyelofibrosis where only mice with functionally normal monocytes and macrophages developed this disease [32].

18.7 Summary

The experimental and clinical data suggest that TGF-β1 might be central to the development of myelofibrosis. In vitro studies have shown that interactions between monocytes and ECM proteins lead to enhanced production of TGF-β1 [3, 15, 30]. In addition, TGF-β1 demonstrates functions possibly associated with BM fibrosis: mitogenic to fibroblasts, induces ECM proteins and the respective receptors [21], induces collagenase inhibitors, which could lead to the accumulation of ECM proteins [8, 21], and the angiogenic effect [1, 8], a typical feature in the BM of patients with myelofibrosis [1].

We have identified at least one adhesion molecule, CD44, that might be partly responsible for the increased induction of IL-1 and TGF-β1 in myelofibrosis monocytes [15]. A subsequent study [30] showed that the role of CD44 is not due to increased membrane expressing receptor. However, the implication of CD44 nonetheless suggests that interactions among fibrogenic cytokines, ECM proteins and their ligands could be contributing to the mechanisms of BM fibrosis (Fig. 18.5). In addition to TGF-β, other soluble factors are also dysregulated in myelofibrosis and, are thought to contribute in the pathophysiology. These include b-FGF [11, 27, 33], IL-1 [3, 15, 29], M-CSF [13], substance P [6] and PDGF [12]. The role of two latter fac-

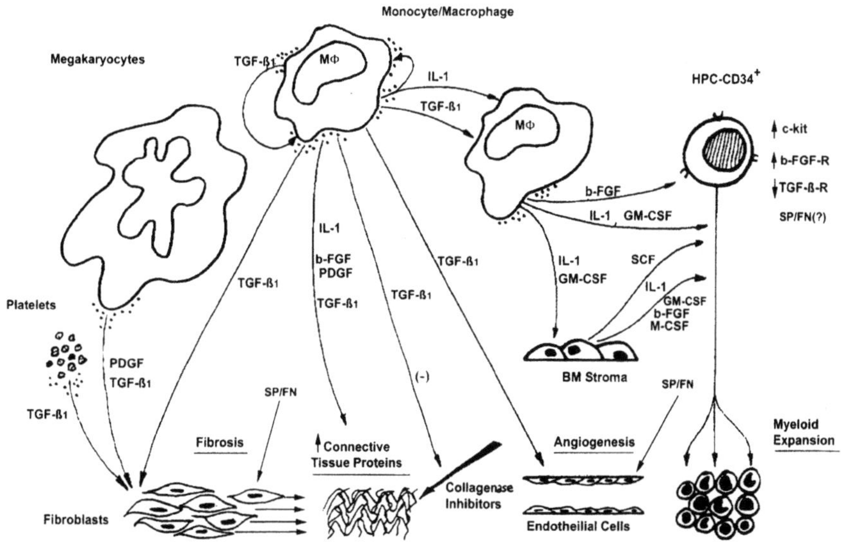

Fig. 18.5. Theoretical model integrating the cells and factors implicated in the mechanisms leading to myelofibrosis

tors is of interest since substance P induces PDGF [24] and both are implicated in myelofibrosis.

Although not limited to monocytes/macrophage and megakaryocytes/platelets, these could be considered as the major cellular sources in the induction of TGF-β1 in myelofibrosis. The clonal hematopoietic progenitors could also be involved in the pathophysiology of secondary BM fibrosis [1, 2, 26] with TGF-β1 being central to the myeloid expansion observed in myelofibrosis [1, 8, 9]. Indication for this is the low expression of TGF-β type II receptor and the high expression of b-FGF types I and II receptors [27]. Other cytokines, IL-1, M-CSF and b-FGF, are also dysregulated in myelofibrosis [3, 11–13, 15, 27, 30], and they could be involved in the myeloid expansion. Overall, the dysfunctions of the TGF-β signaling pathway in patients with BM fibrosis may be used as targets or in combination with other treatments for this disease.

Acknowledgements. This research was supported by grants: HL-54973 and HL-57675 and CA-89868, awarded by National Institutes of Health, and by FIS-00/0679, Fondo de Investigación Sanitaria, Ministerio de Sanidad y Consumo of Spain.

References

1. Barosi B (1999) Myelofibrosis with myeloid metaplasia: diagnostic definition and prognostic classification for clinical studies and treatment guidelines. J Clin Oncol 17:2954–2970
2. Jacobson RJ, Salo A, Fialkow PJ (1978) Agnogenic myeloid metaplasia: a clonal proliferation of haematopoietic stem cells with secondary myelofibrosis. Blood 51:189–194
3. Rameshwar P, Denny T, Stein D, Gascón P (1994) Adhesion of monocytes from patients with bone marrow fibrosis is required for the production of fibrogenic cytokines: potential role for IL-1 and TGF-β. J Immunol 153:2819–2830

4. Martyré MC, Romquin N, Le Bousse-kerdilès C, Chevillard S, Benyahia B, Dupriez B, Demory JL, Bauters F (1994) Transforming growth factor-β and megakaryocytes in the pathogenesis of idiopathic myelofibrosis. Br J Haematol 88:9–16
5. Bosque F, Belkaid Y, Briend E, Hevin B, Lebastard M, Soussi N, Milon G (1997) The biology of macrophages. Pathol Biol 45:103–109
6. Rameshwar P, Joshi DD, Yadav P, Qian J, Gascón P, Chang VT, Anjaria A, Harrison JS, Xiaosong S (2001) Mimicry between neurokinin-1 and fibronectin may explain the transport and stability of increased substance P-immunoreactivity in patients with bone marrow fibrosis. Blood 97:3025–3031
7. Massagué J (1990) The transforming growth factor-β family. Annu Rev Cell Biol 6:597–641
8. Fortunel NO, Hatzfeld A, Hatzfeld JA (2000) Transforming growth factor-β: pleiotropic role in the regulation of hematopoiesis. Blood 96:2022–2036
9. Hooper CW (1991) The role of transforming growth factor-beta in hematopoiesis. A review. Leuk Res 15:179–184
10. Sing GK, Keller JR, Ellingsworth LR, Ruscetti FW (1988) Transforming growth factor-β selectively inhibits normal and leukemic human bone marrow cell growth in vitro. Blood 72:1504–1511
11. Rameshwar P, Chang VT, Thacker UF, Gascón P (1998) Systemic transforming growth factor-β in patients with bone marrow fibrosis: pathological implications. Am J Hematol 59:133–142
12. Martyré MC, Magdelenat H, Bryckaert MC, Laine-Bidron C, Calvo F (1991) Increased intraplatelet levels of platelet-derived growth factor and transforming growth factor-β in patients with myelofibrosis with myeloid metaplasia. Br J Haematol 77:80–86
13. Gilbert HS, Praloran V, Stanley ER (1989) Increased circulating CSF-1 (M-CSF) in myeloproliferative disease: association with myeloid metaplasia and peripheral bone marrow extension. Blood 74:1231–1234
14. Thiele J, Braechel C, Wagner S, Falini B, Dienenmann D, Stein H, Fischer R (1992) Macrophages in normal human bone marrow and in chronic myeloproliferative disorders: an immunohistochemical and morphometric study by a new monoclonal antibody (PG-M1) on trephine biopsies. Virchows Arch A Pathol Anat Histopathol 421:33–39
15. Rameshwar P, Chang VT, Gascón P (1996) Implication of CD44 in adhesion-mediated overproduction of TGF-β and IL-1 in monocytes from patients with bone marrow fibrosis. Br J Haematol 93:22–29
16. Thiele J, Kvasnicka HM, Zankovich R, Diehl V (2000) Relevance of bone marrow features in the differential diagnosis between essential thrombocythemia and early idiopathic myelofibrosis. Haematologica 85:1126–1134
17. Martyré MC (1995) TGF-β and megakaryocytes in the pathogenesis of myelofibrosis in myeloproliferative disorders. Leuk Lymphoma 20:39–44
18. Johnston JB, Dalal BI, Israels SJ, Oh S, McMillan E, Begleiter A, Michaud G, Isreals LG, Greenberg AH (1995) Deposition of transforming growth factor-β in the marrow in myelofibrosis and the intracellular localization and secretion of TGF-β by leukemic cells. Am J Clin Pathol 103:574–582
19. Castro-Malaspina H, Rabelino EM, Yen A, Nachman RL, Moore MAS (1981) Human megakaryocyte stimulation of proliferation of bone marrow fibroblasts. Blood 57:781–787
20. Kimura A, Katoh O, Kuramoto A (1988) Effects of platelet derived growth factor, epidermal growth factor and transforming growth factor-β on the growth of human marrow fibroblasts. Br J Haematol 68:9–12
21. Newman MJ (1993) Transforming growth factor and the cell surface in tumor progression. Cancer Metastasis Rev 12:34–39
22. Hasselbach HC (1993) Idiopathic myelofibrosis. Dan Med Bull 40:39–47
23. Ignotz RA, Massagué J (1987) Cell adhesion protein receptors as targets for transforming growth factor-β action. Cell 51:189–197
24. Fan TP, Hu DE, Guard S, Gresham GA, Watling KJ (1992) Stimulation of angiogenesis by substance P and interleukin-1 and its inhibition by NK1 or interleukin-1 receptor antagonists. Br J Pharmacol 110:43–47
25. Rameshwar P, Poddar A, Zhu G, Gascón P (1997) Receptor induction regulates the synergistic effects of substance P with IL-1 and PDGF on the proliferation of bone marrow fibroblasts. J Immunol 158:3417–3424
26. Douer D, Fabian I, Cline MJ (1983) Circulating pluripotent haemopoietic cells in patients with myeloproliferative disorders. Br J Haematol 54:373–381
27. Le Bousse-Kerdilès MC, Chevillard S, Charpentier A, Romquin N, Clay D, Smadja-Joffe F, Praloran V, Dupriez B, Demory JL, Jasmin C, Martyré MC (1996) Differential expression of transforming growth factor-β, basic fibroblast growth factor, and their receptors in CD34+ hematopoietic progenitor cells from patients with myelofibrosis and myeloid metaplasia. Blood 88:4534–4546

28. Spivak JL, Bender BS, Quinn TC (1984) Hematologic abnormalities in AIDS. Am J Med 77:224–228
29. Rameshwar P, Oh HS, Yook C, Gascon P, Chang VT (2003) Substance P-fibronectin-cytokine interactions in myeloproliferative disorder with bone marrow fibrosis. Acta Haematol 109:1–10
30. Rameshwar P, Ramaswamy N, Qian J, Denny TN, Colon C, Gascón P (2000) NF-kB as a central mediator in the induction of TGF-β in monocytes from patients with idiopathic myelofibrosis: an inflammatory response beyond the realm of homeostasis. J Immunol 165:2271–2277
31. Kaminski NJ, Allard JD, Pittet JF, Zuo F, Griffiths MJD, Morris D, Huang X, Sheppard D, Heller RA (2000) Global analysis of gene expression in pulmonary fibrosis reveals distinct programs regulating lung inflammation and fibrosis. Proc Natl Acad Sci U S A 97:1778–1783
32. Frey BM, Rafii S, Teterson M (1998) Adenovector-mediated expression of human thrombopoietin cDNA in immune-compromised mice: insight in to the pathophysiology of osteomyelofibrosis. J Immunol 160:691–699
33. Martyré MC, Le Bousse-Kerdiles MC, Romquin N, Chevillard S, Pravloran V, Demory JL, Dupriez B (1997) Elevated levels of basic fibroblast growth factor in megakaryocytes and platelets from patients with idiopathic myelofibrosis. Br J Haematol 97:441–448

Idiopathic Myelofibrosis: Evidence for Pathological Crosstalk Between Polymorphonuclear Leukocytes and Megakaryocytes

Alain Schmitt, Arnaud Drouin, Jean-Marc Massé, Josette Guichard, Hedia Shagraoui, Elisabeth M. Cramer

19.1 Introduction

Idiopathic myelofibrosis (MF), also known as primary MF or MF with myeloid metaplasia, is a clonal myeloproliferative disorder characterized by bone marrow fibrosis, extramedullary hematopoiesis, splenomegaly, and an elevated number of peripheral blood hematopoietic precursors [1–3]. It has been shown that an abnormal release of growth factors such as transforming growth factor-β (TGFβ) and platelet-derived growth factor (PDGF) may be responsible for the development of medullary fibrosis [4, 5]. Megakaryocytes (MK) are the principal bone marrow source of these growth factors [6, 7].

Quantitatively and qualitatively abnormal populations of MKs in bone marrow have been described in patients with primary or secondary MF [8]. Indeed, in idiopathic myelofibrosis a major MK proliferation occurs [9]. In addition MF is associated with other myeloproliferative syndromes, such as essential thrombocythemia [10], polycythemia vera [11] and acute megakaryoblastic leukemia (M7) [12] and with MK disorders such as gray platelet syndrome [13, 14] and low expression of GATA1 transcription factor [15]. There is also a topographic relationship between fibrosis and MKs, with a close contact relationship between them [16]. However, the mechanism by which pathological release of growth factors from MK occurs in MF is poorly understood.

Therefore, we investigated the intracellular trafficking pathway of α-granule proteins using immunoelectron microscopy in order to elucidate the mechanism responsible for the abnormal release of α-granular proteins.

19.2 Results

19.2.1 Murine Model for MF

Mice were grafted with bone marrow cells infected with a retrovirus-carrying thrombopoietin (TPO) cDNA. They have previously been shown to develop a disease resembling human idiopathic MF [17, 18]. Morphological examination of the bone marrow from the transgenic mice (TPO mice) showed several striking pathological features.

19.2.1.1
Megakaryocytes

TPO mice presented with a general increase in the number of MKs (up to tenfold), with their regrouping in clusters (composed of three to ten cells). This was associated with an increase in size (two- to threefold the normal size), a mean diameter of 70 μm, and an increased lobularity of the nucleus (Fig. 19.1).

19.2.1.2
Emperipolesis

A pronounced increase in the frequency of emperipolesis within MKs was observed (Fig. 19.2). According to the definition, emperipolesis is the random passage of the different types of bone marrow cells through the MK cytoplasm, but without any significant harm to either host or invading cells [19–21]. It has been shown to occur in normal MKs and to be increased in myeloproliferative disorders [22, 23].

In the TPO mouse model, we found a correlation between the intensity of fibrosis and the degree of emperipolesis in MKs. Three weeks after transplantation, mice showed 25 to 50% MKs showing at least one emperipolesis figure per MK section, and 2 months after transplantation, TPO mice showed more than 60% of MK sections con-

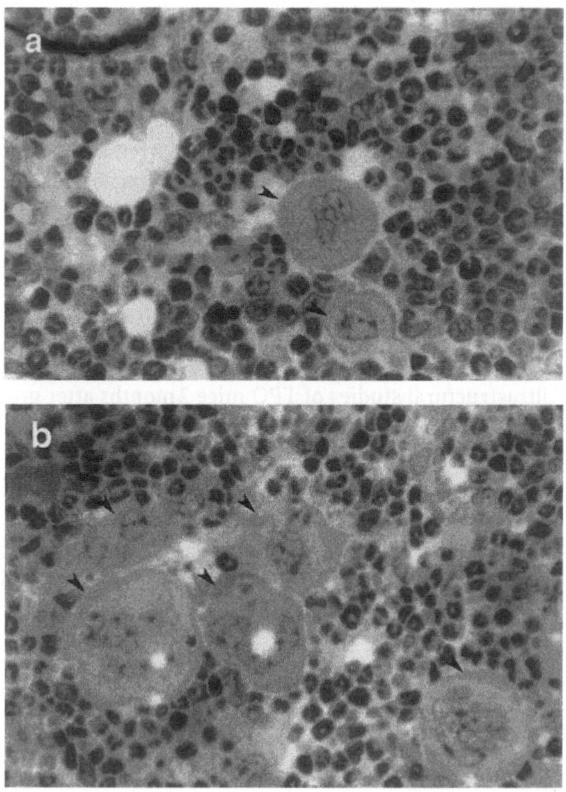

Fig. 19.1 a, b. Light microscopic view of a bone marrow section from a normal mouse (**a**) and from a TPO mouse (**b**). **a** This is a representative field showing the frequency and aspect of the normal MK population. MKs are easily distinguished from the other bone marrow cells by their large size and lobulated nucleus (*arrowheads*). **b** Section from a mouse 3 weeks after transplantation. MKs are more numerous and larger and have more lobulated nuclei than normal. They are often arranged in clusters (*arrowheads*)

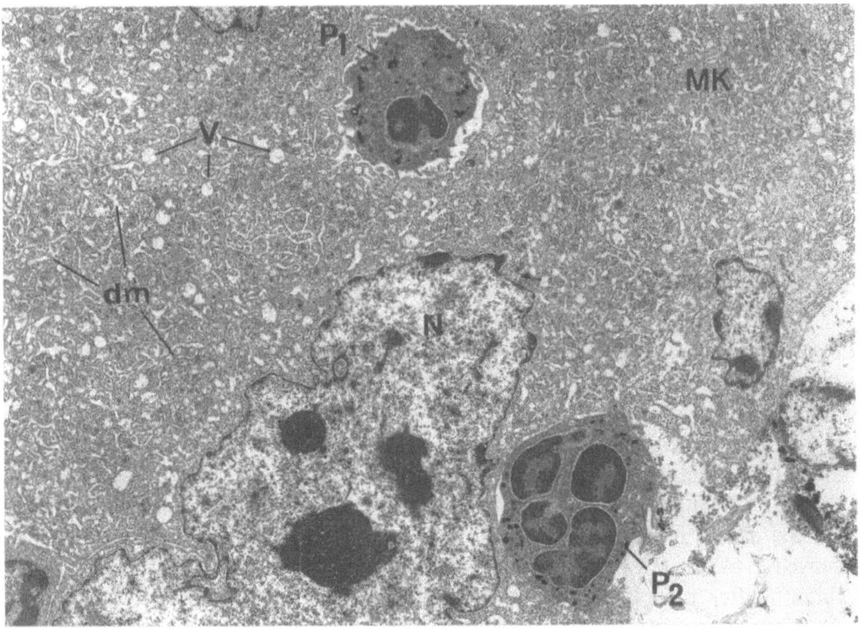

Fig. 19.2. Electron microscopic view of a MK from a TPO mouse. The cytoplasm organelles of the MK show alterations and abnormal vacuoles (*V*). A PMN (*P1*) is trapped between demarcation membranes and shows signs of activation (pseudopods and cytoplasmic vacuoles). In the lower right corner, another PMN (*P2*) is ready to enter the MK (×3300)

taining intracellular foreign cells. Moreover, in TPO mice, cells undergoing emperipolesis were predominantly polymorphonuclear neutrophils (86%) and eosinophils (13%), whereas normally, the type of cells undergoing emperipolesis in MKs is random and reflects the cellular composition of the marrow.

19.2.1.3
Cell Damage

Ultrastructural studies of TPO mice 2 months after grafting demonstrated that both the host MKs and the polymorphonuclear leukocytes (PMNs) located within MKs were significantly altered. PMNs appeared damaged, with apoptotic-like nuclei and disrupted plasma membranes. Myeloperoxidase-positive lysosomal granules from PMNs appeared free, often scattered within the MK cytoplasm. The host MKs also displayed numerous cytoplasmic aberrations including vacuoles, a dystrophic demarcation membrane system (DMS), and ruptured β-granules (Fig. 19.3). Finally, contact fibrosis was found around disrupted MKs.

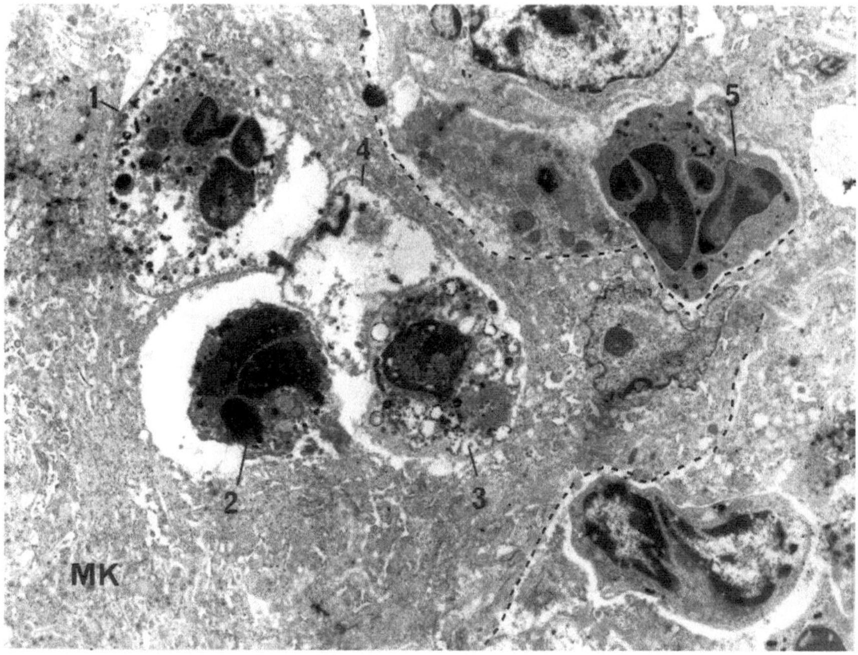

Fig. 19.3. Electron microscopic view of MK from a TPO mouse that shows important signs of alteration, with poorly recognizable organelle limits. Three PMNs (*1*, *2* and *3*) are observed within the dilated DMS. An empty limiting membrane seems to be all that is left of a fourth PMN (*4*). An intact PMN is tethering the MK (*5*). The MK boundary is indicated by a *dotted line* (×3300)

19.2.1.4 P-Selectin

Immunolabeling for a wide range of β-granular proteins was performed. vWF, fibrinogen, αIIbβ3 and TGFβ showed virtually no differences in pattern and density of labeling between control and TPO mice. However, immunolabeling for the specific platelet receptor of leukocytes, P-selectin, which is a component of the β-granule membrane [24, 25] and which is also found associated with the dense granule membrane [26], revealed significant differences. In TPO mice, the overall degree of detected P-selectin was increased, and localized within the membrane of numerous and small intracytoplasmic vacuolar structures in addition to α-granules. P-selectin also appeared to occasionally line the DMS near engulfed PMNs (Fig. 19.4).

19.2.2 Patients with Idiopathic MF

The light microscopic examination of bone marrow biopsies from patients with idiopathic MF, showed characteristic irregular and enlarged MKs with hyperlobulated nuclei. The cells were numerous and arranged in clusters.

Study of paraffin-embedded biopsies from patients with idiopathic MF revealed a

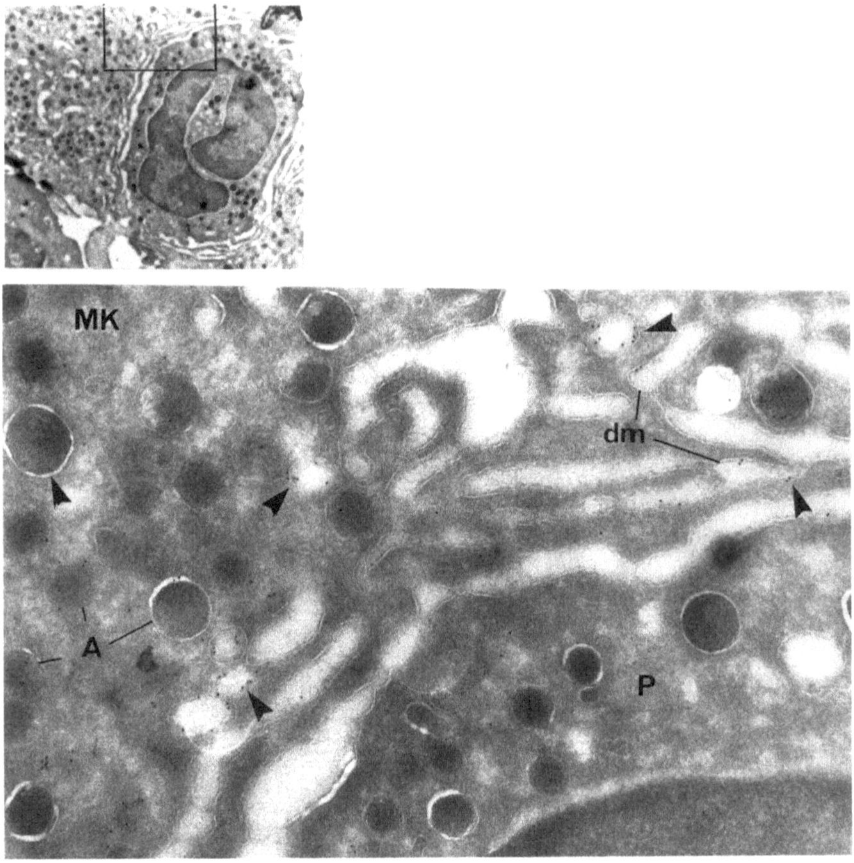

Fig. 19.4. Immunogold labeling for P-selectin performed on a frozen bone marrow section from a TPO mouse. P-selectin (*arrowheads*) is detected in the vicinity of a PMN (*P*) trapped within MK DMS (*dm*) while undergoing emperipolesis. Labeling is located in the α-granular (*A*) membrane, in small cytoplasmic vacuolar structures, and occasionally along demarcation membranes (×38,750). *Inset*: Lower magnification view of the field showing the entire PMN located within the MK (×12,400)

definite and significant increase of the emperipolesis phenomenon: 13.7% of MK sections exhibited at least one emperipolesis image ($n=12$) compared to 2.8% in controls ($n=9$). The use of a specific immunohistochemical staining (by alkaline phosphatase antialkaline phosphatase, APAAP) with specific antibodies to either αIIbβ3 or P-selectin facilitated the recognition of massive hyperplasia of MKs with apparent destruction of their cytoplasm (Fig. 19.5). However, the prominent infiltration of the bone marrow by MK cytoplasmic fragments was not apparent via conventional staining techniques (Fig. 19.1).

Moreover, electron microscopy examination of bone marrows from patients allowed the identification of similar abnormalities to those found in the mouse model. These included: morphological abnormalities of both MKs and the intracellular PMNs, the presence of free PMN-derived myeloperoxidase-positive granules

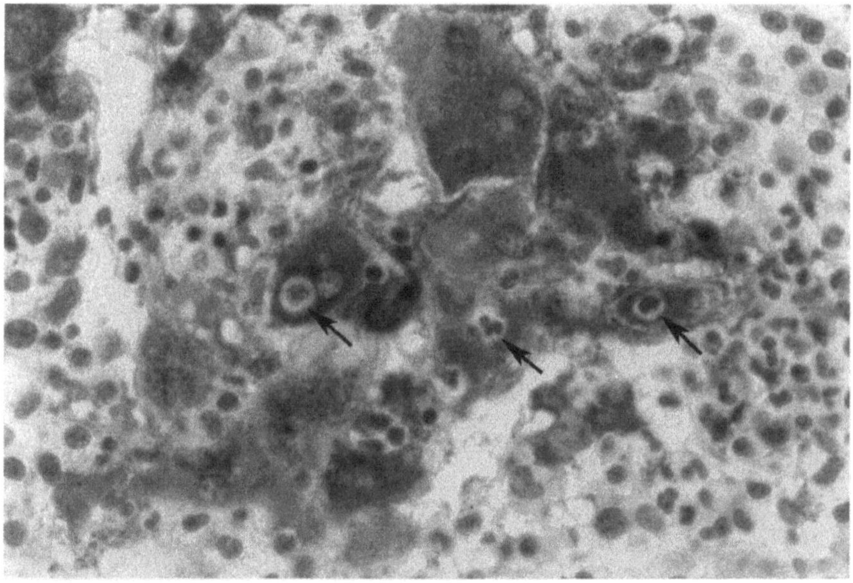

Fig. 19.5. Bone marrow biopsy from a patient with idiopathic MF. MKs are labeled for P-selectin with the APAAP technique and cytoplasm is specifically stained red. MK numbers, size and ploidy are significantly increased, and they are arranged in clusters. Numerous PMNs (*arrows*) are present within the cytoplasm of MKs

within the MK cytoplasm, damaged MKs displaying vacuoles, ruptured α-granules, and contact fibrosis (Fig. 19.6).

Finally, immunolabeling for P-selectin demonstrated not only increased expression but abnormal localization, very similar to the labeling pattern observed in TPO mice. P-selectin was also found within small empty vacuoles scattered throughout the cytoplasm and within the lining of the DMS.

19.3 Discussion

The involvement of MKs in MF development is now well established [1]. Pathological release of growth factors stored in MK granules has been proposed to result in the activation and proliferation of fibroblasts leading to fibrosis [5]. However, the subcellular events which cause the inappropriate release of growth factors from MKs into the extracellular environment are still largely unknown [27, 28].

19.3.1 Pathogenic Interaction Between MKs and PMNs

In TPO mice there is a marked increase in the number of cells undergoing emperipolesis within MKs compared to control mice. The same phenomenon is observed in the bone marrow from patients with idiopathic MF, and its intensity appears to be related

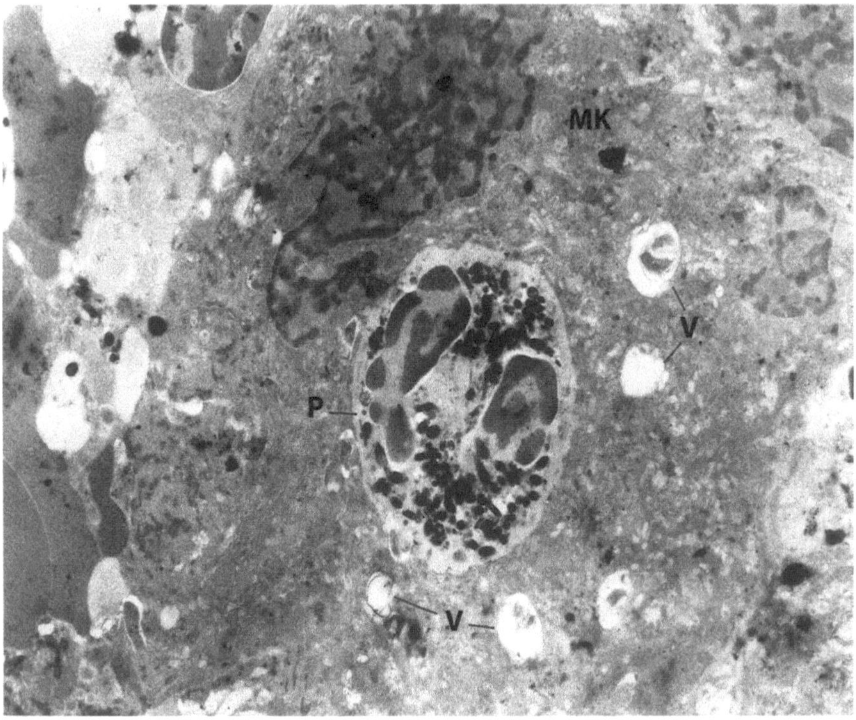

Fig. 19.6. Electron microscopic view of a PMN (*P*) within the DMS. Both cells show important signs of alteration. The cytoplasm from the host MK shows abnormal vacuoles (*V*) and generally damaged organelles including ruptured granules (×3300)

to the severity of the disease. This observation is supported by a correlation between the rate of fibrosis and the intensity of emperipolesis in the TPO mouse model as well as in patients with idiopathic MF.

Nevertheless, there were significant differences in the pathological emperipolesis phenomenon in idiopathic MF patients and in TPO mice and normal emperipolesis as described in the literature. Indeed, the apparent selectivity of the engulfed cells, coupled with the alterations of both the host and the invading cells, indicates that the phenomenon is clearly pathological and differs significantly from the phenomenon usually described.

The presence of foreign cells within the MK cytoplasm had already been observed in myeloproliferative disorders [22, 23]. Here, we correlated the rate of this emperipolesis-like phenomenon with the intensity of fibrosis.

19.3.2
P-Selectin Involvement

There was an increased cytoplasmic immunogold labeling and atypical intracellular distribution of P-selectin observed by electron microscopy in MKs from TPO mice and within the bone marrow from idiopathic MF patients. Indeed, in addition to normal α-granular membrane labeling observed in control mice and in normal subjects, P-selectin appeared to be located within numerous intracytoplasmic vacuoles and within the DMS membranes.

The selectin family is known to mediate leukocyte rolling along the endothelial surface of the vessel wall, which is the initial stage of a multistep process leading to extravasation of blood white cells. It is known that PMNs (neutrophilic and eosinophilic) are known to express the P-selectin ligand 1 (PSGL-1) [29, 30]. Expression of endothelial P-selectin results in binding of PSGL-1, and is the first step that leads to the rolling of neutrophils [31, 32] on the vascular wall. When PMNs penetrate into the DMS of MKs, the binding of PSGL-1 to the abnormally distributed P-selectin could result in irreversible trapping and sequestration of PMNs within DMS. PMNs, abnormally retained within the MK DMS, display activation signs and undergo cell death and breakage, releasing their lysosomes [33] into the MK cytoplasm. This process leads to the progressive destruction of MKs, with α-granular lysis and subsequent release of α-granular growth factors which may induce significant fibroblast activation and proliferation leading to the development of MF.

19.4 Conclusions

Our study performed in a murine model of MF and in patients with idiopathic MF demonstrates a pathological interaction between PMN leukocytes and MKs, correlated with MF development [34]. The results obtained in the animal model of MF revealed a significantly abnormal subcellular P-selectin distribution which appeared to correlate with excessive and pathological emperipolesis of PMN leukocytes within the MKs, leading to MK destruction and leakage of α-granular contents. Similar abnormalities were observed in the bone marrow of patients with idiopathic MF. Therefore, this study provides insight into the possible pathophysiological mechanisms for the genesis of MF. The prominent role of PDGF and TGFβ in the generation of MF has been previously largely documented. These growth factors are both essential for in vitro MK-dependent fibroblast proliferation. Recent work has shown that TGFβ plays a prominent role in TPO-induced myelofibrosis in mice [35]. The intervention of a destructive mutual cellular interaction of MKs and PMNs may lead to the pathological release of PDGF and TGFβ within the bone marrow microenvironment leading, through fibroblast activation, to the generation of MF.

References

1. Reilly JT 1994) Pathogenesis of idiopathic myelofibrosis: present status and future directions. Br J Haematol 88:1
2. Jacobson R, Salo A, Fialkow P (1978) Agnogenic myeloid metaplasia: a clonal proliferation of hematopoietic stem cells with secondary myelofibrosis. Blood 51:189
3. Briere J, Kiladjian J, Peynaud-Debayle E (1996) Dysmegakaryocytopoiesis and dysthrombopoiesis in myeloproliferative syndromes. C R Seances Soc Biol 190:533
4. Martyre MC, Romquin N, Le Bousse-Kerdiles MC, Chevillard S, Benyahia B, Dupriez B, Demory JL, Bauters F (1994) Transforming growth factor-beta and megakaryocytes in the pathogenesis of idiopathic myelofibrosis. Br J Haematol 88:9

5. Reilly JT (1997) Idiopathic myelofibrosis: pathogenesis, natural history and management. Blood Rev 11:233
6. Terui T, Niitsu Y, Mahara K, Fujisaki Y, Urushizaki Y, Mogi Y, Kohgo Y, Watanabe N, Ogura M, Saito H (1990) The production of transforming growth factor-beta in acute megakaryoblastic leukemia and its possible implications in myelofibrosis. Blood 75:1540
7. Wickenhauser C, Hillienhof A, Jungheim K, Lorenzen J, Ruskowski H, Hansmann ML, Thiele J, Fischer R (1995) Detection and quantification of transforming growth factor beta (TGF-β) and platelet-derived growth factor (PDGF) release by normal human megakaryocytes. Leukemia 9:310
8. Michiels JJ, Kutti J, Stark P, Bazzan M, Gugliotta L, Marchioli R, Griesshammer M, van Genderen PJ, Briere J, Kiladjian JJ, Barbui T, Finazzi G, Berlin NI, Pearson TC, Green AC, Fruchtmann SM, Silver RT, Hansmann E, Wehmeier A, Lengfelder E, Landolfi R, Kvasnicka HM, Hasselbalch H, Cervantes F, Thiele J, et al (1999) Diagnosis, pathogenesis and treatment of the myeloproliferative disorders essential thrombocythemia, polycythemia vera and essential megakaryocytic granulocytic metaplasia and myelofibrosis. Neth J Med 54:46
9. Tefferi A (2000) Myelofibrosis with myeloid metaplasia. N Engl J Med 342:1255
10. Ozaki S, Kosaka M, Ozaki K, Wakatsuki S, Hashimoto T, Miyazaki H (1997) Thrombopoietin-responsive essential thrombocythaemia with myelofibrosis. Br J Haematol 97:449
11. Ellis JT, Peterson P, Geller SA, Rappaport H (1986) Studies of the bone marrow in polycythemia vera and the evolution of myelofibrosis and second hematologic malignancies. Semin Hematol 23:144
12. Reilly JT, Barnett D, Dolan G, Forrest P, Eastham J, Smith A (1993) Characterization of an acute micromegakaryocytic leukaemia: evidence for the pathogenesis of myelofibrosis. Br J Haematol 83:58
13. Breton-Gorius J, Vainchenker W, Nurden AT, Levy-Toledano S, Caen JP (1981) Defective alpha-granule production in megakaryocytes from gray platelet syndrome: ultrastructural studies of bone marrow cells and megakaryocytes growing in culture from blood precursors. Am J Pathol 102:10
14. Drouin A, Favier R, Masse JM, Debili N, Schmitt A, Elbim C, Guichard J, Adam M, Gougerot-Pocidalo MA, Cramer EM (2001) Newly recognized cellular abnormalities in the gray platelet syndrome. Blood 98:1382
15. Vannucchi AM, Bianchi L, Cellai C, Paoletti F, Rana RA, Lorenzini R, Migliaccio G, Migliaccio AR (2002) Development of myelofibrosis in mice genetically impaired for GATA-1 expression (GATA-1(low) mice). Blood 100:1123
16. Breton-Gorius J, Bizet M, Reyes F, Dupuy E, Mear C, Vannier JP, Tron P (1982) Myelofibrosis and acute megakaryoblastic leukemia in a child: topographic relationship between fibroblasts and megakaryocytes with an alpha-granule defect. Leuk Res 6:97
17. Villeval JL, Cohen-Solal K, Tulliez M, Giraudier S, Guichard J, Burstein SA, Cramer EM, Vainchenker W, Wendling F (1997) High thrombopoietin production by hematopoietic cells induces a fatal myeloproliferative syndrome in mice. Blood 90:4369
18. Yan XQ, Lacey D, Fletcher F, Hartley C, McElroy P, Sun Y, Xia M, Mu S, Saris C, Hill D, Hawley RG, McNiece IK (1995) Chronic exposure to retroviral vector encoded MGDF (mpl-ligand) induces lineage-specific growth and differentiation of megakaryocytes in mice. Blood 86:4025
19. Breton-Gorius J (1981) On the alleged phagocytosis by megakaryocytes. Br J Haematol 47:635
20. Bobik R, Dabrowski Z (1995) Emperipolesis of marrow cells within megakaryocytes in the bone marrow of sublethally irradiated mice. Ann Hematol 70:91
21. Tanaka M, Aze Y, Shinomiya K, Fujita T (1996) Morphological observations of megakaryocytic emperipolesis in the bone marrow of rats treated with lipopolysaccharide. Vet Med Sci 58:663
22. Thiele J, Kuemmel T, Sander C, Fischer R (1991) Ultrastructure of bone marrow tissue in so-called primary (idiopathic) myelofibrosis-osteomyelosclerosis (agnogenic myeloid metaplasia). I. Abnormalities of megakaryopoiesis and thrombocytes. Submicrosc Cytol Pathol 23:93
23. Cashell AW, Buss DH (1992) The frequency and significance of megakaryocytic emperipolesis in myeloproliferative and reactive states. Ann Hematol 64:273
24. Larsen E, Celi A, Gilbert GE, Furie BC, Erban JK, Bonfanti R, Wagner DD, Furie B (1989) PADGEM protein: a receptor that mediates the interaction of activated platelets with neutrophils and monocytes. Cell 59:305
25. Stenberg PE, McEver RP, Shuman MA, Jacques YV, Bainton DF (1985) A platelet alpha-granule membrane protein (GMP-140) is expressed on the plasma membrane after activation. J Cell Biol 101:880
26. Israels SJ, Gerrard JM, Jacques YV, McNicol A, Cham B, Nishibori M, Bainton DF (1992) Platelet dense granule membranes contain both granulophysin and P-selectin (GMP-140). Blood 80:143
27. Smith MP, Cramer EM, Savidge GF (1997) Megakaryocytes and platelets in alpha-granule disorders. Baillieres Clin Haematol 10:125
28. Yanagida M, Ide Y, Imai A, Toriyama M, Aoki T, Harada K, Izumi H, Uzumaki H, Kusaka M, Tokiwa T (1997) The role of transforming growth factor-beta in PEG-rHuMGDF-induced reversible myelofibrosis in rats. Br J Haematol 99:739

29. Moore KL, Stults NL, Diaz S, Smith DF, Cummings RD, Varki A, McEver RP (1992) Identification of a specific glycoprotein ligand for P-selectin (CD62) on myeloid cells. J Cell Biol 118:445
30. Evangelista V, Manarini S, Sideri R, Rotondo S, Martelli N, Piccoli A, Totani L, Piccardoni P, Vestweber D, de Gaetano G, Cerletti C (1999) Platelet/polymorphonuclear leukocyte interaction: P-selectin triggers protein-tyrosine phosphorylation-dependent CD11b/CD18 adhesion: role of PSGL-1 as a signaling molecule. Blood 93:876
31. Diacovo TG, Roth SJ, Buccola JM, Bainton DF, Springer TA (1996) Neutrophil rolling, arrest, and transmigration across activated, surface-adherent platelets via sequential action of P-selectin and the beta 2-integrin CD11b/CD18. Blood 88:146
32. Broide DH, Humber D, Sriramarao P (1998) Inhibition of eosinophil rolling and recruitment in P-selectin and intracellular adhesion molecule-1-deficient mice. Blood 91:2847
33. Borregaard N, Cowland JB (1997) Granules of the human neutrophilic polymorphonuclear leukocyte. Blood 89:3503
34. Schmitt A, Drouin A, Masse JM, Guichard J, Shagraoui H, Cramer EM (2002) Polymorphonuclear neutrophil and megakaryocyte mutual involvement in myelofibrosis pathogenesis. Leuk Lymph 43:719–724
35. Chagraoui H, Komura E, Tulliez M, Giraudier S, Vainchenker W, Wendling F (2002) Prominent role of TGF-β1 in thrombopoietin-induced myelofibrosis in mice. Blood 100:3495–3503

E Mastocytosis

Chapter 20

C-kit and Mastocytosis

Frédéric Féger, Olivier Hermine, Jean-Jacques Guillosson, Michel Arock

20.1 Introduction

Mast cells (MC) are tissue elements derived from a subset of hematopoietic stem cells expressing CD34, c-kit and CD13 antigens [1] (Fig. 20.1). Immature MC progenitors circulate in the bloodstream then differentiate in tissues under the influence of cytokines, one of utmost importance being stem cell factor (SCF). SCF receptor is encoded by the protooncogene c-kit, belonging to type III receptor tyrosine kinase subfamily [2] (Fig. 20.2). Ligation of the c-kit receptor by SCF induces its dimeriza-

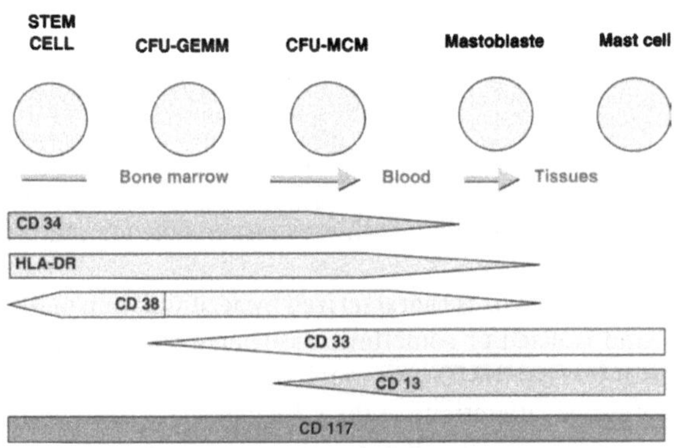

Fig. 20.1. Schematic representation of the differentiation pathways of human mast cells from hematopoietic progenitors

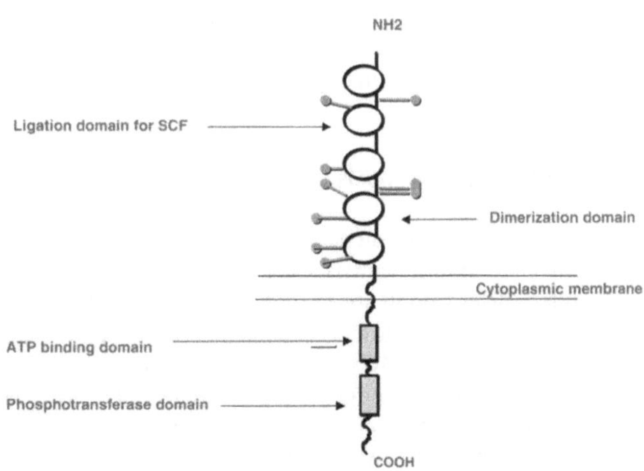

Fig. 20.2. Schematic representation of the structure of the human c-kit receptor

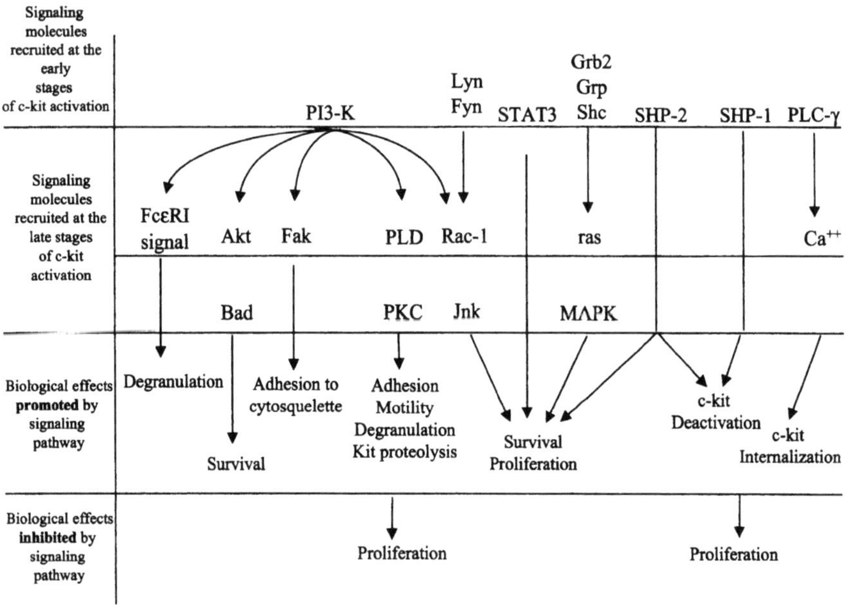

Fig. 20.3. Different intracellular pathways induced by c-Kit activation in human cells

tion followed by its transphosphorylation leading to the recruitment and activation of various intracytoplasmic substrates. These activated substrates induce multiple intracellular signaling pathways responsible for cell proliferation and activation [2] (Fig. 20.3).

Mastocytosis is characterized by accumulation of MC in various tissues, which are found isolated or sometimes associated with hematological clonal non-MC lineage disorders (AHNMD). Although the critical events leading to mastocytosis are not yet unraveled, alterations of the c-kit gene have been described in a significant proportion of the patients. Of particular interest are acquired point mutations resulting in a constitutively activated receptor, possibly involved in the increased numbers of MC in tissues. For this reason, future strategies might target specifically the mutated c-kit and/or its intracellular signaling.

20.2 Classification and Diagnosis of Mastocytosis

Mastocytosis is a heterogeneous group of disorders characterized by abnormal accumulation of MC in different tissues, mainly in the skin and the bone marrow, but also in the spleen, liver, lymph nodes, and gastrointestinal tract, depending on the nature of the disease. These disorders can affect humans of either sex at any age and can be acute or chronic. Acute MC neoplasms are designated as MC leukemia. Chronic MC diseases may be localized or generalized, indolent or aggressive. Cutaneous mastocytosis is the commonest localized neoplasm and is often found in children in whom it frequently remits and never relapses. Mastocytosis diseases usually acquired, but some familial cases have been described. With regard to the heterogeneity of MC neoplasms, several classifications have been proposed. The most used classification [3] distinguishes four types of mastocytosis: type I comprising two subtypes (IA and IB), and types II, III and IV.

Subtype IA includes diseases in which MC infiltration is strictly localized to the skin. This category represents the most frequent type of the disease and includes: (1) urticaria pigmentosa (UP), the most common form of cutaneous mastocytosis, particularly encountered in children, (2) diffuse cutaneous mastocytosis, (3) solitary mastocytoma, and (4) some rare subtypes such as bullous, erythrodermic and telangiectatic mastocytosis. These forms are characterized by their excellent prognosis with spontaneous remissions in children and a very indolent course in adults. Subtype IB is represented by indolent systemic disease (ISM) with or without cutaneous involvement. These forms are much more usual in adults than in children. The course of the disease is often indolent, but sometimes signs of aggressive mastocytosis can occur, leading to progressively impaired organ function.

Type II includes mastocytosis with an associated hematological disorder, such as a myeloproliferative or myelodysplastic syndrome. These malignant mastocytosis diseases do not usually involve the skin. The progression of the disease depends generally on the type of associated hematological disorder that influences the prognosis [4]. Type III is represented by aggressive systemic mastocytosis (ASM) in which the massive infiltration of multiple organs by abnormal MC is common. In these patients, peripheral blood features suggestive of a myeloproliferative disorder are prominent. The progression of the disease can be rapid, similar to acute leukemia, or some patients can show a longer survival time.

Finally, type IV mastocytosis includes MC leukemia (MCL), which is characterized by the presence of circulating MC and MC progenitors representing more than 10% of the white blood cells as well as by a massive infiltration of bone marrow by MC. This entity represents the rarest type of leukemia in humans, and has a very poor prognosis. MCL can occur either de novo or as the terminal phase of urticaria pigmentosa or systemic mastocytosis (SM).

Since types II and III do not differ prognostically, the classification of Metcalfe et al. can be further simplified as shown in Table 20.1 [5].

The diagnosis of mastocytosis is mainly based on histological criteria. The clinical suspicion of mastocytosis is confirmed by histological examination of the skin and bone marrow. Stains such as toluidine blue can be used to identify MC by their metachromatic granules [6]. In addition, immunocytochemistry for tryptase is useful to confirm the nature of the cellular infiltrate. Finally, the diagnosis can be helped by the use of the immunophenotyping of MC in bone marrow aspirate. Indeed, normal as

Table 20.1. Simplified classification of mastocytosis

Localized	Generalized
1. Cutaneous mastocytosis	1. Systemic mastocytosis (with or without cutaneous involvement)
1.1. Solitary mastocytoma	1.1. Indolent
1.2. Urticaria pigmentosa	1.2. Aggressive
	2. Mast cell leukemia

well as mastocytosis-related MC strongly express CD117 antigen [7], and some antigens not found on normal MC can be aberrantly expressed by neoplastic MC, such as CD2 and CD25 [8]. Biochemical determination of MC mediators can also help the diagnosis of mastocytosis: histamine levels in blood and urine, and metabolites of prostaglandin D2 and histamine in the urine are increased in most cases of SM, as well as the level of tryptase in blood [9].

Recently, Longley et al. have proposed including the occurrence of c-kit mutations in the classification of mastocytosis [10].

20.3 Molecular Genetic Lesions in Mastocytosis

20.3.1 In Vitro Data

Most of the present knowledge concerning the consequences of c-kit mutations in hematopoiesis and MC proliferation has been obtained using cell lines bearing different mutations. Four tumoral MC lines have been used to explore the consequences of mutations in the c-kit gene. These MC lines are: (1) P815 and FMA3, two mouse mastocytoma cell lines, in which mutations cause, at codon 814, the substitution of Tyr for Asp in the phosphotransferase domain [11] and, at codons 573 to 579, deletion of seven amino acids in the juxtamembrane domain [12], respectively; (2) RBL-2H3, a rat MC leukemia cell line, in which mutation causes, at codon 817, substitution of Tyr for Asp in the phosphotransferase domain [13]; (3) HMC1, which is the only MC line of human origin derived from a patient with MC leukemia, in which two mutations have been identified, one at codon 560 in the juxtamembrane domain of c-kit causing substitution of Val for Gly and the other at codon 816 in the tyrosine-kinase domain inducing substitution of Asp for Val [14].

The oncogenic potential of c-kit has been primarily studied in these four MC cell lines where c-kit is found constitutively phosphorylated on tyrosine and activated, inducing cell proliferation in the absence of SCF. Nevertheless, the different kit mutations encountered in these cell lines do not have the same biological effects. C-kit-transforming activity is weaker with the mutation in position 560 than with the mutation in position 816 in HMC1 [14]. However, excepted for the deletion of seven amino acids in FMA3, a somatic point mutation in the gene encoding c-kit, resulting in most cases in a change of a single amino acid, is enough to cause c-kit dysregulation.

In order to understand the role of point mutation at codon 814 in the catalytic domain of c-kit, Piao et al. [15] have studied the biological effects of the mutation, after its transfection into IC2 cells, an IL-3-dependent MC line that does not express endogenous wild-type (WT) c-kit. These authors reported three major findings: (1) the mutant was phosphorylated on tyrosine residues in the absence of SCF; (2) the IC2 cells expressing the mutant form of c-kit proliferated for more than 4 weeks in the absence of growth factors and formed SCF-independent colonies in vitro; and finally (3) injection of IC2 cells expressing the mutant form of c-kit into syngenic DBA/2 mice induced the development of hepatic mastocytomas in all mice injected. These observations demonstrate that the expression of this mutant in position 814 is sufficient to confer tumorigenic potential in the context of IC2 cells.

Different molecular dysfunctions related to c-kit mutations have been described. These mutations alter different aspects of c-kit metabolism concerning dimerization, signaling, enzyme expression, and internalization. These changes could explain the oncogenic potential activation of the mutant forms of c-kit.

Tsujimura [12] and Kitayama et al. [16] have performed crosslinking analysis of various c-kit receptors, wild-type and mutated variants, to determine whether the constitutively activated c-kit leads to receptor dimerization or not, in the absence of SCF. They have studied four forms of c-kit: c-kitWT (wild type), c-kitd(573–579) (c-kit with a deletion from codon 573 to 579), c-kitV559G (Val to Gly in codon 559), c-kitD814V (Asp to Val in codon 814). In Ba/F3 cells, they found that activating mutations in the juxtamembrane domain, such as c-kitd(573–579) or c-kitV559G, induces a constitutive dimerization of c-kit in the absence of SCF activation, whereas an activating mutation in the tyrosine kinase domain such as c-kitD814V leads to constitutive activation without dimerization.

In addition, Piao et al. [15] have reported signaling alterations through the c-kitD814Y in the murine MC line IC2, as compared to wild-type c-kit. Indeed, in IC2 cells expressing c-kitD814Y, they detected not only the phosphorylation of a novel substrate, a protein of 130kDa (p130) but also ubiquitin-mediated proteolysis of SHP-1, a tyrosine phosphatase that constitutes a negative regulator of signaling induced by the system SCF/c-kitWT. The differences observed between the two forms of c-kit suggest that the signals transduced by c-kitWT stimulated by SCF and by c-kitD814Y are not equivalent. Recently, the signaling pathways activated by normal and mutated c-kit have been compared two in different studies. Both studies highlight the role of PI3 K which is constitutively tyrosine phosphorylated and associated with the mutated c-kit but not with c-kitwt activated by SCF, both in immortalized murine progenitor cells (MIHCs) expressing c-kitD816V [17] and in BA/F3 cells expressing murine c-kitD814V [18].

Finally, some genetic modifications of c-kit can alter the internalization signal with a prolonged activation of c-kit. The c-kitd(573–579) is not or is poorly internalized in the absence of SCF, whereas the activated c-kitD814V receptor is continuously degraded, even in the absence of SCF [19].

20.3.2 Findings in Patients

The main factors involved in the abnormal proliferation of MC in mastocytosis appear to be SCF and its specific receptor, c-kit. In the skin of some patients with indolent cutaneous mastocytosis, Longley et al. [20] have found increased levels of the soluble form of SCF. In these patients, no mutation of the SCF gene was identified, suggesting an aberrant metabolism of SCF. However, this mechanism is since poorly documented.

By contrast, numerous studies have suggested the presence of genetic abnormalities of c-kit that converts it into an oncoprotein able to induce oncogenic transformation of MC. In most cases, these mutations are found in the catalytic domain of the c-kit and are activating.

In human mastocytosis, a number of studies have been performed to elucidate whether mutations of c-kit are associated with different clinical forms of MC diseases.

Indeed, mutations of c-kit have been described in vivo in various forms of mastocytosis [2]. Among the mutations found, the most common is the activating mutation Asp to Val at codon 816. This mutation has been identified in MC from patients with aggressive SM [21], with indolent cutaneous mastocytosis in adults [22] and in a child [23]. Moreover, other point mutations in the c-kit gene have been reported by Pignon et al. [24] at codon 820, in the tyrosine kinase domain, which resulted in substitution of Asp for Gly in MC from a patient with an aggressive mastocytosis, and by Longley et al. [25] not only at codon 816 causing substitution of tyrosine or phenylalanine for aspartate in a child with sporadic SM or cutaneous mastocytosis, but also at codon 839 with substitution of lysine for glutamic acid (c-kitE839K) in a child with sporadic indolent UP. Furthermore, Longley et al. [25] found evidence that the mutations c-kitD816F and c-kitD816Y, as shown previously for c-kitD816V, caused spontaneous phosphorylation of c-kit, whereas c-kitE839K was not autophosphorylated or phosphorylated after exposure to exogenous SCF, and even inhibited the autophosphorylation of c-kit mutated at the 816 position. Interestingly, a novel mutation of c-kit (F522C), inducing constitutive activation of c-kit, was recently reported in one case of an unusual variant of SM producing normal mature MC [26]. The locations of the different point mutations found in the human c-kit are presented in Fig. 20.4.

Interestingly, the distribution of the Asp816Val mutation among hematopoietic lineages has recently been analyzed by examination of cells bearing differentiation markers for myelomonocytic cells as well as T and B lymphocytes in both peripheral blood and bone marrow obtained from patients with mastocytosis [27]. In this study, the mutation was detectable by PCR in at least one cell lineage in the bone marrow in 7 of 7 patients examined and in the peripheral blood of 11 of 11 adult patients with UP and indolent disease. The mutation was identified most frequently in B cells and myeloid cells. These results are consistent with the conclusion that the c-kit Asp816Val mutation occurs in an early progenitor cell, and not in mature MC since it is carried by myelomonocytic cells, T cells, and B cells in addition to MC. Of note, c-kit mutations at codon 816 have been described in a few patients with mastocytosis associated

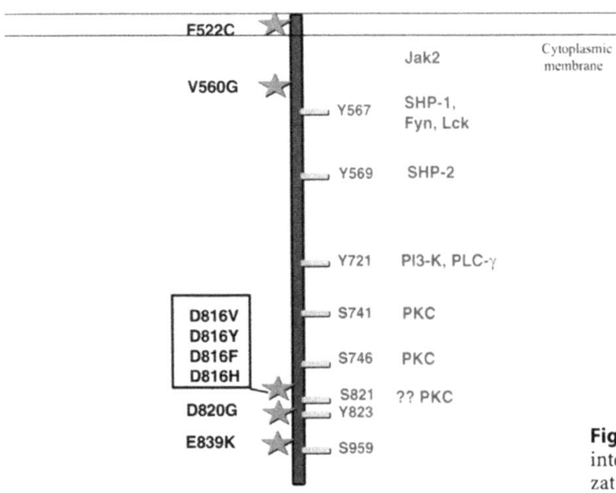

Fig. 20.4. Signaling molecules interacting with c-kit and localization of c-kit mutations

hematological non-MC lineage disorder (AHNMD) [4]: Asp816His in a patient with cutaneous mastocytosis associated with acute myeloid leukemia type 2 (AML2) [28], Asp816Val in a patient with SM associated with AML4 [29], and in a patient with chronic myelomonocytic leukemia [30]. These reports suggest that either SM and AHNMD arise from a common progenitor cell or that the leukemic clone acquires, as a second event, the capability to differentiate along the MC lineage. Recent data support the first hypothesis since evidence for the involvement of a hematopoietic progenitor cell in SM has been reported [31].

The situation observed in the few familial cases reported in the literature seems to be different from that in the sporadic diseases. Longley et al. [25] have reported three patients, members of a kindred with familial cutaneous mastocytosis in a series of 25 patients with mastocytosis: one child and two adults. In these three patients, no mutations of c-kit were found.

In conclusion, with regard to recent progress in c-kit gene analysis, human mastocytosis can be divided in two major groups: a first group representing a significant percentage of patients with activating mutation, representing probably most of the cases of adult SM, and a second group of patients comprising children with cutaneous form of the disease, some adults with systemic disease and the familial cases, where no mutation of c-kit has been demonstrated. However, an inactivating mutation (E839 K) has been reported in three patients from an atypical familial mastocytosis.

20.4 Treatment of Mastocytosis

The treatment of mastocytosis is symptomatic and/or specific, but treatment can be minimal in very indolent non-aggressive forms of the disease.

Symptomatic treatments aim at interfering with adverse effects induced by the abnormal production of mediators by MC [32, 33]. The main drugs used are H1 and H2 antihistamines [34]. H1 antihistamines are usually administered against pruritus and flushing, whereas H2 antihistamines are used to treat gastritis and peptic ulcer. Other drugs such as corticosteroids may be necessary in the case of severe cutaneous symptoms [35]. Anticholinergics are also administered to treat diarrhea and headache. Disodium cromoglycate is used for respiratory symptoms. Acute cardiovascular collapse may require adrenaline and intravenous fluids. It seems likely that bisphosphonates would be useful in patients with osteoporosis and pathological fractures.

Specific treatment must inhibit abnormal proliferation of MC. With this goal, the interferons (INFα and INFγ) are used associated or not with corticosteroids [36–38]. Interferon treatments lead to improvement of the clinical status in some cases. However, recurrence has been noted concomitantly with the appearance of circulating antibody to interferon α [39], and it appears that only a subset of patients respond to IFN-α2b [40]. Therefore, the next question is how "IFN-non-responders" and those with rapidly progressive disease should be treated. For those patients a number of experimental drugs have been suggested. In a few patients with SM, the novel nucleoside 2-chlorodeoxy-adenosine (cladribine, 2-CdA) produces a major response with a significant decrease of bone marrow MC infiltrates [41–43]. In MCL, the most appropriate alternative would be polychemotherapy using drugs that are otherwise used in patients with AML (daunorubicin, cytosine arabinoside, others). If the overall situation allows, and a major response to induction treatment (chemotherapy) is seen, these patients should also be considered for bone marrow transplantation in a way similar to high-risk AML patients. If bone marrow transplantation is not applicable, patients in remission should receive consolidation treatment – again, the standards for AML treatment should be applied. In patients who fail to respond to chemotherapy, palliative cytoreduction with hydroxyurea (or other drugs) seems appropriate.

These different therapies exhibit some interesting activities, but these treatments do not target the initial abnormality, i.e., the presence of activating mutations of c-kit in abnormal MC. Indeed, since it appears that the major forms of the disease are associated with activating mutations of the c-kit in its tyrosine kinase domain, aiming at blocking this abnormal tyrosine kinase activity could be a challenge in the next years for future therapies of SM. In this way, Ma et al. have tested in vitro several indolinone derivatives that are specific tyrosine kinase inhibitors, and found that some of these compounds can inhibit the constitutively activated c-kit mutants and can suppress neoplastic proliferation of MC [44]. Similar studies have been recently conducted by Liao et al. in neoplastic MC lines of murine and canine origin [45], by Fumo et al. in MC lines of human origin [46], and by Zermati et al. in tumoral MC from cell lines and from patients with SM [47]. The findings show a direct correlation between inhibition of constitutively activated c-kit and the death of neoplastic MC, and point to specific tyrosine kinase inhibitors as a potential therapy aimed directly at a cause of mastocytosis. However, in SM without c-kit mutation, molecules able to block the SCF-induced phosphorylation of the wild-type receptor such as STI571 (Gleevec) might have some interesting effects that are currently under investigation.

20.5 Conclusions

MC are implicated in tumoral pathologies, particularly in SM that are hematological diseases. Of interest, mutations of c-kit have been described in vivo in different forms of mastocytosis, and occur in the intracytoplasmic tail of this receptor, mainly in its phosphotransferase domain. Moreover, according to the position of the mutation, its effect on MC proliferation appears to be different. Indeed, these mutations can be found either in aggressive diseases or in indolent mastocytosis. In addition, c-kit mutations can also be found in mastocytosis associated with other malignant hemopathies. However, even if in vitro and in vivo data from the literature using cell lines or animal models are convincing, it remains difficult to conclude that the mutations reported in patients are sufficient by themselves to induce neoplastic transformation of MC or whether other(s) additional abnormality(ies) is(are) required. Additional experiments are required to answer this critical question. Indeed, if mutations of c-kit are shown to be sufficient to induce the disease(s), future therapeutic agents aimed at inhibiting selectively the expression of the mutated c-kit in target cells could be considered and could give rise to promising fields of research for new therapeutic agents in this disease.

20.6 Summary

MC is a tissue-resident granulated cell that releases a number of biologically active mediators (histamine, heparin, protease and cytokines) and that originates from pluripotent hematopoietic progenitor cells. The differentiation processes leading to MC depend greatly on a particular cytokine, SCF, whose receptor is the product of the protooncogene c-kit. Mastocytosis is a rare and heterogeneous group of disorders characterized by abnormal growth and accumulation of MC in skin, bone marrow, gastrointestinal tract, liver, spleen and lymph nodes. With regard to the pathophysiology of mastocytosis, most patients with systemic disease show alterations of the c-kit gene encoding the receptor for SCF. No specific therapy for patients with mastocytosis is today available, but some patients may benefit from corticosteroids and interferon-α treatment. More specific treatment that targets specifically c-kit are currently under investigation.

References

1. Kirshenbaum AS, Goff JP, Semere T, Foster B, Scott LM, Metcalfe DD (1999) Demonstration that human mast cells arise from a progenitor cell population that is CD34(+), c-kit(+), and expresses aminopeptidase N (CD13). Blood 94:2333–2342
2. Feger F, Ribadeau Dumas A, Leriche L, Valent P, Arock M (2002) Kit and c-kit mutations in mastocytosis a short overview with special reference to novel molecular and diagnosis concepts. Int Arch Allergy Immunol 127:110–114
3. Metcalfe DD (1991) Classification and diagnosis of mastocytosis: current status. J Invest Dermatol 96:2S–4S
4. Sperr WR, Horny HP, Valent P (2002) Spectrum of associated clonal hematologic non-mast cell lineage disorders occurring in patients with systemic mastocytosis. Int Arch Allergy Immunol 127:140–142
5. Horny HP, Sillaber C, Menke D, Kaiserling E, Wehrmann M, Stehberger B, Chott A, Lechner K, Lennert K, Valent P (1998) Diagnostic value of immunostaining for Tryptase in patients with mastocytosis. Am J Surg Pathol 22:1132–1140
6. Sperr WR, Escribano L, Jordan JH, Schernthaner GH, Kundi M, Horny HP, Valent P (2001) Morphologic properties of neoplastic mast cells: delineation of stages of maturation and implication for cytological grading of mastocytosis. Leukemia Res 25:529–536
7. Arber DA, Tamayo R, Weiss LM (1998) Paraffin section detection of the c-kit gene product (CD117) in human tissues: value in the diagnosis of mast cell disorders. Hum Pathol 29:498–504
8. Escribano L, Ocqueteau M, Almeida J, Orfao A, San Miguel JF (1998) Expression of the c-kit (CD117) molecule in normal and malignant hematopoiesis. Leuk Lymphoma 30:459–466
9. Granerus G, Lonnqvist B, Wass U (1999) Determination of the histamine metabolite telemethylimidazoleacetic acid and of creatinine in urine by the same HPLC system. Inflamm Res 48:75–80
10. Longley BJ, Reguera MJ, Ma Y (2001) Classes of c-KIT activating mutations: proposed mechanisms of action and implications for disease classification and therapy. Leuk Res 25:571–576
11. Tsujimura T, Furitsu T, Morimoto M, Isozaki K, Nomura S, Matsuzawa Y, Kitamura Y, Kanakura Y (1994) Ligand-independent activation of c-kit receptor tyrosine kinase in a murine mastocytoma cell line P-815 generated by a point mutation. Blood 83:2619–2626
12. Tsujimura T (1996) Role of c-kit receptor tyrosine kinase in the development, survival and neoplastic transformation of mast cells. Pathol Int 46:933–938
13. Tsujimura T, Furitsu T, Morimoto M, Kanayama Y, Nomura S, Matsuzawa Y, Kitamura Y, Kanakura Y (1995) Substitution of an aspartic acid results in constitutive activation of c-kit receptor tyrosine kinase in a rat tumor mast cell line RBL-2H3. Int Arch Allergy Immunol 106:377–385
14. Furitsu T, Tsujimura T, Tono T, Ikeda H, Kitayama H, Koshimizu U, Sugahara H, Butterfield JH, Ashman LK, Kanayama Y, et al (1993) Identification of mutations in the coding sequence of the protooncogene c-kit in a human mast cell leukemia cell line causing ligand-independent activation of c-kit product. J Clin Invest 92:1736–1744

15. Piao X, Paulson R, van der Geer P, Pawson T, Bernstein A (1996) Oncogenic mutation in the Kit receptor tyrosine kinase alters substrate specificity and induces degradation of the protein tyrosine phosphatase SHP-1. Proc Natl Acad Sci U S A 93:14665–14669
16. Kitayama H, Kanakura Y, Furitsu T, Tsujimura T, Oritani K, Ikeda H, Sugahara H, Mitsui H, Kanayama Y, Kitamura Y, et al (1995) Constitutively activating mutations of c-kit receptor tyrosine kinase confer factor-independent growth and tumorigenicity of factor-dependent hematopoietic cell lines. Blood 85:790–798
17. Chian R, Young S, Danilkovitch-Miagkova A, Ronnstrand L, Leonard E, Ferrao P, Ashman L, Linnekin D (2001) Phosphatidylinositol 3 kinase contributes to the transformation of hematopoietic cells by the D816 V c-kit mutant. Blood 98:1365–1373
18. Hashimoto K, Matsumura I, Tsujimura T, Kim DK, Ogihara H, Ikeda H, Ueda S, Mizuki M, Sugahara H, Shibayama H, Kitamura Y, Kanakura Y (2003) Necessity of tyrosine 719 and phosphatidyl 3' kinase-mediated signal pathway in constitutive activation and oncogenic potential of c-kit receptor tyrosine kinase with the Asp814Val mutation. Blood 101:1094–1102
19. Moriyama Y, Tsujimura T, Hashimoto K, Morimoto M, Kitayama H, Matsuzawa, Kitamura Y, Kanakura Y (1996) Role of aspartic acid 814 in the function and expression of c-kit receptor tyrosine kinase. J Biol Chem 271:3347–3350
20. Longley BJ Jr, Morganroth GS, Tyrrell L, Ding TG, Anderson DM, Williams DE, Halaban R (1993) Altered metabolism of mast-cell growth factor (c-kit ligand) in cutaneous mastocytosis. N Engl J Med 328:1302–1307
21. Longley BJ, Tyrrell L, Lu SZ, Ma YS, Langley K, Ding TG, Duffy T, Jacobs P, Tang LH, Modlin I (1996) Somatic c-KIT activating mutation in urticaria pigmentosa and aggressive mastocytosis: establishment of clonality in a human mast cell neoplasm. Nat Genet 12:312–314
22. Buttner C, Henz BM, Welker P, Sepp NT, Grabbe J (1998) Identification of activating c-kit mutations in adult-, but not in childhood-onset indolent mastocytosis: a possible explanation for divergent clinical behavior. J Invest Dermatol 111:1227–1231
23. Nagata H, Okada T, Worobec AS, Semere T, Metcalfe DD (1997) c-kit mutation in a population of patients with mastocytosis. Int Arch Allergy Immunol 113:184–186
24. Pignon JM, Giraudier S, Duquesnoy P, Jouault H, Imbert M, Vainchenker W, Vernant JP, Tulliez M (1997) A new c-kit mutation in a case of aggressive mast cell disease. Br J Haematol 96:374–376
25. Longley BJ Jr, Metcalfe DD, Tharp M, Wang X, Tyrrell L, Lu SZ, Heitjan D, Ma Y (1999) Activating and dominant inactivating c-KIT catalytic domain mutations in distinct clinical forms of human mastocytosis. Proc Natl Acad Sci U S A 96:1609–1614
26. Akin C, Fumo G, Yavuz AS, Lipsky PE, Neckers L, Metcalfe DD (2004) A novel form of mastocytosis associated with a transmembrane c-kit mutation and response to imatinib. Blood 103:3222–3225
27. Akin C, Kirshenbaum AS, Semere T, Worobec AS, Scott LM, Metcalfe DD (2000) Analysis of the surface expression of c-kit and occurrence of the c-kit Asp816Val activating mutation in T cells, B cells, and myelomonocytic cells in patients with mastocytosis. Exp Hematol 28:140–147
28. Pullarkat VA, Pullarkat ST, Calverley DC, Brynes RK (2000) Mast cell disease associated with acute myeloid leukemia: detection of a new c-kit mutation Asp816His. Am J Hematol 65:307–309
29. Sperr WR, Walchshofer S, Horny HP, Fodinger M, Simonitsch I, Fritsche-Polanz R, Schwarzinger I, Tschachler E, Sillaber C, Hagen W, Geissler K, Chott A, Lechner K, Valent P (1998) Systemic mastocytosis associated with acute myeloid leukaemia: report of two cases and detection of the c-kit mutation Asp-816 to Val. Br J Haematol 103:740–749
30. Sotlar K, Marafioti T, Griesser H, Theil J, Aepinus C, Jaussi R, Stein H, Valent P, Horny HP (2000) Detection of c-kit mutation Asp-816-Val in microdissected bone marrow infiltrates in a case of systemic mastocytosis associated with chronic myelomonocytic leukemia. Mol Pathol 53:188–193
31. Yavuz AS, Lipsky PE, Yavuz S, Metcalfe DD, Akin C (2002) Evidence for the involvement of a hematopoietic progenitor cell in systemic mastocytosis from single cell analysis of mutations in the c-kit gene. Blood 100:661–665
32. Worobec AS (2000) Treatment of systemic mast cell disorders. Hematol Oncol Clin North Am 14:659–687
33. Marone G, Spadaro G, Granata F, Triggiani M (2001) Treatment of mastocytosis: pharmacologic basis and current concepts. Leuk Res 25:583–594
34. Gasior-Chrzan B, Falk ES (1992) Systemic mastocytosis treated with histamine H1 and H2 receptors antagonists. Dermatology 184:149–152
35. Burrall BA, Halpern GM, Huntley AC (1990) Chronic urticaria. West J Med 152:268–276
36. Kluin-Nelemans HC, Jansen JH, Breukelman H, Wolthers BG, Kluin PM, Kroon HM, Willemze R (1992) Response to interferon a-2b in a patient with systemic mastocytosis. N Engl J Med 326:619–623
37. Worobec AS, Kirshenbaum AS, Schwartz LB, Metcalfe DD (1996) Treatment of three patients with systemic mastocytosis with interferon alpha-2b. Leuk Lymphoma 22:501–508

38. Delaporte E, Pierard E, Wolthers BG, Desreumaux P, Janin A, Cortot A, Piette F, Bergoend H (1995) Interferon-alpha in combination with corticosteroids improves systemic mast cell disease. Br J Dermatol 132:479–482
39. Fiehn C, Prummer O, Gallati H, Heilig B, Hunstein W (1995) Treatment of systemic mastocytosis with interferon-gamma: failure after appearance of anti-IFN-gamma antibodies. Eur J Clin Invest 25:615–618
40. Hauswirth AW, Simonitsch-Klupp I, Uffmann M, Koller E, Sperr WR, Lechner K, Valent P (2004) Response to therapy with interferon alpha-2b and prednisone in aggressive systemic mastocytosis: report of five cases and review of the literature. Leukemia Res 28:249–257
41. Tefferi A, Li CY, Butterfield JH, Hoagland HC (2001) Treatment of systemic mast-cell disease with cladribine. N Engl J Med 344:307–309
42. Pardanani A, Hoffbrand AV, Butterfield JH, Tefferi A (2004) Treatment of systemic mast cell disease with 2-chorodeoxyadenosine. Leukemia Res 28:127–131
43. Nieva J, Saven A (2004) Cladribine activity in systemic mast cell disease: application of biochemistry in the modern era of molecular biology. Leukemia Res 28:113–114
44. Ma Y, Carter E, Wang X, Shu C, McMahon G, Longley BJ (2000) Indolinone derivatives inhibit constitutively activated KIT mutants and kill neoplastic mast cells. J Invest Dermatol 114:392–394
45. Liao AT, Chien MB, Shenoy N, Mendel DB, McMahon G, Cherrington JM, London CA (2002) Inhibition of constitutively active forms of mutant kit by multitargeted indolinone tyrosine kinase inhibitors. Blood 102:585–593
46. Fumo G, Akin C, Metcalfe DD, Neckers L (2003) 17-Allylamino-17-demethoxygeldanamycin (17-AAG) is effective in down-regulating mutated, constitutively activated KIT protein in human mast cells. Blood 103:1078–1084
47. Zermati Y, De Sepulveda P, Feger F, Letard S, Kersual J, Casteran N, Gorochov G, Dy M, Ribadeau Dumas A, Dorgham K, Parizot C, Bieche Y, Vidaud M, Lortholary O, Arock M, Hermine O, Dubreuil P (2003) Effect of tyrosine inhibitor STI571 on the kinase activity of wild-type and various mutated c-kit receptors found in mast cell neoplasms. Oncogene 22:660–664

Chapter 21

Tryptases, a Marker of Occult Mastocytosis

Dagmar Ludolph-Hauser, Bernhard Przybilla, Christian P. Sommerhoff

21.1 Introduction

Tryptases comprise a family of trypsin-like serine proteinases that are highly and selectively expressed in mast cells and to a lesser extent in basophils. In humans, four family members have been identified, i.e., the tryptases α, β, γ (also called transmembrane tryptase), and δ (or mMCP-7-like) [1–6]. They are derived from four or five genes located within a large serine protease cluster on chromosome 16p13.3 [7, 8]. For each tryptase, two or more allelic variants have been identified, a number that is likely to increase as the tryptase loci appear to be highly polymorphic [9]. Interestingly, α- and β-tryptase alleles compete at least in one of the loci; the resulting α-deficiency affects 29% of all genomes surveyed by Soto et al. and is particularly frequent in Caucasians (45%) [10].

Tryptase β is the most abundant protein present in mast cells, where it is stored in a mature, fully enzymatically active form in secretory granules, comprising up to 25% of the cellular protein [11]. The β-isoenzymes have been well characterized because they are postulated to contribute to the pathogenesis of allergic and inflammatory disorders, most notably asthma [12], a hypothesis recently supported by a clinical trial with a synthetic tryptase inhibitor [13]. In contrast, despite >90% identity in amino acid sequence with the β-isoenzymes, α-tryptase has been considered a nonfunctional protease that is constitutively secreted as a zymogen and has little enzymatic activity even in its (recombinantly produced) mature form [14, 15].

The γ- and δ-tryptases have been identified much later and are thus less well characterized. Tryptase δ is somewhat less closely related to β than α (>80% amino acid sequence identity to both tryptases) and lacks the C-terminal 40 amino acid residues [5, 6]. The expression, stability and features of this truncated protease are still controversial. δ-Tryptase has been produced recombinantly and localized in mast cells by immunohistology whereas in another study transcripts were not detectable [6, 16]. Compared to the other family members, γ-tryptase is only distantly related (about 50% identity with β) and is distinguished by a C-terminal hydrophobic extension that may serve as a membrane anchor [3, 4]. The features and functions of this protease are likely to differ considerably from those of the other tryptases.

21.2 Biochemical and Structural Features

Among the serine proteinases, tryptases are distinguished by several unique features that we have recently explained based on the crystal structures of the human β2- and α1-tryptases [17–19]. Most notably, β-tryptase is enzymatically active only in the form of a tetramer that requires the binding of heparin for stability. The structures reveal that this tetramer resembles a flat rectangular frame that consists of four quasi-equivalent monomers whose active sites are directed towards an oval central pore (Fig. 21.1 left). The tryptase monomer is surprisingly similar in fold to the ancestral proteinase trypsin, but differs in six surface loops (darker grey in Fig. 21.1 left) that are located around the active site and also realize the contacts to its two neighbors in the tetramer. The two distinct monomer–monomer interfaces thus formed differ considerably: the interface between monomers A and D (and their symmetry equivalents B and C) appears quite stable whereas the A–B interface (and its C–D equivalent) is much smaller in area (540 vs 1075 $Å^2$) and exclusively hydrophobic in nature. These A–B and C–D interfaces appear to be the built-in shear points of the tetramer. Heparin that is colocalized with β-tryptase in the secretory granules of mast cells and secreted concomitantly [20] may bridge and thus stabilize this interface by binding to

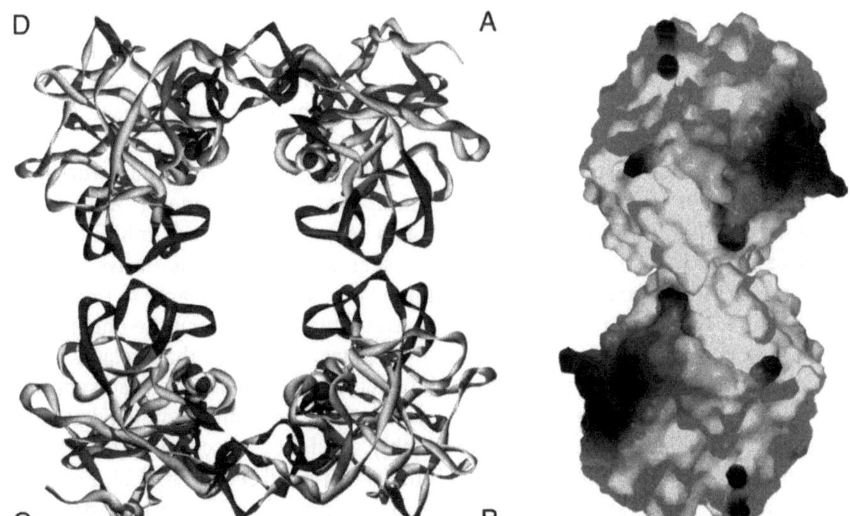

Fig. 21.1. Structure of the human β-tryptase tetramer. *Left* Front view onto the tetramer shown as ribbons. The four monomers (*A–D*) are arranged at the corners of a flat frame-like structure. The four active centers are directed towards the central pore, the catalytic triad residues Ser195, His57, and Asp102 are shown as stick models. At each of them a molecule of the cocrystallized inhibitor 4-amidinophenyl pyruvic acid (shown as CPK model) is bound. The six loops that differ most from the archetypal serine proteinase trypsin and realize the contacts to the neighboring monomers via two distinct interfaces are shown in dark grey. *Right* Side view from the right onto the tetramer shown in a solid-surface representation. The dark patches indicate positive electrostatic potential. A heparin molecule that binds to the clusters of positively charged amino acids on the back of monomer *A* and the front of monomer *B* would bridge the interface between the monomers and thus stabilize the tetramer. Figure produced with Swiss-PdbViewer [37]

an elongated patch of positive charges spanning the two adjacent monomers on their peripheral surface (see dark surface patches in Fig. 21.1 right). In the absence of stabilizing heparin (that may be removed from the tetramer, e.g., due to competition with other heparin binding proteins), the enzymatically active tetramer likely dissociates first into AD and BC dimers and subsequently into monomers, a multistep process thought to regulate the activity of β-tryptase in vivo [21, 22].

The crystal structure also explains the unusual substrate specificity of β-tryptase with its preference for peptidergic over proteinaceous substrates (reviewed in references 12 and 23). β-Tryptase has considerable activity towards neuropeptides such as VIP (vasoactive intestinal peptide) and PHM (peptide histidine methionine). The cleavage of these bronchodilatory peptides (which is particularly relevant due to the close association of mast cells with nerves) has been proposed as a mechanism by which tryptases enhance bronchoconstriction in asthma. Clearly, such peptide substrates are small and flexible enough to enter the tetramer's central pore (approximately 40×15 Å at its entrances) where they can interact with the active sites. On the other hand, tryptase cleaves only a few proteins, thus inactivating, for example, fibrinogen and fibronectin, and activating pro-MMP3 and pro-urokinase. Such macromolecules, as well as the 'protease-activated receptor-2' (PAR-2), a G protein-coupled receptor whose activation by β-tryptase may explain the plethora of cellular effects caused by this protease, are too bulky to enter the central pore and must extend a cleavable surface loop into the central pore. Alternatively, macromolecular substrates may be processed in a coordinated fashion by β-tryptase together with a second proteinase; for example, only high molecular weight kininogen cleaved by neutrophil elastase is processed by β-tryptase to bradykinin, a mechanism thought to activate the kinin system independently of kallikreins at sites of inflammation.

Also the unique resistance of human β-tryptase against endogenous proteinase inhibitors results from the size limitations imposed by the geometry of the tetramer's central pore. The plasma antiproteases (e.g., α1-proteinase inhibitor) that regulate the activity of most trypsin-like proteases and also tissue-derived inhibitors such as MPI (mucus proteinases inhibitor) or elafin are too large to fit into the central pore. In contrast, LDTI (leech-derived tryptase inhibitor), the only known naturally occurring inhibitor of human β-tryptase, is smaller than related Kazal proteins [24] and thus can bind to two of the tetramer's active sites. Also synthetic inhibitors can freely interact with an active site (see the 4-amidinophenyl pyruvic acid [25] molecules in Fig. 21.1a), and suitably sized dibasic compounds can even bind to adjacent monomers, thereby gaining affinity and selectivity [26, 27]. Such synthetic compounds are currently used as tools to investigate the role of β-tryptase in health and disease, and may subsequently have therapeutic potential in mast-cell related disorders.

Compared to the β-tetramer, α-tryptase is quite similar in tetrameric architecture, and the interfaces between the monomers as well as the proposed heparin binding sites are conserved [19]. The α- and β-monomers differ in the Ser214–Gly219 segment that in the α-monomer is unusually kinked probably due to a Gly261Asp exchange [15]. This deformed 214–219 loop blocks the specificity pocket, thus resulting in the observed limited enzymatic activity of this tryptase.

21.3 Diagnostic Applications of Tryptases

Motivated initially by the colocalization of β-tryptase with other preformed mediators (e.g., histamine and heparin proteoglycans) in secretory granules and its presence in virtually all human mast cells, tryptase is increasingly utilized as a marker for the activation and/or presence of mast cells. In addition to mast cells, basophils express β- and predominantly α-tryptase mRNA [28] and need to be considered as a source although transcript and protein levels are orders of magnitude lower. All other normal cells surveyed express no tryptase or only trace amounts. Increased 'total tryptase' levels in the circulation thus primarily reflect mast cell degranulation, e.g., during anaphylaxis. With peak levels after 1–2 hours and a half-time $>$ 1 hour detection is possible even hours after the acute event [29]. Tryptase is also measurable at baseline and appears to reflect the body's mast cell burden, e.g., in patients with mastocytosis [30].

Mastocytosis has been thought to present mostly with easily recognizable cutaneous lesions of urticaria pigmentosa. Recently, however, in a subset of patients with hymenoptera venom anaphylaxis, we have detected occult, i.e., hardly visible, mastocytosis lesions that had been mistaken for nevi during previous examinations [31–33]. Additional assessments revealed systemic mastocytosis in most cases. According to our observations, mastocytosis remains often 'occult' even if urticaria pigmentosa is present, if symptoms in other organs than the skin predominate such as spontaneous fractures and osteoporosis, or gastrointestinal or cardiac complaints. This may happen due to the apparently missing link between frequently severe systemic symptoms and mostly asymptomatic skin lesions imitating nevi, that appear harmless to the nondermatologist. Also diffuse cutaneous mastocytosis of childhood presents with easily missed but characteristic skin lesions. It is frequently missed probably because it is not considered in the differential diagnosis because of its rare occurrence.

Moreover, increased serum levels of tryptase have been found in subsets of patients with AML (particularly FAB classification M0, M2, M3 and M4eo) [34] and myelodysplastic/myeloproliferative syndromes [35, 36]. In these disorders, tryptases may be ectopically produced by myeloblasts or derived from (neoplastic) mast cells and basophils. Based on immunoassays, the predominant form circulating at baseline and in mastocytosis (as well as in AML) was proposed to be α-tryptase [30]. In a recent study, however, total tryptase levels in plasma were found to be similar in healthy subjects with and without the gene for α-tryptase [14]. These results may be indicative of the difficulties in discriminating between tryptases by immunological means. The epitopes recognized by most 'tryptase antibodies' have not been mapped so that it remains unclear whether they recognize all or only some of the closely related tryptases (i.e., α, β, and δ) and their allelic variants.

Thus, further studies are necessary to clarify which tryptases are present in the circulation in different disorders, whether they are useful markers to monitor diseases also in patients with α-deficiency, and subsequently whether tryptases contribute to the pathophysiology or the symptoms of these diseases. Novel assays, e.g., using antibodies that recognize epitopes selected based on the tryptase structures and the increasing information on allelic variants, may allow measurement of all tryptases and their discrimination, and may thus foster this line of research.

Acknowledgements. Christian Sommerhoff is grateful to H. Fritz and W. Bode for friendship and generous support. Supported by SFB 469 of the University of Munich.

References

1. Miller JS, Westin EH, Schwartz LB (1989) Cloning and characterization of complementary DNA for human tryptase. J Clin Invest 84:1188–1195
2. Vanderslice P, Ballinger SM, Tam EK, Goldstein SM, Craik CS, Caughey GH (1990) Human mast cell tryptase: multiple cDNAs and genes reveal a multigene serine protease family. Proc Natl Acad. Sci U S A 87:3811–3815
3. Wong GW, Tang Y, Feyfant E, Sali A, Li L, Li Y, Huang C, Friend DS, Krilis SA, Stevens RL (1999) Identification of a new member of the tryptase family of mouse and human mast cell proteases which possesses a novel COOH-terminal hydrophobic extension. J Biol Chem 274:30784–30793
4. Caughey GH, Raymond WW, Blount JL, Hau LW, Pallaoro M, Wolters PJ, Verghese GM (2000) Characterization of human gamma-tryptases, novel members of the chromosome 16p mast cell tryptase and prostasin gene families. J Immunol 164:6566–6575
5. Pallaoro M, Fejzo MS, Shayesteh L, Blount JL, Caughey GH (1999) Characterization of genes encoding known and novel human mast cell tryptases on chromosome 16p13.3. J Biol Chem 274:3355–3362
6. Wang HW, McNeil HP, Husain A, Liu K, Tedla N, Thomas PS, Raftery M, King GC, Cai ZY, Hunt JE (2002) Delta tryptase is expressed in multiple human tissues, and a recombinant form has proteolytic activity. J Immunol 169:5145–5152
7. Caughey GH (2002) New developments in the genetics and activation of mast cell proteases. Mol Immunol 38:1353–1357
8. Wong GW, Yasuda S, Morokawa N, Li L, Stevens RL (2004) Mouse chromosome 17a3.3 contains thirteen genes that encode functional tryptic-like serine proteases with distinct tissue and cell expression patterns. J Biol Chem 279:2438--2452
9. Guida M, Riedy M, Lee D, Hall J (2000) Characterization of two highly polymorphic human tryptase loci and comparison with a newly discovered monkey tryptase ortholog. Pharmacogenetics 10:389–396
10. Soto D, Malmsten C, Blount JL, Muilenburg DJ, Caughey GH (2002) Genetic deficiency of human mast cell alpha-tryptase. Clin Exp Allergy 32:1000–1006
11. Schwartz LB, Irani AMA, Roller K, Castells MC, Schechter NM (1987) Quantitation of histamine, tryptase and chymase in dispersed human T and TC mast cells. J Immunol 138:2611–2615
12. Sommerhoff CP (2001) Mast cell tryptases and airway remodeling. Am J Respir Crit Care Med 164:S52–58
13. Krishna MT, Chauhan A, Little L, Sampson K, Hawksworth R, Mant T, Djukanovic R, Lee T, Holgate S (2001) Inhibition of mast cell tryptase by inhaled APC 366 attenuates allergen-induced late-phase airway obstruction in asthma. J Allergy Clin Immunol 107:1039–1045
14. Schwartz LB, Min HK, Ren S, Xia HZ, Hu J, Zhao W, Moxley G, Fukuoka Y (2003) Tryptase precursors are preferentially and spontaneously released, whereas mature tryptase is retained by HMC-1 cells, mono-mac-6 cells, and human skin-derived mast cells. J Immunol 170:5667–5673
15. Huang C, Li L, Krilis SA, Chanasyk K, Tang Y, Li Z, Hunt JE, Stevens RL (1999) Human tryptases alpha and beta/II are functionally distinct due, in part, to a single amino acid difference in one of the surface loops that forms the substrate-binding cleft. J Biol Chem 274:19670–19676
16. Min HK, Kambe N, Schwartz LB (2001) Human mouse mast cell protease 7-like tryptase genes are pseudogenes. J Allergy Clin Immunol 107:315–321
17. Pereira PJB, Bergner A, Macedo RS, Huber R, Matschiner G, Fritz H, Sommerhoff CP, Bode W (1998) Human beta-tryptase is a ring-like tetramer with active sites facing a central pore. Nature 392:306–311
18. Sommerhoff CP, Bode W, Pereira PJB, Stubbs MT, Stürzebecher J, Piechottka GP, Matschiner G, Bergner A (1999) The structure of the human betaII-tryptase tetramer: Fo(u)r better or worse. Proc Natl Acad Sci U S A 96:10984–10991
19. Marquardt U, Zettl F, Huber R, Bode W, Sommerhoff CP (2002) The crystal structure of human alpha1-tryptase reveals a blocked substrate-binding region. J Mol Biol 321:491–502
20. Lindstedt KA, Kokkonen JO, Kovanen PT (1998) Regulation of the activity of secreted human lung mast cell tryptase by mast cell proteoglycans. Biochim Biophys Acta 1425:617–627
21. Ren S, Sakai K, Schwartz LB (1998) Regulation of human mast cell beta-tryptase: conversion of inactive monomer to active tetramer at acid pH. J Immunol 160:4561–4569
22. Addington AK, Johnson DA (1996) Inactivation of human lung tryptase: evidence for a re-activatable tetrameric intermediate and active monomers. Biochemistry 35:13511–13518

23. Sommerhoff CP, Bode W, Matschiner G, Bergner A, Fritz H (2000) The human mast cell tryptase tetramer: a fascinating riddle solved by structure. Biochim Biophys Acta 1477:75–89
24. Sommerhoff CP, Söllner C, Mentele R, Piechottka GP, Auerswald EA, Fritz H (1994) A Kazal-type inhibitor of human mast cell tryptase: isolation from the medical leech Hirudo medicinalis, characterization, and sequence analysis. Biol Chem 375:685–694
25. Stürzebecher J, Prasa D, Sommerhoff CP (1992) Inhibition of human mast cells tryptase by benzamidine derivatives. Biol Chem 373:1025–1030
26. Schaschke N, Matschiner G, Zettl F, Marquardt U, Bergner A, Bode W, Sommerhoff CP, Moroder L (2001) Bivalent inhibition of human beta-tryptase. Chem Biol 8:313–327
27. Schaschke N, Dominik A, Matschiner G, Sommerhoff CP (2002) Bivalent inhibition of beta-tryptase: distance scan of neighboring subunits by dibasic inhibitors. Bioorg Med Chem Lett 12:985–988
28. Xia HZ, Kepley CL, Sakai K, Chelliah J, Irani AMA, Schwartz LB (1995) Quantitation of tryptase, chymase, Fc-epsilon-RI-alpha, and Fc-epsilon-RI-gamma mRNAs in human mast cells and basophils by competitive reverse transcription-polymerase chain reaction. J Immunol 154:5472–5480
29. Schwartz LB, Yunginger JW, Miller J, Bokhari R, Dull D (1989) Time course of appearance and disappearance of human mast cell tryptase in the circulation after anaphylaxis. J Clin Invest 83:1551–1555
30. Schwartz LB, Sakai K, Bradford TR, Ren S, Zweiman B, Worobec AS, Metcalfe DD (1995) The alpha form of human tryptase is the predominant type present in blood at baseline in normal subjects and is elevated in those with systemic mastocytosis. J Clin Invest 96:2702–2710
31. Ludolph-Hauser D, Ruëff F, Sommerhoff CP, Przybilla B (1999) Tryptase, ein Marker für die Aktivierung und Lokalisation von Mastzellen. Hautarzt 50:556–561
32. Ludolph-Hauser D, Ruëff F, Fries C, Schoepf P, Przybilla B (2001) Constitutionally elevated serum levels of mast cell tryptase identify patients with mastocytosis and severe anaphylactic reactions to hymenoptera stings. Lancet 357:361–362
33. Biedermann T, Rueff F, Sander CA, Przybilla B (1999) Mastocytosis associated with severe wasp sting anaphylaxis detected by elevated serum mast cell tryptase levels. Br J Dermatol 146:1110–1112
34. Sperr WR, Jordan JH, Baghestanian M, Kiener HP, Samorapoompichit P, Semper H, Hauswirth A, Schernthaner GH, Chott A, Natter S, Kraft D, Valenta R, Schwartz LB, Geissler K, Lechner K, Valent P (2001) Expression of mast cell tryptase by myeloblasts in a group of patients with acute myeloid leukemia. Blood 98:2200–2209
35. Sperr WR, Stehberger B, Wimazal F, Baghestanian M, Schwartz LB, Kundi M, Semper H, Jordan JH, Chott A, Drach J, Jager U, Geissler K, Greschniok A, Horny HP, Lechner K, Valent P (2002) Serum tryptase measurements in patients with myelodysplastic syndromes. Leuk Lymphoma 43:1097–1105
36. Klion AD, Noel P, Akin C, Law MA, Gilliland DG, Cools J, Metcalfe DD, Nutman TB (2003) Elevated serum tryptase levels identify a subset of patients with a myeloproliferative variant of idiopathic hypereosinophilic syndrome associated with tissue fibrosis, poor prognosis, and imatinib responsiveness. Blood 101:4660–4666
37. Guex N, Peitsch MC (1997) Swiss-model and the Swiss-PdbViewer: an environment for comparative protein modeling. Electrophoresis 18:2714–2723

F Hypereosinophilic Syndrome

Chapter 22

Familial Hypereosinophilic Syndrome

Amy D. Klion, John D. Rioux, Melissa Law, Thomas B. Nutman

22.1 Introduction

Idiopathic hypereosinophilic syndrome (HES) is a heterogeneous group of disorders defined as peripheral eosinophilia of > 1500 eosinophils/µl for at least 6 months without discernible cause and the presence of eosinophil-related end-organ dysfunction [1, 2]. HES occurs sporadically in the general population and is most common in men between the ages of 20 and 50 years [3]. End-organ dysfunction frequently involves the heart (myocarditis, cardiomyopathy, endomyocardial fibrosis), the nervous system (peripheral neuropathy, thromboembolism and encephalopathy), the skin (angioedema, urticaria, mucosal ulcerations) and the lungs (chronic cough, infiltrates, pulmonary fibrosis), although any organ can be affected.

The occurrence of unexplained eosinophilia in several members of the same family, although uncommon, has been reported in the literature since 1909 [4] and is felt to represent part of the clinical spectrum of HES. Although many of the early descriptions likely represent undiagnosed parasitic infections or environmental exposures, at least 18 families have been described in which eosinophilia (> 440 eosinophils/µl) is present in at least two generations and common etiologies of eosinophilia have been excluded (familial hypereosinophilia, FE; MIM 131400) [5]. Although clinical illness was often responsible for bringing these families to medical attention, end-organ dysfunction characteristic of HES was not reported.

22.2 Clinical Aspects

We have previously described a large US kindred with an autosomal dominant form of FE [6] (Fig. 22.1). In contrast to the relative paucity of clinical manifestations associated with the other reported cases of FE [5], end-organ involvement typical of HES (endomyocardial fibrosis and neuropathy) was identified in a subset of affected family members at the time of the initial study, and was fatal despite therapy in two individuals.

In order to determine the prevalence of eosinophil-related end-organ damage in FE, a detailed clinical evaluation of 31 family members (15 affected and 16 unaffected) was recently performed at the National Institutes of Health [7]. Study participants ranged in age from 4 months to 76 years and the age and gender distributions were similar between the affected and unaffected groups. Echocardiography, pulmonary function testing, dilated ophthalmologic examination, and a limited radiographic bone survey were performed on all participants in addition to routine labo-

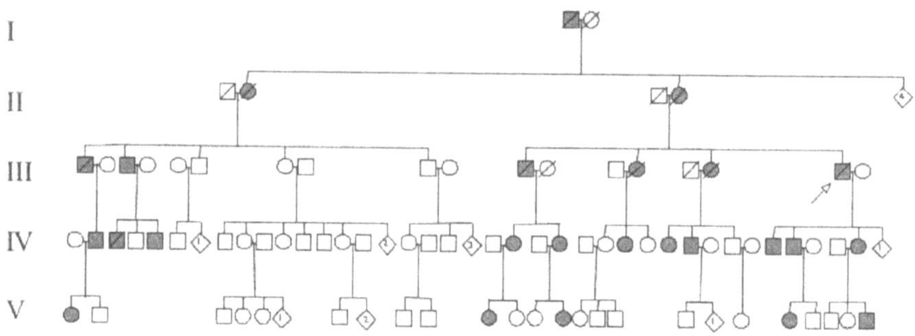

Fig. 22.1. Family pedigree. Affected family members are represented by the *shaded* symbols. The proband, who died of cardiac complications of FE, is indicated by the *arrow*

Table 22.1. Clinical manifestations in patients with family members with familial eosinophilia compared with those in unaffected family members (*NS* $P>0.1$) (from [7], with permission)

Organ system	Clinical manifestation	Affected ($n=15$)	Unaffected ($n=16$)	*P* value
Cardiac	Valvular diseasea	3	2	NS
	AV block	3	1	NS
Neurologic	Peripheral neuropathy	3	2	NS
	TIA/cognitive decline	2	0	NS
	Migraine	2	0	NS
	Tremor	2	2	NS
Pulmonary	Obstructive disease	1	7	<0.001
Skin	Psoriasis	1	2	NS
Psychiatric	Depression	2	2	NS
Ophthalmologic	Cortical cataracts	6	2	NS
	Cortical vacuoles	4	4	NS
	Nuclear cataracts	1	2	NS
	S/P cataract surgery	1	2	NS
	Any abnormality	12	10	NS

[a] Defined as any structural abnormality of a valve seen on echocardiography or mild to severe regurgitant flow as assessed by Doppler

ratory tests and a comprehensive medical history and physical examination. The clinical findings are summarized in Table 22.1.

No clinical abnormalities appeared to be associated with FE. Three affected family members had cardiac abnormalities (mild mitral regurgitation, aortic valvular thickening with moderate aortic regurgitation, and aortic valve replacement 20 years earlier, respectively); however, prior echocardiograms were available in all three cases and demonstrated no progression over a 10-year period, inconsistent with cardiac disease secondary to hypereosinophilia. Similarly, although a mild decrease in vibratory sense, possibly consistent with early peripheral neuropathy, was detected in three affected and two unaffected family members, the clinical significance of this finding is uncertain, as all of the individuals were asymptomatic and had normal nerve conduction velocities. Interestingly, conditions typically associated with eosinophilia (asthma, psoriasis) were less frequent in the affected family members.

Eosinophil counts ranged from 1952 to 4998/μl in affected family members. Eosinophilia was documented as early as 1 week postpartum and remained remarkably stable over time, as had been noted previously [6]. No other hematological abnormalities were apparent, and eosinophil morphology was within normal limits as assessed by both light and electron microscopy [7]. Serum levels of IgE and B12, often elevated in patients with idiopathic HES [3], were not elevated in the affected family members.

22.3 Etiology

Although the etiology of idiopathic HES is unknown, the recent identification of subgroups of HES patients with clonal populations of eosinophils [8, 9] or lymphocytes [10, 11] suggests that patients with HES can be separated into at least three major subgroups: those with a primary disorder of eosinophilopoiesis, those with secondary eosinophilia due to overproduction of eosinophilopoietic cytokines by a clonal population of lymphocytes, and those without evidence of either of the above. Furthermore, the clinical presentation of HES appears to be determined, at least in part, by the underlying etiology, with fibrotic complications (endomyocardial fibrosis, restrictive pulmonary disease and myelofibrosis) more commonly seen in the group with a primary myeloproliferative disorder [12].

Clonality of eosinophils and lymphocytes was excluded by a DNA PCR-based HUMARA assay in four female family members with eosinophilia (Klion AD and Gale RE, unpublished data) and by RT-PCR analysis for the FIP1L1/PDGFRA fusion kinase in two additional affected family members [7]. Furthermore, analysis of lymphocytes from 14 affected family members by flow cytometry failed to demonstrate an increase in any of the lymphocyte subsets reported to be associated with HES (e.g., CD3+CD4−CD8− and CD3−CD4+ [7, 10, 11]. Finally, although a pericentric inversion of chromosome 10 was detected in two affected individuals, no consistent cytogenetic abnormality was observed in the eight affected family members who underwent karyotype analysis [6]. Taken together, these data suggest that FE is the result of a dysregulation of eosinophil homeostasis due to overproduction of a recognized or novel eosinophil growth factor or to an abnormal response to such a factor.

22.4 Genetic Studies

Results of a genome-wide linkage analysis performed using DNA from 53 family members provided evidence that the FE locus is situated on chromosome 5q31–33 between the markers D5S642 and D5S816 (multipoint LOD score of 6.49) [13]. This region contains the human cytokine gene cluster and has been linked to circulating eosinophil levels in normal individuals [14, 15]. It is also a frequent site of translocations and deletions in myeloproliferative disorders with eosinophilia [16–18].

Three members of the chromosome 5q cytokine cluster, IL-5, IL-3 and GM-CSF, have been shown to cause eosinophilia by promoting eosinophilopoiesis and decreasing eosinophil apoptosis in vitro and in vivo [19–21]. Although serum levels of these cytokines were not elevated when compared to the serum of unaffected family members [6], elevations of intracellular IL-5 have been documented in lymphocytes from some patients with HES in the absence of increased serum levels [1]. Consequently,

Table 22.2. Summary of polymorphisms identified in selected genes located on chromosome 5q31–33

Gene	Locations of polymorphisms
IL-5	5'UTR, exon 1
IL-3/GM-CSF	Enhancer
IL-4	Exons 1, 2 and 4, promoter
IL-13	Exons 2 and 3
GRL	Exon 5

the genomic sequences of IL-3, IL-5, GM-CSF and the IL-3/GM-CSF enhancer were obtained for five affected family members and three of their spouses [13]. Three of the polymorphisms were examined in an additional 17 affected and 13 unaffected family members (Table 22.2), but none was found exclusively in the DNA from affected family members. More recently, the genes encoding two additional cytokines important in the Th2 type response, IL-4 and IL-13, have been sequenced in four affected and four unaffected family members with similar results (Table 22.2) (Rioux, unpublished results).

The gene for the glucocorticoid receptor (GRL) has been localized to chromosome 5q31–33 and was of potential interest as a candidate gene for several reasons. First, glucocorticoid receptors are expressed on eosinophils and abnormal receptor function has been described in some steroid-refractory patients with HES [22]. Second, both of the affected family members who died of complications of FE failed to respond to steroid therapy. Finally, although eosinophilia resolved within 12 hours in eight of eight affected patients tested after a single dose of 60 mg prednisone, eosinophil counts had returned to baseline levels by 24 hours. The genomic sequences of GRL exons 2–9 and their flanking regions were determined in seven affected and five unaffected family members; however, none of the polymorphisms identified was restricted to affected family members.

The most recent estimates from the human genome project suggest that the region between markers D5S642 and D5S816 contains between 60 and 80 genes, including numerous cytokines (IL-4, IL-5, IL-3, IL-9, GM-CSF and IL-13), growth factors (e.g., EGR-1, GDF9, CDC23, CDC25C, Smad5 and TCF7), and regulatory molecules (e.g., IRF-1, HSPA9 and RIL) (see http://genome.ucsc.edu/cgi-bin/hgGateway?org=human and http://www.ncbi.nlm.nih.gov/mapview/map_search.cgi?taxid=9606&query=chromosome%205). Although the size of the region precludes sequencing all of the possible candidate genes, studies are currently underway to define patterns of lymphocyte and eosinophil gene expression using microarrays in an attempt to identify the most likely candidate genes for sequence analysis.

22.5 Summary

HES is a rare disorder that occurs sporadically in the general population, and is characterized by eosinophilia (> 1500 eosinophils/μl) of unknown etiology that results in eosinophil-mediated end-organ damage. We previously described a family with autosomal dominant transmission of marked hypereosinophilia. Although the spectrum of clinical findings in familial HES (FE) is similar to that seen in HES and includes cardiac involvement, peripheral neuropathy, and cutaneous manifestations, end-organ sequelae appear to develop in only a minority of affected patients. Clonality of lymphocytes or eosinophils could not be demonstrated by either quantification of X-chromosome inactivation using a DNA PCR-based HUMARA assay, RT-PCR for the FIP1L1/PDGFRA fusion kinase or flow cytometry. Using standard genetic linkage techniques, the gene responsible for FE has been mapped to chromosome 5q31–q33. However, sequence analysis of the most likely candidate genes in this region, including IL-5, IL-3 and GM-CSF, did not identify any differences between affected and unaffected family members. It is likely, therefore, that delineation of the genetic basis of FE will lead to the identification of a previously unrecognized gene or mechanism involved in the regulation of eosinophilia.

Acknowledgements. The authors would like to thank the family members for their participation in these studies, Ms. Laura Fontaine for administrative assistance in recontacting the family members, and the many consultants, nurses and laboratory staff members from the National Institutes of Health Clinical Center who were involved in their evaluation.

References

1. Chusid MJ, Dale DC, West BC, Wolff SM (1975) The hypereosinophilic syndrome. Medicine 54:1–27
2. Fauci AS, Harley JB, Roberts WC, Ferrans VJ, Gralnick HR, Bjornson BH (1982) The idiopathic hypereosinophilic syndrome. Ann Intern Med 97:78–92
3. Weller PF, Bubley GJ (1994) The idiopathic hypereosinophilic syndrome. Blood 83:2759–2779
4. Gaugain M (1909) Un cas d'eosinophilie familiale. Sem Med 29:329
5. Naiman JL, Oski FA, Allen FH Jr, Diamond LK (1964) Hereditary eosinophilia: report of a family and review of the literature. Am J Hum Genet 16:195–203
6. Lin AY, Nutman TB, Kaslow D, Mulvihill JJ, Fontaine L, White BJ, Knutsen T, Theil KS, Raghuprasad PK, Goldstein AM, Tucker MA (1998) Familial eosinophilia: clinical and laboratory results of an US kindred. Am J Med Genet 76:229–237
7. Klion AD, Law MA, Riemenschneider W, McMaster ML, Brown MR, Horne M, Karp B, Robinson M, Sachdev V, Tucker E, Turner M, Nutman TB (2004) Familial eosinophilia: a benign disorder? Blood 103:4050–4055
8. Chang HW, Leong KH, Koh DR, Lee SH (1999) Clonality of isolated eosinophils in the hypereosinophilic syndrome. Blood 93:1651–1657
9. Cools J, DeAngelo DJ, Gotlib J, Stover EH, Legare RD, Cortes J, Kutok J, Clark J, Galinsky I, Griffin JD, Cross NC, Tefferi A, Malone J, Alam R, Schrier SL, Schmid J, Rose M, Vandenberghe P, Verhoef G, Boogaerts M, Wlodarska I, Kantarjian H, Marynen P, Coutre SE, Stone R, Gilliland DG (2003) A novel tyrosine kinase created by the fusion of the PDGFRA and FIP1L1 genes is a therapeutic target of imatinib in idiopathic hypereosinophilic syndrome. N Engl J Med 348:1201–1214
10. Simon HU, Plotz SG, Dummer R, Blaser K (1999) Abnormal clones of T cells producing interleukin-5 in idiopathic eosinophilia. N Engl J Med 341:1112–1120
11. Roufosse F, Schandené L, Sibille C, Willard-Gallo K, Kennes B, Efira A, Goldman M, Cogan E (2000) Clonal Th2 lymphocytes in patients with the idiopathic hypereosinophilic syndrome. Br J Haematol 109:540–548
12. Klion AD, Noel P, Akin C, Law MA, Gilliland DG, Cools J, Metcalfe DD, Nutman TB (2003) Elevated serum tryptase levels identify a subset of patients with a myeloproliferative variant of idiopathic hypereosinophilic syndrome associated with tissue fibrosis, poor prognosis and imatinib responsiveness. Blood 101:4660–4666
13. Rioux JD, Stone VA, Daly MJ, Cargill M, Green T, Nguyen H, Nutman T, Zimmerman PA, Tucker MA, Hudson T, Goldstein AM, Lander E, Lin AY (1998) Familial eosinophilia maps to the cytokine gene cluster on human chromosomal region 5q31–q33. Am J Hum Genet 63:1086–1094
14. Martinez FD, Solomon S, Holberg CJ, Graves PE, Baldini M, Erickson RP (1998) Linkage of circulating eosinophils to markers of chromosome 5q. Am J Respir Crit Care Med 158:1739–1744

15. Holberg CJ, Halonen M, Wright AL, Martinez FD (1999) Familial aggregation and segregation analysis of eosinophil levels. Am J Respir Crit Care Med 160:1604–1610
16. Le Beau MM, Espinosa R 3rd, Neuman WL, Stock W, Roulston D, Larson RA, Keinanen M, Westbrook CA (1993) Cytogenetic and molecular delineation of the smallest commonly deleted region of chromosome 5 in malignant myeloid disease. Proc Natl Acad Sci U S A 90:5484–5488
17. Baranger L, Szapiro N, Gardais J, Hillion J, Derre J, Francois S, Blanchet O, Boasson M, Berger B (1994) Translocation of t(5,12)(q31-q33;p12–13): a non-random translocation associated with a myeloid disorder with eosinophilia. Br J Haematol 88:343–347
18. Yagasaki F, Jinnai I, Yoshida S, Yokoyama Y, Matsuda A, Kusumoto S, Kobayashi H, Terasaki H, Ohyashiki K, Asou N, Murohashi I, Bessho M, Hirashima K (1999) Fusion of TEL/ETV 6 to a novel ACS2 in myelodysplastic syndrome with acute myelogenous leukaemia with t(5;12)(q31;p13). Genes Chromosomes Cancer 26:192–202
19. Rothenberg ME, Owen WF Jr, Silberstein DS, Woods J, Soberman RJ, Austen KF, Stevens RL (1988) Human eosinophils have prolonged survival, enhanced functional properties and become hypodense when exposed to human interleukin 3. J Clin Invest 81:1986–1992
20. Owen WF Jr, Rothenberg ME, Silberstein DS, Gasson JC, Stevens RL, Austen KF, Soberman RJ (1987) Regulation of humans eosinophil viability, density and function by GM-CSF in the presence of 3T3 fibroblasts. J Exp Med 166:129–141
21. Dent LA, Strath M, Mellor AL, Sanderson CJ (1990) Eosinophilia in transgenic mice expressing interleukin-5. J Exp Med 172:1425–1431
22. Prin L, Lefebvre P, Gruart V, Capron M, Storme L, Formstecher P, Loiseau S, Capron A (1989) Heterogeneity of human eosinophil glucocorticoid receptor expression in hypereosinophilic patients: absence of a detectable receptor correlates with resistance to glucocorticoid therapy. Clin Exp Immunol 78:383–389

Mononuclear Cell Preparations from Patients with Idiopathic Hypereosinophilic Syndromes Do Not Express the Wilms' Tumor Gene

Hans D. Menssen, A. Schmidt, Eckart Thiel

23.1 Introduction

The Wilms' tumor gene (wt1) is located on chromosome 11p13 [1]. Due to alternate splicing it is translated into at least four major WT1 proteins. These zinc finger-containing proteins are transcription factors which are involved in the regulation of growth and differentiation of various normal and malignant cell types (ovarian cancer, breast cancer, melanoma, mesothelioma, desmoplastic round cell tumor, renal cell carcinoma, colorectal cancer, lung cancer, gastric cancer, and glioblastoma). The biological function of WT1 proteins depends on interactions with other transcription factors (e.g., p53, PAX2, NF-kB), the promoter structure of the target genes, and on the presence or absence of the adenovirus E1B gene product. Depending on these circumstances, WT1 proteins activate or suppress transcription of target growth factor genes or their receptors (IGF-II, IGF-I receptor, PDGF-A, EGF, CSF-1, and TGF-β). They also regulate the expression of bcl-2 and c-myc. Further, wt1 expression is negatively autoregulated [2]. Expression of wt1 was found in blasts of almost all acute leukemia patients, irrespective of their morphologic or immunologic phenotype [3–6]. Normal blood mononuclear cells (MNCs) and CD34+ hematopoietic progenitors express wt1 on a far lower level [4] or not at all [5, 6] depending on the RT-PCR protocol used. Consequently, WT1-RT-PCR has been suggested as a diagnostic tool to detect minimal residual disease and imminent relapses in acute leukemia patients [7].

Here, we demonstrate and discuss the usefulness of testing for wt1 expression to discriminate patients with acute eosinophilic leukemia (EoL) from those suffering from idiopathic HES, a notoriously difficult differential diagnosis.

23.2 Continuous Overexpression of WT1 in Blasts of Patients with Acute Leukemia

Many authors have shown wt1 expression in cell lines and blasts of acute leukemia patients, using differing detection systems. Implementing qualitative RT-PCR protocols, wt1 mRNA transcripts could be found in up to 97% of acute myeloid leukemia (AML) and in up to 88% of acute lymphoblastic leukemia (ALL) samples [6]. In contrast, Northern blot analysis showed wt1 expression in only 59% and 40%, respectively [3]. Blasts of all subgroups of AML patients (according to the FAB classification) express wt1 in a comparable fashion. More mature and myeloblastic differentiated AML-M5 leukemia samples seem to have a lower wt1 expression level as compared to minimally differentiated AML-M0/1 blasts [3]. For ALL patients, a higher frequency of wt1 expression was found in blasts of pre-pre B-ALL and common ALL

Table 23.1. Expression of wt-1 in leukemia patients [2] (*sqRT-PCR* semiquantitative RT-PCR, *IMFL* indirect immunofluorescence using mAb H2)

Diagnosis	Patients (*n*)	wt1 gene expression N (%)	Material and method	Reference
De novo AML				
All	22	15 (68)	BM MNC; RT-PCR	[3]
All	45	45 (100)	MNC; sqRT-PCR	[4]
All	52	41 (79)	MNC; RT-PCR	[6]
All	57	53 (97)	MNC; RT-PCR	[5]
All	83	67 (81)	MNC; RT-PCR	[5]
All	64	41 (64)	BM MNC; IMFL	[9]
All	161	124 (77)	BM MNC; RT-PCR	[5]
All	125	91 (73)	BM MNC; RT-PCR	[2]
CML				
Chronic phase	4	0	BM-MNCs; Northern	[3]
	23	0	MNC; sqRT-PCR	[4]
	3	0	BM-MNC; RT-PCR	[6]
Blast crisis	10	8 (80)	BM-MNC; Northern	[3]
	2	2 (100)	MNC; sqRT-PCR	[8]
	4	4 (100)	BM-MNC; RT-PCR	[6]
ALL				
All	16	7 (44)	BM-MNC; Northern	[5]
All	22	22 (100)	BM-MNC; sqRT-PCR	[8]
ppB-ALL	14	12 (96)	BM-MNC; RT-PCR	[6]
c-ALL	41	33 (80)	BM-MNC; RT-PCR	[6]
T-ALL	31	23 (74)	BM-MNC; RT-PCR	[6]
NHL				
Mature	18	0	MNC; Northern	[3]
Mature	24	0	MNC; sqRT-PCR	[4]
Mature	20	0	MNC; RT-PCR	[2]
Controls				
Healthy	Not disclosed	0	PB MNC; sqRT-PCR	[4]
Healthy	13	0	MNCs; RT-PCR	[5]
Healthy	20	0	All blood cells; RT-PCR	[9, 10]
Fetal anemia	6	5 (83)	Fetal blood cells; RT-PCR	[9, 10]
Healthy	Not disclosed	0	BM-MNC; sqRT-PCR	[4]
Healthy	Not disclosed	0	BM-MNC; RT-PCR	[5]
Solid cancer	10	0	BM-MNC; RT-PCR	[9]
Solid cancer	6	0	$CD34^+$ MNC; RT-PCR	[6]
Healthy	Not disclosed	Positive	$CD34^+$ MNC; IMF	[14]
Healthy	Not disclosed	Positive	$CD34^+CD38^-$ subsets; RT-PCR	[14]
Healthy	Not disclosed	0	$CD34^-$ BM MNC; RT-PCR	[14]
Healthy	4	4 (100)	$CD34^+CD33^-$ MNC; RT-PCR	[13]
Healthy	Not disclosed	0	FACS-sorted subsets[a]; sqRT-PCR	[8]

[a] Various $CD34^+$ and $CD34^-$ BM-MNC subsets

as compared to T-ALL (Table 23.1). Normal maturing blood cells or physiologically maturing bone marrow cells do not express wt1 at significant levels [8, 9].

23.3 Translation of WT1 Nuclear Proteins in Blasts of Acute Leukemia Patients but Not in Normal Mononuclear Cells

In leukemic blasts wt1 is translated into a protein and its isoforms, which are strictly localized to the nucleus [10] and to distinct subnuclear regions [11, 12]. Using indirect immunofluorescence with WT1 protein-specific mAb H2, we detected WT1 nuclear fluorescence in leukemic blasts in varying proportions of cells (10–85%) and in differing intensities, indicating a heterogeneous WT1 expression pattern within a given malignant clone and from patient to patient. No WT1 immunofluorescence was detectable in CD34+ progenitor-enriched MNCs from patients with solid cancer prepared to receive autologous peripheral hematopoietic stem cell support [12]. Although not all blasts of a given leukemia patient disclose WT1 nuclear fluorescence, it can be summarized that WT1 translation is a characteristic feature of leukemic blasts.

23.4 Transient Expression of WT1 in Normal CD34+ Hematopoietic Progenitor Cells

Physiologic CD34+ progenitor cells express wt1 under not yet fully understood circumstances. Using nested primer RT-PCR, we detected wt1 expression in umbilical cord blood cells of human fetuses ($n=6$) aged between 19 and 34 weeks of gestation (Table 23.1). In clonal growth assays we found wt1 expression in normal hematopoietic progenitors to be restricted to the early exponential growth phase. Colonies containing between 100 and 1000 vital cells (trypan blue uptake in less than 5% of cells) were separately analyzed in this study, using qualitative WT1-RT-PCR [9]. In almost all colonies picked on day 14 (100–300 cells per colony) wt1 expression was found irrespective of lineage, whereas no wt1 transcripts were detected in colonies picked on day 21 or later. MNC preparations (106 cells) from leukapheresis products of patients with limited-disease solid cancer ($n=10$; CD34+ progenitor content 0.5–6.6%) did not express wt1.

Using more sensitive RT-PCR protocols such as the semiquantitative RT-PCR protocol of Inoue et al. [7] and the RT-PCR protocols of Maurer et al. [13] and Baird and Simmons [14], wt1 expression was found in normal CD34+ progenitors. Whereas some authors have detected very low wt1 expression levels in various FACS-sorted subsets of normal hematopoietic progenitors [8], others have found strong wt1 expression in cells bearing the CD34+ phenotype but not in progenitors lacking CD34+ expression [13, 14]. Using single-cell RT-PCR analysis, Baird and Simmons [14] found wt1 expression in the candidate stem cell-containing populations of CD34+CD38– hematopoietic progenitors. We could not detect the nuclear WT1 protein in CD34+ hematopoietic progenitors [10], possibly due to the limited sensitivity of indirect immunofluorescence as compared to PCR. Taken together, these data suggest that physiologic wt1 expression is limited to very early progenitors of the human blood cell system, implying its critical role in normal hematopoiesis. Thus, deregulated wt1 expression in hematopoietic progenitors such as continuing overexpression possibly causes or maintains acute leukemia. This hypothesis is supported by wt1 antisense experiments, which show that wt1 antisense oligomers inhibit growth of K562 blasts, MM6 blasts and clonogenic leukemia blasts obtained from AML patients [15, 16].

23.5 Analysis of wt1 Expression in Mononuclear Cells from Patients with Eosinophilic Leukemia, Idiopathic Eosinophilic Syndromes, and Reactive Eosinophilia

EoL is a rare form of acute myelogenous leukemia. In addition to clinical and pathological features such as hepatosplenomegaly, anemia, and thrombocytopenia, it presents with a substantially increased series of left-shifted but maturing eosinophilic precursors and an increased number of blasts in bone marrow [17]. Frequently in this male-dominant disorder, organ infiltrations by immature eosinophilic cells result in organ enlargement (spleen, liver), as well as pulmonary, pericardial, lymph node, and CNS involvement. Sometimes, a short chronic phase precedes the ultimate acute transformation in EoL patients [17]. In contrast, the idiopathic hypereosinophilic syndrome (HES) describes a heterogeneous group of non-malignant leukoproliferative disorders of unknown origin which are marked by sustained overproduction of mature and sometimes immature eosinophilic cells, leukocytosis, and multiple eosinophilic organ infiltrations predominantly involving the heart, skin, lungs, spleen, and liver [18]. Finally, reactive eosinophilia (REo), which like HES is mediated by factors originating from T cells [19, 20], can be found in a variety of diseases including protozoan and metazoan infections, allergic disorders, dermatitis, chronic inflammatory bowel disease, cutaneous T cell lymphomas, and other malignant tumors.

REo usually is not mixed with EoL, but the distinction between the truly malignant EoL and the non-neoplastic HES is notoriously difficult, especially if the bone marrow contains few blasts (< 10%) only [18]. In many cases with unaltered cytogenetics, the diagnosis of HES is one of exclusion, since clinical and hematological features do not necessarily differ between EoL and HES patients. We analyzed MNCs of three patients with EoL, seven patients with HES and four patients with REo and found wt1 expression only in MNCs of EoL patients (Table 23.2) [2]. These results need to be confirmed in a larger series of EoL and HES patients.

23.6 Conclusions

Permanent overexpression of wt1 is a characteristic feature of acute leukemic blasts, irrespective of lineage differentiation. Normal immature subsets of CD34+ hematopoietic progenitors express substantially lower wt1 levels than leukemic blasts, whereas committed hematopoietic progenitors and mature blood cells lack wt1 expression. MNCs from patients with HES do not express wt1. Thus, testing for wt1 expression using RT-PCR qualifies as a powerful complementary diagnostic tool to distinguish acute EoL from idiopathic HES.

Table 23.2. Expression of wt1 gene in patients with acute eosinophilic leukemia (EoL), idiopathic hypereosinophilic syndrome (HES) and reactive eosinophilia (REo)

Patient	Diagnosis	Clinical state	MNC source	wt1 expression
FE	EoL	At diagnosis in 7/95	PB	+
			BM	+
		CR in 10/95	BM	–
		CR in 12/95	BM	+
		CR in 2/96	BM	+
		CNS relapse in 2/96	CSF	+
		Hematological relapse in 3/96	BM	+
		CR after allo-BMT in 10/96	BM	–
SCH	EoL	At diagnosis in 8/95	BM	+
KS	EoL	At diagnosis in 2/97	BM	+
RE	HES	8 months after diagnosis	BM	–
SE	HES	3 years after diagnosis	BM	–
SMF	HES	2 years after diagnosis	PB	–
EM	HES	2 years after diagnosis	PB	–
ET	HES	4 years after diagnosis	BM	–
HC	HES	6 years after diagnosis	PB	–
JPK	HES	2 years after diagnosis	BM	–
			PB	–
IK	REo	Pleomorphic carcinoma	PB	–
CT	REo	Churg-Strauss syndrome	BM	–
			PB	–
HF	REo	Mycosis fungoides	PB	–
KR	REo	Eosinophilic cellulitis/HIV	PB	–
10 patients	Leukapheresis products	Limited-disease solid cancer	PB	–

All samples were tested positive for expression of the c-ABL protooncogene to verify RNA integrity

References

1. Gessler M, Poustka A, Cavenee W, Neve RL, Orkin SH, Bruns GAP (1990) Homozygous deletions in Wilms' tumours of a zinc-finger gene identified by chromosome jumping. Nature 343:774–778
2. Menssen HD, Schmidt A, Bartelt S, et al (2000) Analysis of Wilms tumor gene (WT1) expression in acute leukemia patients with special reference to the differential diagnosis between eosinophilic leukemia and idiopathic hypereosinophilic syndromes. Leuk Lymphoma 36:285–294
3. Miwa H, Beran M, Saunders GF (1992) Expression of the Wilms' tumor gene (WT1) in human leukemias. Leukemia 6:405–409
4. Inoue K, Sugiyama H, Ogawa H, et al (1994) WT1 as a new prognostic factor and a new marker for the detection of minimal residual disease in acute leukemia. Blood 84:3071–3079
5. Brieger J, Weidmann E, Fenchel K, Mitrou PS, Hoelzer D, Bergmann L (1994) The expression of the Wilms' tumor gene in acute myelocytic leukemias as a possible marker for leukemic blast cells. Leukemia 8:2138–2143
6. Menssen HD, Renkl HJ, Rodeck U, et al (1995) Presence of Wilms' tumor gene (wt1) transcripts and the WT1 nuclear protein in the majority of human acute leukemias. Leukemia 9:1060–1067
7. Inoue K, Ogawa H, Yamagami T, et al (1996) Long-term follow-up of minimal residual disease in leukemia patients by monitoring WT1 (Wilms tumor gene) expression levels. Blood 88:2267–2278
8. Inoue K, Ogawa H, Sonoda Y, et al (1997) Aberrant overexpression of the Wilms tumor gene (WT1) in human leukemia. Blood 89:1405–1412
9. Menssen HD, Renkl H-J, Entezami M, Thiel E (1997) Wilms' tumor gene expression in human CD34+ hematopoietic progenitors during fetal development and early growth (letter). Blood 89:3486–3487
10. Menssen HD, Renkl HJ, Rodeck U, Kari C, Schwartz S, Thiel E (1997) Detection by monoclonal antibodies of the Wilms' tumor (WT1) nuclear protein in patients with acute leukemia. Int J Cancer 70:518–523
11. Englert C, Vidal M, Maheswaran S, et al (1995) Truncated WT1 mutants alter the subnuclear localization of the wild-type protein. Proc Natl Acad Sci U S A 92:11960–11964

12. Larsson SH, Charlieu JP, Miyagawa K, et al (1995) Subnuclear localization of WT1 in splicing or transcription factor domains is regulated by alternative splicing. Cell 81:391–401
13. Maurer U, Weidmann E, Karakas T, Hoelzer D, Bergmann L (1997) Wilms tumor gene (wt1) mRNA is equally expressed in blast cells from acute myeloid leukemia and normal CD34+ progenitors (letter). Blood 90:4230–4232
14. Baird PN, Simmons PJ (1997) Expression of the Wilms' tumor gene (WT1) in normal hemopoiesis [see comments]. Exp Hematol 25:312–320
15. Yamagami T, Sugiyama H, Inoue K, et al (1996) Growth inhibition of human leukemic cells by WT1 (Wilms tumor gene) antisense oligodeoxynucleotides: implications for the involvement of WT1 in leukemogenesis. Blood 87:2878–2884
16. Algar EM, Khromykh T, Smith SI, Blackburn DM, Bryson GJ, Smith PJ (1996) A WT1 antisense oligonucleotide inhibits proliferation and induces apoptosis in myeloid leukaemia cell lines. Oncogene 12:1005–1014
17. Bain BJ (1996) Eosinophilic leukaemias and the idiopathic hypereosinophilic syndrome. Br J Haematol 95:2–9
18. Weller PF, Bubley GJ (1994) The idiopathic hypereosinophilic syndrome. Blood 83:2759–2779
19. Raghavachar A, Fleischer S, Frickhofen N, Heimpel H, Fleischer B (1987) T lymphocyte control of human eosinophilic granulopoiesis. Clonal analysis in an idiopathic hypereosinophilic syndrome. J Immunol 139:3753–3758
20. Owen WF, Rothenberg ME, Petersen J, et al (1989) Interleukin 5 and phenotypically altered eosinophils in the blood of patients with the idiopathic hypereosinophilic syndrome. J Exp Med 170:343–348

Chapter 24

Clonality Analysis and Hypereosinophilia

Szu-Hee Lee, Hsiao-Wen Chang

24.1 Introduction

Eosinophils are differentiated leukocytes in the peripheral blood and tissues that play an important role in inflammatory and immune responses in a number of disease states. Peripheral blood eosinophilia is commonly associated with parasitic infections, allergic and hypersensitivity reactions, and less commonly with autoimmune vasculitic disorders, some malignant tumors, and hematological malignancies. The causes of hypereosinophilia are generally classified into three groups: reactive eosinophilias, eosinophilic leukemias, and unexplained or idiopathic hypereosinophilias. The diagnosis of idiopathic hypereosinophilia is based on the exclusion of other causes of eosinophilia [1]. It must be distinguished from reactive, clinically benign eosinophilia (discrimination possible through PDGFA/FIP1L1 fusion gene test, see Chap. 1) and also from eosinophilic leukemias associated with increased blast cells and karyotypic abnormalities. However, in the absence of such abnormalities, the distinction between idiopathic hypereosinophilia and entities such as chronic eosinophilic leukemia, myelodysplastic syndromes or myeloproliferative disorders may be problematical. A specific test for eosinophil clonality would clarify the pathogenesis of the idiopathic hypereosinophilias and result in more precise diagnosis of patients presenting with this disorder.

24.2 Idiopathic Hypereosinophilic Syndrome

The idiopathic hypereosinophilic syndrome (IHES) is a rare disorder characterized by unexplained, persistent eosinophilia associated with multiple-organ dysfunction due to eosinophilic tissue infiltration [2, 3].

Until recently, there was no specific test diagnostic for IHES. Rather the syndrome was defined as the combination of unexplained prolonged eosinophilia and evidence of organ involvement [2, 4] (see also Chap. 1).

The term "hypereosinophilic syndrome" (HES) was first used to describe three patients with hypereosinophilia, cardiac and pulmonary symptoms and hepatosplenomegaly [5]. In 1975, Chusid et al. [2] described 14 patients with hematological, cardiac and neurological abnormalities attributable to hypereosinophilia, and reviewed 57 other published cases. Their criteria for inclusion were (1) a persistent eosinophilia of > 1500/μl for more than 6 months, (2) a lack of evidence of parasitic, allergic or other known causes of eosinophilia, and (3) presumptive signs and symptoms of organ involvement, including hepatosplenomegaly, cardiac, nervous system or pulmonary involvement, and fever, weight loss and anemia. Subsequently, further series of patients with HES were reported [6–8]. It is likely that with present-day karyotyping techniques, a number of the patients reported in earlier published series would today be diagnosed as eosinophilic leukemias, myelodysplastic syndromes or myeloproliferative disorders.

The term "IHES" is usually applied to distinguish HES from reactive eosinophilias associated with known causes of eosinophilia such as parasitic infections, allergies, drug reactions, some malignant tumors, cutaneous, gastrointestinal or connective tissue disorders on the one hand, and the eosinophilic leukemias on the other. Patients with IHES usually present in middle age, and between 84% and 91% of the reported patients are male. Cardiovascular, central and peripheral nervous system, gastrointestinal, joint, skin, muscle and retinal involvement have been described [4]. Common presenting symptoms are fever, nocturnal sweats, nonproductive and nocturnal cough, symptoms of cardiovascular disease, anorexia and weight loss. Other symptoms include neurological and gastrointestinal symptoms and pruritic rashes. Some patients with IHES may show features usually associated with myeloproliferative syndromes such as splenomegaly and thrombocytopenia [3, 8, 9]. Hepatomegaly and lymphadenopathy may also be present in some patients. Anemia and folate deficiency are common. While the syndrome may have some distinctive features, there is no question that IHES is a heterogeneous group of disorders whose common denominator is persistent eosinophilia with organ system involvement, dysfunction or both, related either to infiltration of eosinophils or secondary to an eosinophil-associated damage to tissues [3].

Eosinophilic proliferation and differentiation is promoted by several cytokines, including interleukin-3 (IL-3), granulocyte-macrophage colony-stimulating factor and IL-5 which is the most important and, in humans, restricted to stimulating eosinophil production [10]. Reactive causes of eosinophilia such as infections, allergies, drug reactions, skin diseases and connective tissue diseases are due to stimulation of eosinophil production by IL-5 secreted by T cells. Clonal populations of T cells, of unusual phenotype, that are capable of IL-5 secretion, have been reported in the peripheral blood of some patients with idiopathic hypereosinophilias [11, 12]. In these patients, apparently idiopathic hypereosinophilia is secondary to the proliferation of an abnormal clone of IL-5-secreting T cells.

In the study of Chusid et al. [2], the average length of survival in HES was 9 months, with a 3-year survival of only 12%. Factors associated with a poor prognosis were a high peripheral leukocyte count, peripheral blood myeloblasts and congestive heart failure. Subsequently, in a prospective study of 26 patients with HES, Parillo et al. [13] found a 3-year mortality of 4% in patients treated with corticosteroids, or hydroxyurea in steroid-resistant cases, thus demonstrating a marked improvement in long-term survival with these therapies. In patients with IHES who have high levels of IgE, it has been proposed that hypereosinophilia may result from an IgE-mediated hypersensitivity response to an as-yet-unidentified antigen or antigens [14]. This subgroup of patients is characterized by responsiveness to corticosteroid therapy and a good prognosis.

24.3 Analysis of X-Chromosome Inactivation Patterns in Hypereosinophilias (XCIP)

Analysis of maternal and paternal X-chromosome activation status has been utilized as a means of determining whether certain proliferative disorders are clonal in origin [15]. These methods are based on the assumption that random inactivation of one X-chromosome occurs in each somatic cell during early embryogenic development, and that this is passed on to the progeny of the cell in a stable fashion [16–18]. Therefore, some cells from a normal female carry active maternal X-chromosome while others cells carry active paternal X-chromosome. Differential methylation patterns between the active and inactive X-chromosome have been documented at several loci such as the phosphoglycerate kinase (PGK), hypoxanthine phosphoribosyl transferase (HPRT) and the hypervariable DXS255 (M27ß) loci [19]. Digestion of DNA with a methylation-sensitive restriction endonuclease such as *HpaII* permits the distinction of the active (unmethylated) from the inactive (methylated) X-chromosome.

An important finding was reported by Luppi et al. [20], who analyzed the methylation status of the PGK gene in unseparated granulocytes from a female patient with IHES with 70% eosinophilia and found this to show a clonal pattern by Southern hybridization. Clonality analysis of the PGK gene is restricted by a low incidence of constitutional heterozygosity of approximately 40% in the general female population [21]. Allen et al. [22] have shown that methylation of *HpaII* and *HhaI* restriction endonuclease sites near the polymorphic trinucleotide CAG repeat of the human androgen receptor gene (HUMARA) also correlates with X-inactivation. The HUMARA loci show a high incidence of constitutional heterozygosity of approximately 90% [22, 23], and are therefore highly informative in clonality analysis.

Human eosinophils emit marked fluorescence at 520 nm when excited at 450 nm due to their fluorescent granule contents, and this property may be used to purify eosinophils for study [24]. By isolating eosinophils, it is feasible to extend clonality studies to samples with smaller proportions of eosinophils in the blood. Eosinophils can be purified from peripheral blood samples by flow cytometric sorting based on their autofluorescence and granularity, to >90% purity [25]. Therefore one strategy to determine whether eosinophils from female patients with IHES are clonal would be to analyze the X-inactivation patterns of the HUMARA loci in eosinophils purified by flow cytometric sorting [25].

24.4 Clonal and Nonclonal Hypereosinophilias

By HUMARA analysis of purified eosinophils, Chang et al. [25] found clonal eosinophilia in a female patient with IHES, whereas purified eosinophils were nonclonal in a patient with Churg-Strauss syndrome, and also in patients with reactive eosinophilias (Table 24.1). Further, in the patient with IHES, analysis of eosinophil-depleted leukocytes revealed a nonclonal pattern of X-inactivation, indicating that the clonality of purified eosinophils was not due to skewed random X-inactivation.

A major vasculitic disorder that is associated with eosinophilia is the Churg-Strauss syndrome [26]. A history of asthma, nonfixed pulmonary infiltrates, blood eosinophilia >10%, paranasal sinus abnormalities, mononeuropathy or polyneuro-

Table 24.1. Clonality analysis of eosinophils in hypereosinophilias

Patient	Age (years)	AEC (× 109/l)[a]	Cause of eosinophilia	Amplification pattern at the HUMARA locus
1	50	5.4	IHES	Clonal
2	43	11.6	Churg-Strauss syndrome	Nonclonal
3	65	13.4	Reaction to phenytoin	Nonclonal
4	55	2.0	*Strongyloides* infection	Nonclonal
5	41	1.3	Atopic eczema, house-dust mite allergy	Nonclonal
6	40	1.2	Asthma, house-dust mite allergy	Nonclonal
7	46	3.1	Asthma, allergen unknown	Nonclonal
8	48	3.0	Asthma, allergen unknown	Nonclonal

[a] Absolute eosinophil count at presentation.

athy, and a biopsied blood vessel demonstrating extravascular eosinophils are features of this syndrome [26, 27]. In some patients, clear distinction on clinical grounds between IHES and the Churg-Strauss syndrome may be difficult. However, in a female patient with characteristic features of this syndrome, eosinophils were found to be nonclonal [25], thus providing definitive evidence that eosinophilia is reactive in nature in the Churg-Strauss syndrome.

Two cases of IHES with clonal eosinophilia detected by analysis of X-linked polymorphisms have so far been described [20, 25]. These patients show certain similarities: evidence of organ damage associated with sustained eosinophilia, a normal karyotype in bone marrow cells, an absence of features associated with myeloproliferative disorders, asthmatic symptoms, a mild to moderate increase in polyclonal IgE, and corticosteroid-responsiveness with a favorable outcome. In these patients, it appears that a primary dysregulation of eosinophil production had occurred, resulting in autonomous replication of a clonal population of eosinophils, and that the patients had, in reality, a low-grade clonal myeloproliferative disorder. Several hypotheses for the pathogenesis of dysregulated eosinophil production in IHES have been proposed, such as an acquired somatic mutation affecting eosinophil production [25], or defects in cytokine receptors, or in their signal transduction or suppressor regulatory pathways [4, 28], but these at present remain speculative.

The purification of blood eosinophils for HUMARA analysis allows the determination of eosinophil clonality when the proportion of peripheral blood eosinophils is low. This should, in principle, permit detection of clonal relapse in IHES and facilitate the monitoring of therapeutic responses. However, it should be noted that an absence of clonal eosinophilia by this method of analysis cannot completely exclude the possibility that a minor clonal population of eosinophils may persist. A further limitation of the test is that only a small minority of patients with IHES may be analyzed, as clonality analysis of X-linked polymorphisms may only be applied to females.

Clonality analysis of purified eosinophils can be applied to distinguish clonal from nonclonal eosinophilias in patients presenting with idiopathic hypereosinophilia. This test could facilitate a rational classification of the hypereosinophilias into disorders of clonal or nonclonal origin.

Acknowledgements. This work was supported by grant no. R-170-000-016-213 from the National Medical Research Council, Singapore. Hsiao-Wen Chang was a recipient of a Medical Research Scientist Award from the National Medical Research Council, Singapore.

References

1. Bain BJ (2000) Hypereosinophilia. Curr Opin Hematol 7:21–25
2. Chusid MJ, Dale DC, West BC, Wolff SM (1975) The hypereosinophilic syndrome: analysis of 14 cases with review of the literature. Medicine (Baltimore) 54:1–27
3. Fauci AS Harley JB, Roberts WC, Ferrans VJ, Gralnick HR, Bjornson BH (1982) The idiopathic hypereosinophilic syndrome. Clinical, pathophysiologic, and therapeutic considerations. Ann Intern Med 97:78–92
4. Weller PF, Bubley GJ (1994) The idiopathic hypereosinophilic syndrome. Blood 83:2759–2779
5. Hardy WR, Anderson RE (1968) The hypereosinophilic syndromes. Ann Intern Med 68:1220–1229
6. Parrillo JE, Borer JS, Henry WL, Wolff SM, Fauci AS (1979) Cardiovascular manifestations of the hypereosinophilic syndrome: prospective study of 26 patients, with review of the literature. Am J Med 67:572–582
7. Spry CJF, Davies J, Tai PC, Olsen EGJ, Oakley CM, Goodwin JF (1983) Clinical features of fifteen patients with the hypereosinophilic syndrome. Q J Med 205:1–22
8. Lefebvre C, Bletry O, Degoulet P, Guillevin L, Bentata-Pesyre M, Le Thi HD, Godeau P (1989) Facteurs pronostiques du syndrome hyperéosinophilique. Étude de 40 observations. Ann Med Interne (Paris) 140:253–257
9. Schooley RT, Flaum MA, Gralnick HR, Fauci AS (1981) A clinico-pathological correlation of the idiopathic hypereosinophilic syndrome. II. Clinical manifestations. Blood 58:1021–1026
10. Sanderson CJ (1992) Interleukin 5, eosinophil and disease. Blood 79:3101–3109
11. Cogan E, Schandené L, Crusiaux A, Cochaux P, Velu T, Goldman M (1994) Clonal proliferation of type 2 helper T cells in a man with hypereosinophilic syndrome. New Engl J Med 330:535
12. Simon HU, Plotz SG, Dummer R, Blaser K (1999) Abnormal clones of T cells producing interleukin-5 in idiopathic eosinophilia. New Engl J Med 341:1112–1120
13. Parillo JE, Fauci AS, Wolff SM (1978) Therapy of the hypereosinophilic syndrome. Ann Intern Med 89:167–172
14. Parillo JE, Lawley TJ, Frank MM, Kaplan AP, Fauci AS (1979) Immunologic reactivity in the hypereosinophilic syndrome. J Allergy Clin Immunol 64:113–121
15. Vogelstein B, Fearon ER, Hamilton SR, Preisinger AC, Willard HF, Michelson AM, Riggs AD, Orkin SH (1987) Clonal analysis using recombinant DNA probes from the X-chromosome. Cancer Res 47:4806–4813
16. Lyon MF (1972) X-chromosome inactivation and developmental patterns in mammals. Biol Rev Camb Philos Soc 47:1–35
17. Riggs AD (1975) X-inactivation, differentiation and DNA-methylation. Cytogenet Cell Genet 14:9–25
18. Martin GR, Epstein CJ, Travis B, Tucker G, Yatziv S, Martin DW Jr, Clift C, Cohen S (1978) X-chromosome inactivation during differentiation of female teratocarcinoma stem cells in vitro. Nature 271:329–333
19. Busque L, Gilliland G (1993) Clonal evolution in acute myeloid leukemia. Blood 82:337–342
20. Luppi M, Marasca R, Morselli M, Barozzi P, Torelli G (1994) Clonal nature of the hypereosinophilic syndrome. Blood 84:349–350
21. Gale RE, Wainscoat JS (1993) Clonal analysis using X-linked DNA polymorphisms. Br J Haematol 85:2–8
22. Allen CR, Zoghbi HY, Moseley AB, Rosenblatt HM, Belmont JW (1992) Methylation of HpaII and HhaI sites near the polymorphic CAG repeat in the human androgen receptor gene correlates with X-chromosome inactivation. Am J Hum Genet 51:1229–1239
23. Gale RE, Mein CA, Linch DC (1996) Quantification of X-chromosome inactivation patterns in haematological samples using the DNA PCR-based HUMARA assay. Leukemia 10:362–367
24. Weil GJ, Chused TM (1981) Eosinophil autofluorescence and its use in isolation and analysis of human eosinophils using flow microfluorometry. Blood 57:1099–1104
25. Chang HW, Leong KH, Koh DR, Lee SH (1999) Clonality of isolated eosinophils in the hypereosinophilic syndrome. Blood 93:1651–1657
26. Churg J, Strauss L (1951) Allergic granulomatosis, allergic angiitis and periarteritis nodosa. Am J Pathol 27:277–301

27. Masi AT, Hunder GG, Lie JT, Michael BA, Bloch DA, Arend WP, Calabrese LH, Edworthy SM, Fauci AS, Leavitt RY, Lightfoot RWJ, McShane DJ, Mills JA, Stevens MB, Wallace SL, Zvaifler NJ (1990) The American College of Rheumatology 1990 criteria for the classification of Churg-Strauss syndrome (allergic granulomatosis and angiitis). Arthritis Rheum 33:1094–1100
28. Spry CJF (1992) Idiopathic hypereosinophilic syndrome. In: Makino T, Fukuda S (eds) Eosinophils: biological and clinical aspects. CRC Press, Boca Raton, FL, p 403

Chapter 25

Clonal Lymphocytes in Patients with Idiopathic Hypereosinophilic Syndrome

Florence Roufosse, L. Schandené, A. de Lavareille, E. Cogan, M. Goldman

25.1 Introduction

The idiopathic hypereosinophilic syndrome (IHES) is defined as persistent hypereosinophilia of unknown origin complicated by organ damage or dysfunction. Although this entity was introduced in an attempt to standardize management of such patients, the heterogeneous nature of the hypereosinophilic syndrome rapidly emerged with regard to clinical and biological parameters, disease course, and response to therapy. Patients with clinical and biological markers reminiscent of myeloproliferative disorders generally responded poorly to glucocorticoids and presented life-threatening cardiac complications. In contrast, high IgE levels and polyclonal hypergammaglobulinemia were considered as markers of good prognosis as they were frequently associated with restriction of clinical manifestations to the skin and favorable response to glucocorticoids [1].

Interleukin-5 (IL-5) is a highly specific eosinophilopoietic cytokine which increases eosinophil levels both by stimulating their differentiation from bone marrow precursors and by inhibiting peripheral apoptosis [2–4]. IL-5 overproduction by Th2-type lymphocytes has been demonstrated in a variety of hypereosinophilic disorders including parasitic or allergic diseases and Omenn's syndrome [5]. Th2-type cells also secrete IL-4 and IL-13, which are responsible for the overproduction of IgE often associated with hypereosinophilia. As mentioned, this association is encountered in a subgroup of patients with the IHES, suggesting that Th2 cells may be involved in the pathogenesis of this disease.

25.2 T-Cell Immunophenotyping in Patients with Hypereosinophilia

To investigate this possibility, we systematically performed T-cell immunophenotyping, a search for T-cell clonality, and analysis of cytokine production by peripheral blood T cells in patients with persistent idiopathic hypereosinophilia. We identified four patients with an underlying T-cell disorder characterized by monoclonal expansion of an aberrant CD3–CD4+-T-cell population producing high levels of IL-5, IL-4 and IL-13 indicative of a Th2 profile [6, 7]. The clonal T cells were further characterized by their production of variable amounts of IL-2, an activated memory phenotype (HLA-DR+, CD45RO+), high-level expression of the Fas-receptor (CD95) and their lack of membrane expression of CD7 and CD27. Although T-cell clonality was easily demonstrated on peripheral blood samples from three of the patients, it could only be detected after in vitro purification of the CD3–CD4+ cell population in one patient because of the small proportion of aberrant T cells.

25.3
Clinical Characteristics of Patients with Clonal T Cells

We compared the clinical and biological features of these four patients with those of five other patients fulfilling the diagnostic criteria of IHES in whom no aberrant T-cell subset was detected [7]. We observed a homogeneous profile among those with clonal CD3–CD4+ Th2 cells consisting predominantly of cutaneous manifestations (including pruritus, eczema and urticaria) with lack of severe end-organ involvement, elevated serum IgE levels and polyclonal hypergammaglobulinemia involving either IgM or IgG. Although vitamin B12 is classically considered as a marker of the myeloproliferative variant of IHES, we observed elevated serum levels in one patient with T-cell clonality. Moreover, serum levels of IL-5 and soluble CD25 were of no help in the discrimination of patients with an underlying clonal T-cell disorder in our series.

25.4
Premalignant Nature of Aberrant T Cells

Aberrant IL-5-producing T-cell populations in the setting of IHES have been reported by several independent groups and appear to be related to protracted development of T-cell lymphoma in some cases (Table 25.1) [8–12]. Importantly, 3 of 16 hypereosinophilic patients with an aberrant T-cell population developed T-cell lymphoma that conserved the abnormal surface phenotype initially observed, suggesting that the aberrant cells could be the precursors of malignant T cells [13]. The malignant potential of the CD3–CD4+ cell population in our patients is suggested by the development of anaplastic null-cell lymphoma in one patient, and of peripheral T-cell lymphoma which conserved the CD3–CD4+ phenotype in another. Furthermore, chromosomal abnormalities including partial deletions on chromosomes 6 and 10 were detected in CD3–CD4+ cells from two of the four patients.

Table 25.1. Overview of reports of IHES patients with an aberrant population of circulating T cells (*ND* not determined)

Reference	No. of patients	Characteristics of aberrant T cell populations			Development of lymphoma
		Surface phenotype	Cytokine profile	Clonality	
[8]	2	$CD3^-CD4^+$	ND	ND	+ (2/2)
[9]	1	$CD3^-CD4^+$	ND	+	+
[6]	1	$CD3^-CD4^+$	IL-4, IL-5	+	+
[10]	1	$CD3^-CD4^+$	IL-5	–	-
[27]	2	$CD3^+CD4^-CD8^-$	IL-5, IL-3, IL-2 (1/2)	Mono-/ oligoclonal	-
[11]	1	$CD3^+CD4^-CD8^-$	IL-5	+	–
[12]	1	$CD3^-CD4^+$	IL-4	ND	–
[13]	16/60	$CD3^+CD4^-CD8^-$ (3/16), $CD3^-CD4^+$ (2/16), ...	IL-5 (13/16), IL-4 (4/16)	+ (8/16)	+ (3/16)
[28]	1	$CD3^-CD4^+$	ND	+	–
[7]	4/9	$CD3^-CD4^+$	IL-4, IL-5, IL-13, IL-2	+ (4/4)	+ (2/4)

25.5 Activation and Expansion of Aberrant T Cells

Given the apparently premalignant nature of the aberrant T-cell populations underlying the IHES in some patients, we next studied the factors involved in activation and expansion of these cells. The absence of spontaneous activation in vitro contrasted with clinical evidence that the clonal T cells were in an activated state in vivo. Indeed, the long-standing hypereosinophilia observed in our patients indicated persistent secretion of Th2-type cytokines, since eosinophils quickly undergo apoptosis in the absence of specific survival-promoting cytokines such as IL-5 [4]. Furthermore, the monoclonality of these cells suggested constant expansion of the cell population. The divergence between in vivo and in vitro behavior of the CD3–CD4+ cells argues against constitutional activation of signaling pathways within the clonal T cells, but suggests on the contrary that they remain dependent upon exogenous signals for both proliferation and cytokine production.

We sought to determine whether costimulatory signals provided by antigen-presenting cells (APC) could lead to activation of the clonal Th2 cells in absence of signaling through the TCR/CD3 complex. To this end, we cocultured CD3–CD4+ T cells from two patients with IHES with mature dendritic cells (DC) in a series of mixed leukocyte cultures (MLC) [14]. We observed that DC did indeed stimulate CD3–CD4+ cells to proliferate, to upregulate their expression of the IL-2R-α chain (CD25) and to produce Th2 cytokines. To investigate the nature of the activation signals delivered by DC to clonal T cells, blocking monoclonal antibodies (mAbs) to B7-1, B7-2, CD2 or CD40 were added to MLCs. These experiments established that B7/CD28 and LFA-3/CD2 interactions are critically involved in their TCR-independent activation, as indicated by profound inhibition of proliferation and cytokine production when cocultures were performed in the presence of blocking antibodies that interfered with these costimulatory pathways. These effects were in part related to CD28/CD2-dependence of CD25 upregulation on clonal T cells. In contrast, addition of a blocking anti-CD40 mAb had no significant effect in this system.

The role of endogenous IL-2 production in the activation of CD3–CD4+ T cells during MLCs was investigated using a blocking anti-IL-2R-α (CD25) mAb. The addition of anti-IL-2R-α to cocultures dramatically decreased proliferative responses of the CD3–CD4+ cells and enhanced their apoptosis rate. In parallel, secretion of both IL-5 and IL-13 was profoundly inhibited. To investigate the effects of IL-2 on the synthesis of Th2 cytokines independently from its effects on survival and proliferation, cocultures were prepared in the presence of exogenous IL-15, a T-cell survival-promoting factor. Under these conditions, anti-IL-2Rα specifically inhibited cytokine production without affecting T-cell survival or proliferation. Taken together, these experiments establish that costimulatory signals delivered by DC initiate an IL-2/IL-2R autocrine loop which is critically involved in the survival and proliferation of the CD3–CD4+ cells as well as in their secretion of cytokines (Fig. 25.1).

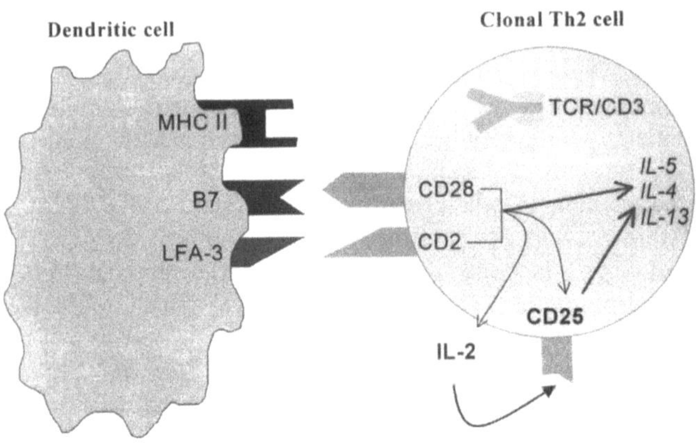

Fig. 25.1. Activation pathways of clonal CD3–CD4+ Th2 cells encountered in patients with the idiopathic hypereosinophilic syndrome. The clonal Th2 cells are activated by antigen-presenting cells, in the absence of TCR/CD3 engagement. Signaling through CD2 and CD28 on the CD3–CD4+ cells leads to production of IL-2 and upregulation of surface CD25 (the high-affinity IL2-Rα chain) expression, resulting in the initiation of an autocrine IL-2-dependent loop. The combined engagement of CD2, CD28 and CD25 induces production and secretion of the Th2-type cytokines, IL-5, IL-4 and IL-13

25.6 Chemokine Receptor Expression by Aberrant T Cells

Current knowledge on chemokine receptor expression patterns on T-cell subsets is predominantly based on studies performed on in vitro polarized or expanded Th1 and Th2 cells. Thus, CCR5 and CXCR3 appear to be preferentially expressed by Th1 cells whereas CCR3, CCR4 and CCR8 are found on Th2 cells [15–18]. The CD3–CD4+ cell population provided us with a unique opportunity to study the pattern of chemokine receptor expression on an "in vivo generated clone" of Th2 cells. We studied surface expression of chemokine receptors by the clonal CD3–CD4+ cells from two patients both immediately after purification and following a 24-hour culture in human serum-free medium. CCR5 and CXCR4 were detected on freshly isolated cells from both patients. Surprisingly, the clonal Th2 cells expressed neither CCR3 nor CCR4. In contrast to CCR3 which remained undetectable when clonal cells were maintained in human serum-free culture, CCR4 progressively appeared on their surface.

As CCR4 only appeared on the CD3–CD4+ cells after ex vivo culture, we reasoned that the continuous exposure of these cells to factor(s) present in patient blood might be responsible for CCR4 downregulation. Indeed, we found that the addition of patient serum to clonal Th2 cells that had been precultured in FCS-containing medium for 2 days was rapidly followed by CCR4 downregulation, whereas the addition of serum from healthy individuals barely affected CCR4 expression. As TARC (thymus and activation regulated chemokine) and MDC (macrophage-derived chemokine) are the two major CCR4 ligands, we measured serum levels of these chemokines in four patients with clonal CD3–CD4+ cells. We found that the serum of patients with IHES with circulating clonal Th2 cells contained much higher levels of TARC, but not of MDC, than serum of IHES patients without T-cell abnormalities or serum of healthy donors. We therefore suggest that the level of circulating TARC could be discriminatory of the IHES variant with Th2 clonality. We further demonstrated that interaction of TARC with its receptor in vivo could be responsible for CCR4 internalization, explaining lack of CCR4 expression on freshly isolated clonal cells. Indeed, downregulation of CCR4 expression by the clonal cells in the presence of autologous serum was inhibited by a mAb against TARC. The persistence of clonal Th2 cells in high numbers in peripheral blood of IHES patients such as ours could be related to TARC-induced CCR4 downregulation in vivo.

TARC has been shown to be produced by monocytes and monocyte-derived dendritic cells, especially in the presence of IL-4 and GM-CSF [19, 20]. As clonal Th2 cells from our patients were able to produce these cytokines upon stimulation, we investigated whether these cells could induce TARC production by dendritic cells. During cocultures between dendritic cells and T cells, much higher levels of TARC were produced in the presence of clonal Th2 cells than in the presence of T cells from healthy donors. We also demonstrated that this induction was dependent on IL-4 receptor signaling. Taken together our data suggest that the cross-talk between Th2 cells and dendritic cells results not only in the induction of cytokine production by T cells but also in the production of TARC by dendritic cells.

25.7 Effects of Interferon-α on Clonal T Cells

Finally, as interferon-α (IFN-α) is used in the therapy of the IHES [21, 22], we determined the effects of this cytokine on clonal Th2 cells from two of our patients. Initially, the rationale for the use of IFN-α in the management of IHES was based on its beneficial effects in patients with cMPDs such as chronic myelogenous leukemia, polycythemia vera or essential thrombocythemia, and the fact that some patients with IHES showed several features suggestive of a chronic myeloproliferative disease. The beneficial effects observed with IFN-α in such patients may result from its direct actions on eosinophils, including inhibition of eosinophilopoiesis, of several effector functions of eosinophils, and of their recruitment into tissues [23, 24]. The notion that clonal Th2 cells play a pathogenic role in a subgroup of patients with chronic hypereosinophilia has emerged only recently, and most studies in which favorable effects of IFN-α have been found in the setting of the IHS have been conducted in patients with no evidence of an underlying T-cell disorder. The long-term effects of IFN-α in patients with an aberrant T-cell population are therefore unclear. To address this issue, we investigated the direct effects of IFN-α on the clonal Th2 cytokine-producing cells in vitro.

We first demonstrated that IFN-α is a potent inhibitor of IL-5 synthesis by differentiated human Th2 clones, including CD3–CD4+ cells obtained from two IHES patients [25], providing a rationale for treatment of such patients with this molecule. However, as previously mentioned, the premalignant nature of clonal Th2 cells found in some patients with IHES has been suggested by the subsequent development of T-cell lymphoma. We therefore focused our attention on the influence of IFN-α on the survival of CD3–CD4+ cells. We observed that these clonal T cells were highly prone to undergoing apoptosis when cultured in cytokine-free medium. This increased susceptibility to apoptosis was associated with a low level of bcl-2 expression, whereas bcl-xL expression was similar to that of control CD4+ memory T cells. Furthermore, the CD3–CD4+ cells showed high-level expression of CD95 and underwent apoptosis following ligation of this receptor by soluble Fas-ligand. The addition of IFN-α to cultures significantly reduced spontaneous apoptosis of the clonal Th2 cells in a dose-dependent manner, and a protective effect was observed at a concentrations as low as 1 IU/ml. Contrasting with the inhibitory effects on spontaneous apoptosis, IFN-α did not affect Fas-induced apoptosis of the clonal T cells.

The spontaneous apoptosis of the Th2-like cells during in vitro culture contrasts with their persistence in vivo, and their lack of any sign of apoptosis immediately after purification, suggesting that they are not yet committed to death. This might be related to their in vivo exposure to survival factors such as IL-2, IL-4 or IL-15. An autocrine loop promoting Th2 cell survival might be operative in vivo as a consequence of their contact with antigen-presenting cells and their subsequent production of IL-2 and IL-4. Our data suggest that IFN-α represents another survival factor of Th2 cells which might be operative in vivo in a paracrine fashion.

These findings suggest that the long-term effects of IFN-α therapy in IHES might depend on the subtype of the syndrome considered. Indeed, we observed development of peripheral T-cell lymphoma in two out of four patients in our series, both of whom had received IFN-α for more than 1 year. In view of the antiapoptotic effects of IFN-α on clonal Th2-type CD3–CD4+ cells, we would advise great caution when administering this molecule as monotherapy in the context of the lymphocytic variant of the IHES.

25.8 Conclusions

We and others have identified a subgroup of IHES patients with an underlying T-cell disorder. The premalignant nature of the disease presented by these patients is suggested by the protracted development of lymphoma in some cases, and the occasional detection of chromosomal abnormalities in purified cells. Our data suggest that in addition to careful lymphocyte phenotyping, TCR gene rearrangement analysis and search for chromosomal abnormalities, the measurement of serum levels of the chemokine TARC could help in the identification of such patients. Furthermore, IFN-α should be used with caution in this setting, as it has been shown to prevent apoptosis of clonal Th2 cells in our patients, and could thus favor further expansion. Future proposals for management of hypereosinophilic patients such as ours could include anti-IL-2R-α and CTLA4-Ig, given that both proliferation and Th2 cytokine production are dependent on engagement of CD28 by B7 molecules and the integrity of an autocrine IL-2-dependent loop [26].

Acknowledgements. We would like to thank all the clinicians without whom this work would not have been possible, in particular Bernard Kennes and André Efira. We are also grateful to Martine Ducarme and Alain Crusiaux for excellent technical assistance.

References

1. Weller PF, Bubley GJ (1994) The idiopathic hypereosinophilic syndrome. Blood 83:2759–2779
2. Wardlaw AJ (1994) Eosinophils in the 1990s: new perspectives on their role in health and disease. Postgrad Med J 70:536–552
3. Walsh GM (1997) Human eosinophils: their accumulation, activation and fate. Br J Haematol 97:701–709
4. Simon HU, Blaser K (1995) Inhibition of programmed eosinophil death: a key pathogenic event for eosinophilia? Immunol Today 16:53–55
5. Romagnani S (1996) Th1 and Th2 in human diseases. Clin Immunol Immunopathol 80:225–235
6. Cogan E, Schandené L, Crusiaux A, Cochaux P, Velu T, Goldman M (1994) Brief report: clonal proliferation of type 2 helper T cells in a man with the hypereosinophilic syndrome. N Engl J Med 330:535–538
7. Roufosse F, Schandené L, Sibille C, Willard-Gallo K, Kennes B, Efira A, Goldman M, Cogan E (2000) Clonal Th2 lymphocytes in patients with the idiopathic hypereosinophilic syndrome. Br J Haematol *109:540–548*
8. O'Shea JJ, Jaffe ES, Lane HC, MacDermott RP, Fauci AS (1987) Peripheral T cell lymphoma presenting as hypereosinophilia with vasculitis. Clinical, pathologic, and immunologic features. Am J Med 82:539–545
9. Bagot M, Bodemer C, Wechsler J, Divine M, Haioun C, Capesius C, Saal F, Cabotin P, Roubertie E, de Prost Y, Lorette G, Revuz J (1990) Non epidermotropic T lymphoma preceded for several years by hypereosinophilic syndrome. Ann Dermatol Venereol 117:883–885
10. Brugnoni D, Airo P, Rossi G, Bettinardi A, Simon HU, Garza L, Tosoni C, Cattaneo R, Blaser K, Tucci A (1996) A case of hypereosinophilic syndrome is associated with the expansion of a CD3–CD4+ T-cell population able to secrete large amounts of interleukin-5. Blood 87:1416–1422
11. Kitano K, Ichikawa N, Mahbub B, Ueno M, Ito T, Shimodaira S, Kodaira H, Ishida F, Kobayashi H, Saito H, Okubo Y, Enokihara H, Kiyosawa K (1996) Eosinophilia associated with proliferation of CD(3+)4-(8-) alpha beta+ T cells with chromosome 16 anomalies. Br J Haematol 92:315–317
12. Bank I, Reshef A, Beniaminov M, Rosenthal E, Rechavi G, Monselise Y (1998) Role of gamma/delta T cells in a patient with CD4+CD3- lymphocytosis, hypereosinophilia, and high levels of IgE. J Allergy Clin Immunol 102:621–630
13. Simon HU, Plotz SG, Dummer R, Blaser K (1999) Abnormal clones of T cells producing interleukin-5 in idiopathic eosinophilia. N Engl J Med 341:1112–1120
14. Roufosse F, Schandené L, Sibille C, Kennes B, Efira A, Cogan E, Goldman M (1999) T-cell receptor-independent activation of clonal Th2 cells associated with chronic hypereosinophilia. Blood 94:994–1002
15. Sallusto F, Mackay CR, Lanzavecchia A (1997) Selective expression of the eotaxin receptor CCR3 by human T helper 2 cells. Science 277:2005–2007
16. Zingoni A, Soto H, Hedrick JA, Stoppacciaro A, Storlazzi CT, Sinigaglia F, D'Ambrosio D, O'Garra A, Robinson D, Rocchi M, Santoni A, Zlotnik A, Napolitano M (1998) The chemokine receptor CCR8 is preferentially expressed in Th2 but not Th1 cells. J Immunol 161:547–551
17. Bonecchi R, Bianchi G, Bordignon PP, D'Ambrosio D, Lang R, Borsatti A, Sozzani S, Allavena P, Gray PA, Mantovani A, Sinigaglia F (1998) Differential expression of chemokine receptors and chemotactic responsiveness of type 1 T helper cells (Th1s) and Th2s. J Exp Med 187:129–134
18. Andrew DP, Chang MS, McNinch J, Wathen ST, Rihanek M, Tseng J, Spellberg JP, Elias CG (1998) STCP-1 (MDC) CC chemokine acts specifically on chronically activated Th2 lymphocytes and is produced by monocytes on stimulation with Th2 cytokines IL-4 and IL-13. J Immunol 16:5027-5038
19. Imai T, Nagira M, Takagi S, Kakizaki M, Nishimura M, Wang J, Gray PW, Matsushima K, Yoshie O (1999) Selective recruitment of CCR4-bearing Th2 cells toward antigen-presenting cells by the CC chemokines thymus and activation-regulated chemokine and macrophage-derived chemokine. Int Immunol *11:81–88*
20. Hashimoto S, Suzuki T, Dong HY, Nagai S, Yamazaki N, Matsushima K (1999) Serial analysis of gene expression in human monocyte-derived dendritic cells. Blood. *94:845–852*
21. Bockenstedt PL, Santinga JT, Bolling SF (1994) Alpha-interferon treatment for idiopathic hypereosinophilic syndrome. Am J Hematol 45:248–251
22. Butterfield JH, Gleich GJ (1994) Interferon-alpha treatment of six patients with the idiopathic hypereosinophilic syndrome. Ann Intern Med 121:648–653
23. Aldebert D, Lamkhioued B, Desaint C, Gounni AS, Goldman M, Capron A, Prin L, Capron M (1996) Eosinophils express a functional receptor for interferon alpha: inhibitory role of interferon alpha on the release of mediators. Blood 87:2354–2360
24. Morita M, Lamkhioued B, Soussi Gounni A, Aldebert D, Delaporte E, Capron A, Capron M (1996) Induction by interferons of human eosinophil apoptosis and regulation by interleukin-3, granulocyte/macrophage-colony stimulating factor and interleukin-5. Eur Cytokine Netw 7:725–732

25. Schandené L, Del Prete GF, Cogan E, Stordeur P, Crusiaux A, Kennes B, Romagnani S, Goldman M (1996) Recombinant interferon-alpha selectively inhibits the production of interleukin-5 by human CD4+ T cells. J Clin Invest 97:309–315
26. Rouffosse F, Cogan E, Goldman M (2003) The hypereosinophilic syndrome revisited. Annu Rev Med 54:169–184
27. Simon HU, Yousefi S, Dommann-Scherrer CC, Zimmermann DR, Bauer S, Barandun J, Blaser K (1996) Expansion of cytokine-producing CD4-CD8- T cells associated with abnormal Fas expression and hypereosinophilia. J Exp Med 183:1071–1082
28. Zenone T, Felman P, Malcus C, Durieu I, Durand DV (1999) Indolent course of a patient with hypereosinophilic syndrome associated with clonal T-cell proliferation. Am J Med 107:509–111

Subject Index

Printing: Saladruck, Berlin
Binding: Stein+Lehmann, Berlin

MIX
Papier aus verantwortungsvollen Quellen
Paper from responsible sources
FSC® C105338

If you have any concerns about our products,
you can contact us on
ProductSafety@springernature.com

In case Publisher is established outside the EU,
the EU authorized representative is:
Springer Nature Customer Service Center GmbH
Europaplatz 3, 69115 Heidelberg, Germany

Printed by Libri Plureos GmbH
in Hamburg, Germany